MEDICAL TRANSCRIPTION

–

ONE BOOK
TO MAKE YOU
GENIUS

by

VIRUTI SHIVAN

PREFACE: A JOURNEY INTO MEDICAL TRANSCRIPTION

Welcome to the exciting world of medical transcription! This is a very important job in the healthcare industry. I did not plan to become a medical transcriptionist. I started learning about it, then it became my job, and now, I love it!

At first, medical transcription looked very difficult. There were so many medical words and short forms to learn. But as I learnt more, I found that it's like learning a new language. It's a very special job because it helps doctors and nurses do their jobs better. This helps patients get better treatment.

Over the years, medical transcription has changed a lot. Earlier, doctors used to record their notes and someone had to write them down. But now, we use computers and smart programs to do this job. Medical transcription has become very important now because doctors need correct and detailed patient records.

I wrote this book "Medical Transcription - One Book to Make You Genius by VIRUTI SHIVAN" to make it easy for everyone to understand medical transcription. This book is for everyone - people who are just starting to learn about this job or people who have been doing it for many years and want to improve their skills.

This book has 15 chapters. Each chapter talks about one part of medical transcription. The first chapter is an introduction. After that, we will learn about what skills are needed, how to understand medical words, English language rules, and many other things. We will learn new things in each chapter.

Furthermore, to facilitate your learning process, this guide comes with Weekly Transcription Masterclasses. These masterclasses delve into core areas including the 'Comprehensive Guide to Medical Terminology', 'Deep Dive into Different Medical Specialties', and 'Conforming to Transcription Guidelines for Accuracy'. Scheduled throughout your study plan, these classes provide you with the opportunity to consolidate what you've learnt in each chapter, clarify doubts and engage in valuable discussions.

I have tried to write this book in a simple and easy-to-understand way. I have also included examples from real life and exercises for practice. At the end of the book, there are some extra pages where you can find practice transcription files, common errors, and helpful resources.

To get the most from this book, I suggest starting from the first page and reading all the way to the end of chapter 15. Then, you should do masterclass daily or weekly one-by-one. But if you are already working as a medical transcriptionist and you want to learn about something specific, you can go directly to that masterclass.

Remember, it is normal to find learning something new a bit hard at first. But don't worry, with time and practice, you can become very good at it. I hope this book will be helpful to you in your journey.

Viruti Shivan

Table of Contents

CHAPTER 1: INTRODUCTION TO MEDICAL TRANSCRIPTION

Definition and Scope of Medical Transcription

Medical transcription is a vital part of healthcare service. It involves converting the spoken words of doctors, nurses, and other healthcare professionals into written form. It is a specialized job that requires a deep understanding of medical terminology, attention to detail, and a high level of accuracy. This role is fulfilled by an individual known as a medical transcriptionist.

Imagine a doctor speaking into a device about a patient's health condition, diagnosis, treatment plan, and other relevant details. The doctor is busy and can't write all this down. So, it is the medical transcriptionist's job to listen to this audio recording and create a written document out of it.

This written record, known as a medical transcript, serves many purposes. It forms a part of the patient's permanent medical record, helps in insurance processes, and is useful for future reference by the doctor or other medical staff.

The scope of medical transcription is vast. Medical transcriptionists can work in various healthcare settings, including hospitals, clinics, physician's offices, transcription service organizations, insurance companies, home healthcare agencies, and public health agencies. With the rise of technology, many medical transcriptionists are now able to work remotely from their homes.

The Evolution of Medical Transcription Over the Years

Medical transcription has a long history, and its evolution is fascinating. It has come a long way from its humble beginnings, adapting to technological changes, and transforming itself to meet the needs of the growing healthcare sector.

Years ago, medical transcription was a manual and laborious process. Doctors would dictate their notes into a tape recorder. These tapes were then handed over to the transcriptionist who would listen carefully and type out the dictated notes into a written document. The transcriptionist would use a typewriter, making it a slow and meticulous task. Errors had to be corrected by hand, and the documents were stored as hard copies, requiring a lot of physical storage space.

Then came the advent of computers and word processors, which brought a significant change in the field of medical transcription. With the ability to edit and format text easily, correcting mistakes became simpler and the overall transcription process became quicker.

With the rise of the internet, the process of medical transcription underwent another major shift. Doctors could now dictate their notes into digital recorders, and these audio files could be sent over the internet to the transcriptionist, irrespective of their location. This made it possible for transcriptionists to work remotely and allowed for the expansion of transcription services.

More recently, the field of medical transcription has been transformed by advanced technologies such as speech recognition software. This software can automatically convert spoken words into written text. However, these transcriptions still require human oversight for error correction and editing, maintaining the need for skilled medical transcriptionists.

Looking ahead, the field of medical transcription is set to evolve further with advancements in artificial intelligence and machine learning. But no matter how advanced technology becomes, the role of medical transcriptionists will always be crucial due to the need for accuracy and human judgment in transcribing critical medical information.

Importance of Medical Transcription in Modern Healthcare

The role of medical transcription in modern healthcare can't be underestimated. Its impact is huge and multifaceted, contributing to various aspects of patient care, administrative work, and overall healthcare delivery.

1. **Creates Permanent Medical Records:** Medical transcription helps create a permanent record of each patient's medical history, treatment details, lab results, and other relevant information. This information is vital for doctors to provide appropriate treatment and follow-up care.
2. **Facilitates Communication Among Healthcare Professionals:** Transcriptions serve as a communication tool among doctors, nurses, and other healthcare professionals. They can review the patient's records to understand the treatment provided, the medications prescribed, and the patient's progress. This ensures seamless care, especially when a patient is referred to a specialist or transferred to another facility.
3. **Aids in Research and Studies:** Medical records are a treasure trove of data. Researchers and medical professionals often rely on these records for conducting health studies, tracking disease patterns, and developing new treatment methods.
4. **Useful for Legal and Insurance Purposes:** In case of any legal or insurance claim, the transcribed medical records serve as an important piece of evidence. They can prove what care was given to a patient and whether all necessary protocols were followed.
5. **Helps in Billing and Coding:** Medical transcriptions are used by medical coders and billers to understand the services provided to the patient. This helps them to correctly code the services for insurance reimbursement.
6. **Improves Patient Care:** Most importantly, medical transcription contributes to improved patient care. With clear and accurate transcriptions, doctors can make better-informed decisions, avoid harmful drug interactions, and provide targeted treatment.

To sum it up, medical transcription plays a critical role in maintaining the integrity of patient information, facilitating effective communication among healthcare professionals, ensuring smooth administrative functions, and ultimately, enhancing patient care. This is why the demand for skilled and accurate medical transcriptionists remains high in the healthcare industry.

Real-life examples and case studies help us understand better. Let's take a look at two case studies to highlight the significance of medical transcription in healthcare.

Case Study 1: Patient Ram

Consider a patient named Ram, who has been experiencing frequent headaches. He visits his local physician, Dr. Gupta, for a checkup. Dr. Gupta examines Ram and suspects he might have migraines. He advises Ram about lifestyle modifications and prescribes medication for headache relief.

This entire interaction, including the medical history discussion, physical examination findings, and the treatment plan, is recorded. A medical transcriptionist transcribes this conversation. The transcribed record includes important details like Ram's symptoms, Dr. Gupta's clinical observations, prescribed medication, and follow-up instructions.

A few weeks later, Ram moves to another city. He experiences a severe headache and visits a new doctor, Dr. Verma. Dr. Verma can quickly read through Ram's transcribed medical records. These records provide him with a clear understanding of Ram's past medical history, his symptoms, and the treatment given by Dr. Gupta. Dr. Verma can then make an informed decision about Ram's ongoing care.

Without the medical transcription, the new doctor would lack this valuable insight into Ram's health.

Case Study 2: Multi-Specialty Healthcare Approach

Now, imagine a patient, Sita, who is diagnosed with diabetes. Her primary care physician refers her to various specialists - an endocrinologist for diabetes management, a dietitian for nutritional advice, and a podiatrist for foot care.

Each healthcare provider examines Sita and provides specific care instructions. All these conversations are recorded and transcribed. The medical transcription provides a comprehensive view of Sita's health status, the various specialists involved in her care, and the multifaceted approach taken to manage her diabetes.

If Sita visits a new healthcare provider, they can read the transcribed records and understand the full extent of Sita's health journey. They can also see what each specialist has contributed to Sita's care.

These case studies illustrate the indispensable role of medical transcription in maintaining continuity of care, ensuring seamless communication among various healthcare providers, and ultimately enhancing patient outcomes.

I hope this gives you a good idea about medical transcription. In the next chapter, we will talk about the person who does this job - the medical transcriptionist.

CHAPTER 2: THE MEDICAL TRANSCRIPTIONIST

Necessary Skills for a Successful Transcriptionist

Indeed, to become a successful medical transcriptionist, certain skills are essential. Let's discuss them in more detail.

1. Good Listening Skills: Medical transcription involves converting voice-recorded reports into text format. For this, one needs to have excellent listening skills. You should be able to understand the doctor's voice clearly, even if they have an accent or speak quickly.

2. Fast and Accurate Typing Skills: Typing speed is also very important for this job. A medical transcriptionist should be able to type quickly without making mistakes. On average, a good typing speed is around 60-70 words per minute.

3. Computer Skills: You should be comfortable using computers, as you'll be using them all the time. This includes knowledge of word processing software like Microsoft Word, and transcription software if required.

4. Knowledge of Medical Terminology: Medical transcriptionists deal with medical terms every day. They need to understand medical jargon, abbreviations, and names of medicines. For this, having some background in biology or healthcare can be helpful.

5. Good English Language Skills: This job requires a strong grasp of English grammar and spelling rules. You should be able to understand the doctor's sentences and write them correctly. This is very important for making clear and accurate medical reports.

6. Attention to Detail: Medical transcriptionists should be good at spotting and correcting errors. They should pay attention to every little detail. Even small mistakes can lead to serious problems. For example, a wrong number in a patient's drug dose can be dangerous.

7. Confidentiality: Medical transcriptionists often deal with private patient information. So, they need to respect the confidentiality rules and keep this information safe.

These are the basic skills needed for this job. But remember, skills can be improved with practice. So, don't worry if you're not perfect at first. With time and effort, you can become a great medical transcriptionist!

Educational Requirements and Additional Qualifications

In order to become a medical transcriptionist, you need to fulfil some educational requirements and possibly gain additional qualifications. Let's see what they are:

1. Basic Education: The first step is to complete your schooling. You need to have passed at least the high school. Having good grades in English and Biology will be helpful but is not mandatory. Students from any stream can do transcription work.

2. Medical Transcription Training: Next, you need to undergo a training course in medical transcription. These courses are offered by many institutions, and they can be done either in-person or online. They teach you all the necessary skills for this job. These include typing, listening skills, use of transcription tools, and most importantly, knowledge of medical terminology.

3. Certification: After finishing the training course, some people choose to get certified. This is not a must, but it can help you in your job search. There are two main certifications for medical transcriptionists:

      - Certificate in Medical Transcription (CMT): This is for those who are just starting their career. It covers the basic skills needed for this job.

      - Diploma in Medical Transcriptionist (DMT): This is for those who have more experience. It covers more advanced knowledge, including different medical specialties.

These certifications are offered by the Association for Healthcare Documentation Integrity (AHDI) in the United States. In India, there may be similar associations offering certifications. Getting certified shows that you have a good understanding of medical transcription. This can impress employers and help you get better job offers.

Remember, becoming a medical transcriptionist is a journey. It starts with education, but it doesn't end there. You will need to keep learning and improving your skills throughout your career.

Detailed Job Responsibilities

A medical transcriptionist has various job responsibilities. Let's explore them in more detail:

1. Listening to Medical Dictations: The main part of a medical transcriptionist's job is to listen to dictations. These dictations are typically audio recordings made by doctors or other healthcare workers. The medical transcriptionist needs to listen to these recordings carefully and understand what is being said.

2. Transcribing Medical Dictations: After listening to the dictation, the medical transcriptionist has to type out what they heard. They need to type it word for word, exactly as it was said in the recording. This is done on a computer, using a special transcription software.

3. Reviewing and Editing Transcripts: Once the transcription is done, the next step is to review it. The medical transcriptionist needs to read through the typed document and check for any mistakes. They need to correct spelling errors, punctuation mistakes, or any other errors that they find. They also need to make sure that the medical terms and abbreviations are used correctly.

4. Researching Unclear Information: Sometimes, the recording may not be clear. The doctor's voice might be muffled, or they might use a term that the transcriptionist does not know. In such cases, the transcriptionist needs to research the unclear information. They might need to listen to the recording again, look up medical terms, or consult with others to understand what was said.

5. Formatting and Submitting Transcripts: After the transcription is reviewed and edited, it needs to be formatted. The medical transcriptionist has to make sure that it follows the correct format for medical records. This can include adding headings, bullet points, or other formatting elements. Once the transcript is ready, the transcriptionist has to submit it to the doctor or healthcare provider who made the dictation.

So, as you can see, the job of a medical transcriptionist involves more than just typing. They need to have good listening skills, attention to detail, and a strong knowledge of medical terminology. They also need to be comfortable with using computers and doing research.

Career Path and Growth Opportunities

Starting as a medical transcriptionist can open many doors for career growth. Let's explore some of these opportunities:

1. Experienced Medical Transcriptionist: With years of experience and consistent high-quality work, a medical transcriptionist can become a senior or an experienced medical transcriptionist. In this role, they can handle more complex medical cases or work with highly specialized areas of medicine. Experienced medical transcriptionists are often more in demand and have a higher pay scale.

2. Specialized Medical Transcriptionist: Medical transcriptionists can choose to specialize in a specific area of medicine, such as cardiology, neurology, or orthopedics. This requires further study and understanding of the particular medical field. Specialized medical transcriptionists often have higher earning potential because of their specialized skills and knowledge.

3. Quality Analyst/Editor: After gaining substantial experience, a medical transcriptionist can move into quality analysis or editing roles. Quality analysts or editors review and edit the work done by other transcriptionists, ensuring accuracy and adherence to format standards. This role requires a high level of expertise and a keen eye for detail.

4. Training and Teaching: Experienced medical transcriptionists can also become trainers or teachers, helping to train new entrants in the field of medical transcription. This could involve working with a training institute or offering freelance training courses.

5. Management Roles: With the right skills and experience, a medical transcriptionist can also move into management roles. This could include managing a team of transcriptionists, overseeing the transcription operations of a healthcare facility, or even starting their own medical transcription service.

6. Consulting: Experienced transcriptionists with a deep understanding of the medical transcription industry can become consultants. They can advise healthcare providers on improving their transcription processes, implementing new transcription technologies, or adhering to regulations related to medical documentation.

As you can see, a career in medical transcription offers several paths for growth and advancement.

That's the end of Chapter 2. We will now move on to the next chapter.

CHAPTER 3: UNDERSTANDING MEDICAL TERMINOLOGY

Fundamentals of Medical Terminology

Medical terminology is a specific language used in healthcare to ensure precise communication. It is primarily derived from Latin and Greek. Understanding the basics of medical terminology is crucial in the healthcare field, including for medical transcriptionists.

Here are the main components of medical terms:

1. **Root Words:** Root words are the basic parts of a word and provide the general meaning of the term. For example, in the term 'cardiology,' the root word is 'cardi' which means heart.

2. **Prefixes:** A prefix is placed at the beginning of a word to modify or change its meaning. For instance, in the term 'hypoglycemia,' the prefix 'hypo-' means under or below.

3. **Suffixes:** A suffix is added at the end of a word to change its meaning. For example, in the term 'cardiology,' the suffix '-logy' means study of.

4. **Combining Vowels:** A combining vowel (often 'o') is used to ease pronunciation between a word root and a suffix, or between two word roots. For example, in the term 'gastroenterology,' the combining vowel 'o' is used between 'gastro' (stomach) and 'entero' (intestines).

Here are a few general rules about medical terminology:

- Words are usually broken down into their root components to understand their meaning.

- Many medical terms can be understood by understanding the individual components of the term.

- Certain terms have common prefixes and suffixes. For example, terms ending in '-itis' (like arthritis, bronchitis) refer to conditions involving inflammation.

Understanding medical terminology requires practice and time, but a solid foundation in these basics can make the process much easier. As a medical transcriptionist, it's essential to have a strong grasp of medical terminology to ensure accuracy in transcribing medical reports.

Understanding Medical Abbreviations and Jargon

Medical language is full of abbreviations and special words. These can seem hard to understand. But with practice, you can learn them.

1. Abbreviations: These are short forms of long words or phrases. For example, 'BP' stands for 'blood pressure' and 'OPD' stands for 'outpatient department'. Doctors use these abbreviations to save time. As a medical transcriptionist, you need to know these abbreviations and what they stand for.

2. Jargon: Jargon is special words used in a particular field. Medical jargon includes words like 'diagnosis', 'prognosis', 'acute', 'chronic', and so on. Knowing these words will help you understand what the doctor is saying.

To help you get started, we will give lists of common abbreviations and jargon in the next section. We will also explain what they mean and how they are used. This will help you build your medical vocabulary.

Note: Be careful while transcribing abbreviations. Some abbreviations can have more than one meaning. The meaning can change based on the context in which it is used. Always check the context if you are not sure.

The Etymology of Medical Terms

Etymology is the study of the origins of words and how their meanings have evolved over time. Many medical terms have their roots in Latin or Greek. Understanding the etymology of medical terms can make them easier to understand and remember. Here are some examples:

1. Cardio-: This prefix comes from the Greek word 'kardia', which means heart. So, any term starting with 'cardio-' is related to the heart. For example, 'cardiology' is the study of the heart and its functions.

2. Hepato-: This prefix comes from the Greek word 'hepar', which means liver. So, any term starting with 'hepato-' is related to the liver. For example, 'hepatitis' is inflammation of the liver.

3. Neuro-: This prefix comes from the Greek word 'neuron', which means nerve. So, any term starting with 'neuro-' is related to the nerves or the nervous system. For example, 'neurology' is the study of the nervous system and its disorders.

4. -itis: This suffix comes from the Greek word 'itis', which means inflammation. So, any term ending in '-itis' refers to an inflammatory condition. For example, 'arthritis' is inflammation of the joints.

5. -logy: This suffix comes from the Greek word 'logia', which means study of. So, any term ending in '-logy' refers to the study of a specific field. For example, 'biology' is the study of living organisms.

Understanding the roots of medical terminology not only enhances your vocabulary but also gives you a deeper understanding of the medical field.

Now, let's look at some common prefixes, suffixes, and root words. These can help you understand many medical terms.

Prefixes:

1. **'Hyper-'** means 'over' or 'too much'. For example, 'hyperactive' means 'too active'.

2. **'Hypo-'** means 'under' or 'too little'. For example, 'hypoglycemia' means 'too little sugar in the blood'.

3. **'Anti-'** means 'against'. For example, 'antibiotic' means 'against life'. It refers to medicines that kill bacteria.

Suffixes:

1. **'-itis'** means 'inflammation'. For example, 'arthritis' means 'inflammation of the joints'.

2. **'-ology'** means 'study of'. For example, 'biology' means 'study of life'.

3. **'-ectomy'** means 'removal'. For example, 'appendectomy' means 'removal of the appendix'.

Root words:

1. **'Cardio-'** refers to the heart. For example, 'cardiology' means 'study of the heart'.

2. **'Gastro-'** refers to the stomach. For example, 'gastroenteritis' means 'inflammation of the stomach and intestines'.

3. **'Hepato-'** refers to the liver. For example, 'hepatitis' means 'inflammation of the liver'.

Remember, these are just examples. There are many more prefixes, suffixes, and root words in medical language. The more you learn, the easier it will be for you to understand medical terms. As you move forward in the book, you will learn more complex medical terms that combine these prefixes, root words, and suffixes.

This is the end of Chapter 3. In the next chapter, we'll delve into the basics of human anatomy and physiology, and how it relates to medical transcription. Stay tuned!

CHAPTER 4: ANATOMY AND PHYSIOLOGY FOR MEDICAL TRANSCRIPTION

Basic Concepts in Human Anatomy and Physiology

In anatomy, we learn about different parts of the body. These parts are arranged into different systems, each with a unique function. Here are some key body systems:

1. Skeletal System: This is made up of bones. It gives shape to our body. It also protects important parts like the brain, heart, and lungs.

2. Muscular System: This is made up of muscles. It helps us move. There are three types of muscles: skeletal, smooth, and cardiac.

3. Digestive System: This is made up of organs like the stomach and intestines. It helps to break down food and take out nutrients.

4. Respiratory System: This includes the nose, windpipe, and lungs. It helps us breathe.

5. Circulatory System: This includes the heart and blood vessels. It carries blood to all parts of the body.

6. Nervous System: This includes the brain, spinal cord, and nerves. It carries messages from one part of the body to another.

In physiology, we learn how these systems work. For example, we learn how food moves through the digestive system. Or how the heart pumps blood around the body. As a medical transcriptionist, this knowledge is very useful. It helps you understand what a doctor is saying in a recording. It also helps you make sure that what you type makes sense.

In the following sections, we will learn more about each body system. We will also learn about common diseases and conditions related to each system. And we will learn how to transcribe medical reports about these systems.

Introduction to Anatomy

Anatomy studies the structure of the human body - how it is built. Here are the main areas:

- **Cells:** The smallest unit of life. They come together to form tissues.

- **Tissues:** A group of similar cells working together. For example, muscle tissue helps us move.

- **Organs:** A group of tissues working together to perform a specific function. For example, the heart pumps blood.

- **Body systems:** Organs working together to achieve a common goal. For example, the digestive system helps us digest food.

Introduction to Physiology

Physiology is all about understanding how the body works. It looks at how different parts of the body function and how they work together. Each body system has its own set of tasks. For example, when you eat food, it goes through many stages. It is chewed, swallowed, digested, and finally, it gives energy to the body. This is all a part of physiology.

Let's talk about the main body systems and their jobs:

1. **Circulatory System:** This system is like a transport service. It carries blood, oxygen, and nutrients to all parts of the body. The heart, blood vessels, and blood are all part of this system.

2. **Respiratory System:** This system helps us breathe. It takes in oxygen and lets out carbon dioxide. The main parts of this system are the nose, throat, windpipe, and lungs.

3. **Digestive System:** This system breaks down the food we eat. It turns food into nutrients that the body can use. It includes the mouth, stomach, liver, and intestines.

4. **Nervous System:** This system carries messages to and from the brain. It helps us think, feel, and move. It includes the brain, spinal cord, and nerves.

5. **Musculoskeletal System:** This system supports the body and helps it move. It includes the bones, muscles, and joints.

6. **Endocrine System:** This system makes hormones. Hormones are special chemicals that control many body functions. The glands, such as the thyroid gland and the adrenal glands, are part of this system.

As a medical transcriptionist, you need to know these body systems well. You will hear about them a lot in medical reports.

Detailed Study of Different Body Systems

The Circulatory System

The circulatory system is like a transport system in our body. It carries blood, oxygen, and nutrients to all parts of the body. The main parts are the heart, blood vessels, and blood.

In medical reports, you may come across words like 'cardiac' (related to the heart), 'vascular' (related to blood vessels), or 'hemoglobin' (a protein in red blood cells that carries oxygen).

The Respiratory System

The respiratory system helps us breathe. It takes in oxygen and lets out carbon dioxide. The main parts are the nose, throat, windpipe, and lungs.

You might hear words like 'pulmonary' (related to lungs), 'bronchitis' (an inflammation of the bronchial tubes in the lungs), or 'asthma' (a condition that causes difficulty in breathing).

The Digestive System

The digestive system breaks down the food we eat. It turns food into nutrients that our body can use. It includes parts like the mouth, stomach, liver, and intestines.

Words related to this system could be 'gastric' (related to the stomach), 'hepatic' (related to the liver), or 'colitis' (an inflammation of the colon).

The Nervous System

The nervous system carries messages to and from the brain. It helps us think, feel, and move. It includes the brain, spinal cord, and nerves.

You might encounter terms like 'neurology' (the study of the nervous system), 'cerebral' (related to the brain), or 'paralysis' (loss of muscle function).

The Musculoskeletal System

The musculoskeletal system supports the body and helps it move. It includes bones, muscles, and joints.

Terms you may find could include 'osteo' (related to bones), 'muscular' (related to muscles), or 'arthritis' (inflammation of joints).

The Urinary System

The urinary system removes waste from the body. It includes parts like kidneys, bladder, and urethra.

Words related to this system might be 'renal' (related to kidneys), 'cystitis' (bladder inflammation), or 'urinalysis' (a test of urine to detect and manage a range of disorders).

The Reproductive System

The reproductive system includes organs like the ovaries in females and testes in males. It is responsible for creating new life.

You might encounter words like 'gynecology' (the study of female reproductive system), 'obstetrics' (care of women during pregnancy and childbirth), or 'andrology' (the study of male reproductive system).

Knowing these systems well will help you in medical transcription. In the next section, we will discuss common medical procedures and tests.

Common Diseases and Conditions Related to Each System

Circulatory System Diseases and Conditions

- **Hypertension:** Also known as high blood pressure, it can strain the heart and damage blood vessels, leading to heart attacks, stroke, or kidney problems.

- **Heart Disease:** This can refer to several types of heart conditions, like coronary artery disease, arrhythmias (irregular heartbeats), and heart failure.

- **Anemia:** This condition occurs when the body doesn't have enough red blood cells or hemoglobin. This can make you feel tired or weak because your body isn't getting the oxygen it needs.

Respiratory System Diseases and Conditions

- **Asthma:** This condition causes the airways to swell and narrow, which can make breathing difficult.

- **Pneumonia:** This is an infection in one or both lungs. It's usually caused by bacteria, viruses, or fungi.

- **Chronic Obstructive Pulmonary Disease (COPD):** This is a group of diseases that cause airflow blockage and breathing-related problems. It includes conditions like emphysema and chronic bronchitis.

Digestive System Diseases and Conditions

- **Gastritis:** This condition involves inflammation, irritation, or erosion of the stomach lining. It can occur suddenly or gradually.

- **Hepatitis:** This is an inflammation of the liver, often caused by viruses like hepatitis A, B, and C.

- **Colitis:** This is an inflammation of the colon, the longest part of the large intestine.

Nervous System Diseases and Conditions

- **Neurological Disorders:** These are diseases of the brain, spine, and the nerves that connect them. There are more than 600 diseases of the nervous system, such as Alzheimer's disease, Parkinson's disease, stroke, and epilepsy.

- **Paralysis:** This condition involves the loss of muscle function in part of your body.

Musculoskeletal System Diseases and Conditions

- **Arthritis:** This condition involves inflammation of one or more joints, causing pain and stiffness.

- **Osteoporosis:** This is a condition that weakens bones, making them fragile and more likely to break.

- **Muscular Dystrophy:** This is a group of diseases that cause progressive weakness and loss of muscle mass.

Urinary System Diseases and Conditions

- **Kidney Disease:** This includes conditions that cause your kidneys to not function as well as they should. It can range from mild to severe and can progress over time.

- **Urinary Tract Infections (UTIs):** These are infections that can occur anywhere along the urinary tract, which includes the kidneys, bladder, and urethra.

Reproductive System Diseases and Conditions

- **Polycystic Ovary Syndrome (PCOS):** This is a hormonal disorder common among women of reproductive age.

- **Prostate Cancer:** This is a common type of cancer in men, where cells in the prostate gland start to grow uncontrollably.

- **Infertility:** This is a condition that affects a person's ability to reproduce.

Understanding these common diseases and conditions will help you to comprehend and transcribe medical records more accurately.

Medical Procedures and Their Transcription

There are many medical procedures doctors do. They can be related to any body system. Common procedures are surgeries, diagnostic tests, and therapies. Let's understand some examples:

Circulatory System Procedures

- **Heart Bypass Surgery:** This is a major surgery. It is done when the heart's blood vessels are blocked. In this surgery, the doctor takes a blood vessel from another part of the body and uses it to bypass the blocked vessel.

- **Blood Tests:** This is a common test. It is done to check different things in the blood. For example, it can check if a person has anemia.

Respiratory System Procedures

- **Lung Biopsy:** In this procedure, a small piece of lung tissue is taken out. It is then checked under a microscope for disease.

- **Lung Function Tests:** These tests measure how well your lungs work. They are often done to check for diseases like asthma or COPD.

Musculoskeletal System Procedures

- **Physical Therapy:** This is a treatment that helps people move better and feel less pain. It is often used after surgery or injury.

- **Joint Replacement Surgery:** In this surgery, a damaged joint is replaced with an artificial one. It is often done for damaged knee or hip joints.

Urinary System Procedures

- **Dialysis:** This is a treatment for people with kidney failure. It helps remove waste products from the body.

In medical transcription, you will come across these and many more procedures. You need to know the name of the procedure, what it involves, and why it is done. This will help you to write it down correctly.

That's the end of Chapter 4. In the next chapter, we will study pharmacology for medical transcription. Stay tuned!

CHAPTER 5: PHARMACOLOGY FOR MEDICAL TRANSCRIPTION

Understanding Different Categories of Drugs

In the world of medicine, drugs play a big role. They are used to treat many health problems. Drugs can be put into different categories based on what they do. Let's understand some main drug categories:

Pain Killers (Analgesics): These are drugs that help to reduce pain. Paracetamol and ibuprofen are common examples. They can be used for different kinds of pain like headache, body ache, etc.

Infection Fighters (Antibiotics): These drugs are used to kill bacteria in the body. They are used when a person has an infection. Penicillin and amoxicillin are common examples. They can be used for many different bacterial infections.

Virus Killers (Antivirals): These drugs are used to kill viruses in the body. They are used when a person has a viral infection. Acyclovir and oseltamivir are common examples. They can be used for many different viral infections.

Pressure Controllers (Antihypertensives): These drugs are used to lower high blood pressure. They help the heart and blood vessels to work better. Amlodipine and lisinopril are common examples.

Sugar Controllers (Antidiabetics): These drugs are used to control the level of sugar in the blood. They are used by people with diabetes. Metformin and insulin are common examples.

As a medical transcriptionist, you need to know these drug categories. You will come across them many times in your work. Understanding them will help you to do your job well.

Medical Implications of Common Drugs

Each drug has a special effect on the body. For example, pain killers reduce pain. Infection fighters kill bacteria. But, drugs can also have other effects. These are called side effects. Let's understand this better:

Pain Killers (Analgesics): These drugs reduce pain. But, they can also have side effects. For example, they can cause stomach upset or dizziness.

Infection Fighters (Antibiotics): These drugs kill bacteria. But, they can also have side effects. For example, they can cause allergies in some people.

Virus Killers (Antivirals): These drugs kill viruses. But, they can also have side effects. For example, they can cause nausea or headache.

Pressure Controllers (Antihypertensives): These drugs lower high blood pressure. But, they can also have side effects. For example, they can cause tiredness or swelling in the feet.

Sugar Controllers (Antidiabetics): These drugs control the level of sugar in the blood. But, they can also have side effects. For example, they can cause low blood sugar levels or skin rash.

As a medical transcriptionist, you need to know these effects and side effects. This will help you to understand and write about drugs better.

Decoding Pharmaceutical Jargon

Pharmaceutical jargon is a language within itself, used by healthcare professionals to ensure precise communication regarding medications. Here are some common terms and abbreviations you may encounter as a medical transcriptionist:

1. Dosage Forms:

- Tablet (tab)

- Capsule (cap)

- Injection (Inj)

- Syrup (syp)

- Suspension (susp)

2. Frequency:

- Once daily (qd)

- Twice daily (bid)

- Three times daily (tid)

- Four times daily (qid)

3. Routes of Administration:

- Oral (PO)

- Intravenous (IV)

- Subcutaneous (SC)

- Intramuscular (IM)

- Topical (top)

4. As Needed:

- Pro re nata (PRN): This Latin term means "as needed." For example, a pain medication might be prescribed "PRN" for a patient to take when their pain becomes unmanageable.

5. Units of Measurement:

- Milligram (mg)

- Gram (g)

- Microgram (mcg)

- Liter (L)

- Milliliter (mL)

6. Drug Classes:

- Antibiotics: Drugs that fight bacterial infections (e.g., amoxicillin).

- Antivirals: Drugs that fight viral infections (e.g., oseltamivir).

- Analgesics: Drugs that relieve pain (e.g., paracetamol).

- Antipyretics: Drugs that reduce fever (e.g., ibuprofen).

These are just some of the many terms you might encounter when dealing with pharmaceutical jargon. It's crucial to familiarize yourself with these terms as a medical transcriptionist, to ensure accuracy in transcription and prevent potentially harmful errors.

Dealing with Pharmaceutical Abbreviations in Transcription

Pharmaceutical abbreviations are frequently used in medical prescriptions and reports. When transcribing, it's crucial to accurately interpret these abbreviations because they can greatly affect a patient's treatment plan.

Here are some common pharmaceutical abbreviations that you should know:

- bid: This is an abbreviation for 'bis in die', which is Latin for twice a day. This instructs the patient to take the prescribed medication twice daily.

- tid: 'Ter in die' or three times a day. Medication should be taken three times daily.

- qid: 'Quater in die', which means the medication should be taken four times a day.

- hs: This stands for 'hora somni', meaning at bedtime.

- prn: 'Pro re nata', or as needed. The medication should be taken when required, for example, for pain relief.

- pc: 'Post cibum', or after meals.

- ac: 'Ante cibum', meaning before meals.

- mg: Milligrams, a unit of measurement for medication dosage.

- mcg: Micrograms, another unit of measurement for medication dosage.

- cc: Cubic centimeters, often used to measure liquid medication.

- PO: 'Per os', or by mouth. The medication should be taken orally.

- IV: Intravenous, meaning the medication should be administered through the vein.

Remember, when in doubt, it's always better to ask for clarification than to make an error in the transcription. Medical professionals will appreciate the diligence, and patients' safety could depend on it.

That's the end of Chapter 5. In the next chapter, we will learn about understanding American English for medical transcription. Stay tuned!

CHAPTER 6: UNDERSTANDING AMERICAN ENGLISH FOR MEDICAL TRANSCRIPTION

Basics of American English Grammar

When you transcribe, most of the time you will be using American English. American English is a bit different from British English. There are some changes in spelling, pronunciation, and sometimes even meaning of words. Here are some basics of American English grammar:

- **Nouns:** Nouns are words that tell us about people, places, things, or ideas. For example, doctor, hospital, medicine, and health.

- **Verbs:** Verbs are words that tell us what is happening. For example, is, eat, run, and examine.

- **Adjectives:** Adjectives are words that describe nouns. For example, big, healthy, quick, and blue.

- **Adverbs:** Adverbs are words that describe verbs. They tell us how, when, where, or why something happens. For example, quickly, daily, outside, and well.

- **Prepositions:** Prepositions are words that tell us about time, place, or direction. For example, in, at, on, and from.

- **Conjunctions:** Conjunctions are words that join words or groups of words together. For example, and, or, but, because.

Sentence structure: A sentence in English usually has a subject (the doer), a verb (the action), and an object (the receiver of the action). For example, in the sentence "The doctor examines the patient," "The doctor" is the subject, "examines" is the verb, and "the patient" is the object.

Knowing these basics will help you a lot in your transcription work.

Differences between British and American English

As a medical transcriptionist, you will need to be aware of the differences between British and American English. Here are some of the most important differences:

- **Spelling Differences:** Some words are spelled differently in American and British English. For instance, words that end in "or" in American English often end in "our" in British English. Examples include color/colour, labor/labour, and honor/honour. Similarly, words that end in "er" in American English often end in "re" in British English. Examples include center/centre, meter/metre, and fiber/fibre.

- **Vocabulary Differences:** There are some words that are used differently in American and British English. For example, the word 'truck' in American English is equivalent to 'lorry' in British English. Similarly, 'elevator' in American English is 'lift' in British English. Even in medical terms, there can be differences. For example, the American 'pediatrician' is 'paediatrician' in British English.

- **Pronunciation Differences:** The pronunciation of some words is also different in American and British English. For example, the word 'vitamin' is pronounced 'vahy-tuh-min' in American English and 'vit-uh-min' in British English. Another example is the word 'garage' which is pronounced 'gə-ˈräzh' in American English and ''ga-rij' or 'gə-ˈräj' in British English.

- **Grammar Differences:** There are also some differences in grammar between the two versions of English. For example, in American English, collective nouns are usually treated as singular (the team is winning), while in British English, they are often treated as plural (the team are winning).

Remember, the goal in medical transcription is clarity and accuracy. It's important to use the form of English that your client or employer prefers and is most suitable for the patients' understanding.

Understanding Colloquialisms and Slang in Medical Dictation

Colloquialisms and slang often pop up in spoken language, which includes the dictations you'll be transcribing. While medical professionals strive for clarity and accuracy in their communication, they're also human and might occasionally use informal speech patterns, abbreviations, or slang terms.

In the context of medical transcription, understanding colloquialisms and slang terms becomes essential, especially when they're commonly used in the healthcare field. For example, 'BP' is a standard abbreviation for blood pressure, 'ER' stands for the emergency room, and 'CABG' (pronounced as 'cabbage') refers to Coronary Artery Bypass Grafting, a type of heart surgery.

It's crucial to keep in mind that these informal terms or abbreviations must be transcribed into their formal versions unless the context or transcription guidelines specify otherwise. In the above examples, 'BP' would be transcribed as 'blood pressure', 'ER' as 'emergency room', and 'CABG' as 'Coronary Artery Bypass Grafting'.

Always make sure to clarify any colloquialisms or slang terms you're unsure about to ensure accuracy in the transcribed medical records. The healthcare field has zero tolerance for guesswork. As a medical transcriptionist, you're part of the healthcare team, contributing to patient safety and care by providing clear and accurate transcriptions.

Importance and Rules of Punctuation in Medical Transcription

Punctuation is absolutely crucial in medical transcription for several reasons:

1. Clarity: Proper punctuation helps convey the correct meaning of a sentence. For example, the sentence "Let's eat, Grandma" has a vastly different meaning from "Let's eat Grandma." In the context of medical transcription, this could be the difference between correct and incorrect treatment instructions.

2. Flow: Punctuation aids in the flow of reading, helping the reader to understand where pauses, emphasis, or certain tonal inflections should occur. This can help healthcare providers understand the nuances of a patient's medical history or treatment instructions.

3. Accuracy: Certain abbreviations or medical terms may require specific punctuation. Misplaced or missing punctuation could lead to misunderstandings or errors in transcription.

Here are the main punctuation marks used in medical transcription and their rules:

- **Comma (,):** This punctuation mark is used to separate items in a list, clauses in a sentence, or to indicate a pause in speech.

- **Period (.):** This is used at the end of a complete sentence. In medical transcription, it is also used after many abbreviations.

- **Semicolon (;):** This is used to separate two closely related independent clauses within the same sentence. It can also be used to separate items in a list if the items themselves contain commas.

- **Colon (:):** This is used to introduce a list, an explanation, or a definition. It should always follow a complete sentence.

- **Hyphen (-):** This is used to connect two words that function as a single concept. It's often used in compound words or to connect prefixes to certain words.

- **Apostrophe ('):** This is used to show possession or to form a contraction. In medical transcription, it's often used in anatomical terms or to indicate missing numbers or letters in dates and abbreviations.

Remember, each healthcare institution may have its own style guide, so it's essential to adapt to those specific guidelines when performing medical transcription.

In the next chapter, we will learn about Advanced English for Medical Transcription. Let's continue our journey!

CHAPTER 7: ADVANCED ENGLISH FOR MEDICAL TRANSCRIPTION

Advanced Rules and Exceptions in English Grammar

English grammar is indeed quite complex and is filled with rules and exceptions. Here are a few advanced aspects of English grammar that you might find useful:

- Irregular verbs: English has many verbs that don't follow the regular conjugation rules. These are known as irregular verbs. For example, the past tense of "go" is "went," not "goed."

- Conditional sentences: These are sentences that express certain conditions. The result of the condition is usually indicated in the latter part of the sentence. For example, "If you study hard, you will pass the exam."

- The passive voice: In English, sentences can be expressed in active or passive voice. In passive sentences, the subject is acted upon by the verb. For example, "The ball was thrown by John" is a passive sentence.

- Modal verbs: These are special types of verbs that express necessity, possibility, permission, or ability. Examples include can, could, may, might, will, would, shall, should, and must.

- Indirect speech: When we report what someone else has said, we usually shift the tenses back. For example, "He said he was tired."

- Complex sentences: These are sentences that contain one independent clause and at least one dependent clause. The dependent clause can be a noun clause, an adjective clause, or an adverb clause.

It's important to have a good understanding of these and other rules to ensure accuracy in your transcriptions. And, as with all rules, remember there can be exceptions.

Enhancing Vocabulary for Medical Transcription

Absolutely, having a robust medical vocabulary is crucial for any medical transcriptionist. Here are a few strategies that can be used to enhance your medical vocabulary:

1. Use Medical Dictionaries and Textbooks: Medical dictionaries and textbooks can be a valuable resource for learning medical terms. They typically provide definitions and context for each term.

2. Online Courses and Quizzes: There are many online courses and quizzes specifically designed to enhance medical vocabulary. They can be interactive and engaging, making learning easier.

3. Flashcards: Creating flashcards with medical terms on one side and their meanings on the other can be a great way to memorize new words.

4. Reading Medical Journals and Articles: Regularly reading medical journals and articles not only keeps you updated on the latest medical advancements but also helps in learning new medical terms and their usage.

5. Practice: Try to use new medical terms in your work or discussions. The more you use these terms, the more familiar they will become.

6. Continuous Learning: Medicine is a field that is constantly evolving. New terms and procedures are being added regularly. Therefore, it's important to continue learning and stay updated.

Remember, it's not just about knowing the terms, but also understanding their meanings, usage, and implications in different medical contexts.

Sound-alikes and Their Proper Usage

In medical transcription, sound-alikes or homophones are words that sound similar but have different meanings and spellings. Using the wrong sound-alike can change the meaning of a medical report, leading to miscommunication or even medical errors. Therefore, it's crucial to understand and use these words properly.

Here are some examples of common sound-alikes in medical transcription:

1. Affect/Effect: "Affect" is usually a verb meaning to influence something, while "effect" is usually a noun meaning the result of an action. However, "effect" can also be used as a verb meaning to bring about, and "affect" can be a noun in psychology referring to emotion.

2. Complement/Compliment: "Complement" means to complete or enhance something. In medicine, it refers to a part of the immune system. On the other hand, "compliment" refers to a nice thing said about someone.

3. Discrete/Discreet: "Discrete" means separate or distinct, while "discreet" means careful or unobtrusive.

4. Principle/Principal: "Principle" is a noun meaning a fundamental truth or law, while "principal" can be a noun meaning the most important person or thing, or an adjective meaning main or most important.

5. Prostate/Prostrate: "Prostate" is a gland in the male reproductive system, while "prostrate" is an adjective meaning lying flat or overcome.

6. Illicit/Elicit: "Illicit" means forbidden by law or rules, while "elicit" means to draw out a response or answer.

It's important to use the right word based on the context. If you're unsure about a word, it's always best to check its spelling and meaning. Using a medical dictionary can be very helpful in this case.

Dealing with regional accents and dialects can be challenging in medical transcription, but it's an essential skill. Speakers from different regions, countries, or cultural backgrounds may pronounce words differently or use different vocabulary. Here are some tips to help you deal with accents and dialects:

1. Familiarize Yourself: Take the time to familiarize yourself with different accents and dialects. Watch movies, listen to radio broadcasts, or use language learning tools that feature speakers from different regions.

2. Research Common Terms and Phrases: Different regions may use different terms for the same concept. For example, the same disease might have different names in different regions. If you're transcribing dictations from a particular region, try to learn some common terms and phrases from that region.

3. Use Context Clues: If a word is unclear due to an accent, try to use the context to figure out what the word might be. Consider the overall topic of the dictation and the words surrounding the unclear word.

4. Slow Down: If you're having trouble understanding an accent, try slowing down the playback speed of the dictation. This can give you more time to process what's being said.

5. Don't Hesitate to Ask for Clarification: If you're still unsure about a word after trying the above strategies, don't hesitate to ask the speaker for clarification, if possible. It's better to be sure than to risk making a mistake in the transcription.

6. Use a Good Quality Headset: A good quality headset can make it easier to hear subtle differences in pronunciation, making it easier to understand different accents.

Remember, it takes time to become comfortable with different accents and dialects, so be patient with yourself. Practice is key when it comes to understanding and transcribing various accents accurately.

In the next chapter, we will learn about Medical Specialties and their Transcription. Let's move forward in our learning journey!

CHAPTER 8: MEDICAL SPECIALTIES AND THEIR TRANSCRIPTION

Medical transcriptionists must often adapt their practices according to the specialty of the physician or healthcare provider they're transcribing for. Each medical specialty has its own unique terminology, diagnostic procedures, treatment options, and potential complications. Here are a few examples of transcription rules and practices for different medical specialties:

1. Cardiology: Transcriptionists working with cardiologists must be familiar with terms relating to the heart and the circulatory system. This includes the names of various heart diseases (like myocardial infarction or atherosclerosis), diagnostic procedures (like EKG or cardiac catheterization), and treatment options (like bypass surgery or angioplasty).

2. Radiology: Radiologists often describe images in their reports, so transcriptionists must understand the terms used to describe body positions, views, and anomalies. It's also important to know the terminology related to various imaging techniques like MRI, CT scan, ultrasound, and X-rays.

3. Orthopedics: Transcriptionists in this field need to know terminology related to the musculoskeletal system, including terms for bones, muscles, and connective tissues. They must also be familiar with terms related to trauma, fractures, orthopedic surgeries, and prosthetics.

4. Oncology: In oncology, transcriptionists must be familiar with a wide range of terms related to cancer types, stages, and treatments. This includes terms related to chemotherapy, radiation therapy, immunotherapy, surgical procedures, and more.

5. Psychiatry: Transcriptionists working in psychiatry need to understand terms related to mental health disorders, psychological assessments, psychotherapy, and psychotropic medications.

6. Pediatrics: Transcriptionists transcribing pediatric notes should be aware of terms related to growth and development, common childhood illnesses, vaccinations, and developmental milestones.

It's also essential for transcriptionists to follow privacy laws and ethical guidelines, regardless of the medical specialty they're working in. All patient information must be treated as confidential, and it should only be shared with individuals who have a legitimate need to know.

Each medical specialty has unique terminology and jargon that are important for a medical transcriptionist to understand. Here are examples from several specialties:

1. Cardiology: Terms such as "myocardial infarction" (heart attack), "angioplasty" (a procedure to open blocked or narrowed coronary arteries), "stent placement" (a device used to keep the artery open), and "arrhythmia" (irregular heartbeat) are unique to this specialty.

2. Radiology: Radiologists use terms like "radiolucent" (an area appearing dark on a radiograph, indicating penetration of x-rays), "radiopaque" (appearing white or light on a radiograph), "contrast" (a substance used to make certain structures or tissues more visible on the scans), and specific types of imaging like "MRI", "CT", or "ultrasound".

3. Orthopedics: Terms such as "arthroscopy" (a procedure for diagnosing and treating joint problems), "osteoarthritis" (degeneration of joint cartilage and the underlying bone), "prosthesis" (an artificial body part), and "fracture" (a break in a bone) are common.

4. Oncology: Oncologists use terms like "carcinoma" (cancer that starts in the skin or the tissues that line other organs), "metastasis" (cancer spread to other parts of the body), "chemotherapy", "radiation", and specific cancer types like "leukemia" or "melanoma".

5. Psychiatry: Psychiatry has unique terms such as "schizophrenia" (a mental disorder characterized by abnormal behavior, strange speech, and a decreased ability to understand reality), "bipolar disorder", "psychotherapy" (a range of treatments that can help with mental health problems), and "antidepressants".

6. Pediatrics: Pediatricians often refer to terms like "neonate" (a newborn child), "pediatric milestones" (key skills expected to be achieved by certain ages), "immunization", and specific childhood diseases like "chickenpox" or "measles".

Knowing the terminology and jargon of each specialty not only allows medical transcriptionists to accurately transcribe reports, but it also helps in understanding the context of the reports, which contributes to their overall quality and reliability.

Understanding Different Types of Reports in Each Specialty

Medical transcription involves working with many different types of reports, and each medical specialty tends to have specific types of reports that are most commonly used. Here are examples of some report types you may encounter in different specialties:

1. Operative Reports: In specialties such as General Surgery, Orthopedics, and Obstetrics and Gynecology, you'll encounter operative reports. These describe the details of a surgical procedure, including the preoperative and postoperative diagnoses, the procedure performed, the findings during the surgery, and any specimens taken.

2. Radiology Reports: In Radiology, radiologists generate reports detailing their interpretation of imaging studies like X-rays, CT scans, MRIs, ultrasounds, and others. The report will typically include the reason for the study, a description of the findings, and an interpretation or conclusion.

3. Discharge Summaries: In Internal Medicine and Family Practice, discharge summaries are common. These provide a complete picture of a patient's hospital stay, including the reason for admission, the findings, the course in the hospital, the treatment provided, the condition of the patient at discharge, and the plan for follow-up.

4. Pathology Reports: In Pathology, you will encounter pathology reports. These detail the findings of a pathologist's microscopic examination of tissue samples, such as from a biopsy. The report will include a description of the sample, the microscopic findings, and a diagnosis.

5. Psychiatric Evaluations: In Psychiatry, you'll often transcribe psychiatric evaluations. These reports include the patient's mental status examination, which assesses appearance, behavior, thought processes, mood and affect, cognitive abilities, and insight and judgment.

6. Progress Notes: In nearly every specialty, you'll transcribe progress notes. These are ongoing records of a patient's condition, treatment, and progress.

Knowing the format and content expected in each type of report will help ensure your transcriptions are accurate and complete.

Case Studies and Examples

Let's look at a couple of examples that you might encounter in medical transcription:

Case Study 1: Cardiology

Consider a patient who had a cardiac catheterization procedure due to complaints of chest pain. The transcription might read as follows:

The patient, a 65-year-old male with a history of hypertension and hyperlipidemia, presented with recurrent episodes of chest pain. He was scheduled for a cardiac catheterization to evaluate the status of his coronary arteries. The procedure was uneventful, and the patient tolerated it well. The left main coronary artery was normal. The left anterior descending artery had a 40% stenosis in the proximal segment. The left circumflex and the right coronary artery were normal. The ejection fraction was 60%. The patient will be started on optimal medical management and will be scheduled for a stress test to evaluate the significance of the lesion in the left anterior descending artery.

Case Study 2: Neurology

Consider a patient who presented with symptoms of a stroke. The transcription might read as follows:

The patient, a 70-year-old female, was brought to the emergency department with sudden onset of right-sided weakness and slurred speech. A CT scan of the brain was performed, which showed a large left middle cerebral artery infarction. The patient was immediately started on intravenous thrombolytic therapy. Neurological examination revealed a right hemiparesis with a National Institutes of Health Stroke Scale (NIHSS) score of 10. The patient was subsequently admitted to the stroke unit for further management. The plan is to start the patient on occupational and physical therapy as soon as she is medically stable.

In both these examples, the transcriptionist would need to understand the medical terminology, abbreviations, and the nature of the procedures described in order to accurately transcribe the report.

In the next chapter, we will delve into different types of medical reports and their transcription. Let's continue our journey in understanding the intricacies of medical transcription!

CHAPTER 9: TYPES OF MEDICAL REPORTS AND THEIR TRANSCRIPTION

Different Types of Medical Reports and Their Formats

There are several types of medical reports and each has its own format. Here are some common ones:

1. History and Physical Examination (H&P): This is often the first document created in a patient's medical record when they are admitted to a hospital. It contains the patient's medical history, a review of systems, and the findings from a physical examination. It is used to identify the patient's primary and secondary diagnoses and to develop a plan of care.

2. Consultation Report: This is a document written by a specialist, who has been asked to evaluate a patient. It usually includes the reason for the consultation, a brief history, the specialist's findings, and suggestions for further treatment or tests.

3. Operative Report: This is a detailed report written by a surgeon after a surgical procedure. It includes information about the patient before the operation, a detailed description of the procedure and findings, the status of the patient after surgery, and the names of the primary and assisting surgeons.

4. Discharge Summary: This report is created when a patient is discharged from the hospital. It summarizes the patient's stay, including the reason for admission, significant findings, procedures performed, treatment given, the condition of the patient at discharge, and instructions for follow-up care.

5. Radiology Report: This report is created by a radiologist after interpreting an imaging study, such as an X-ray, CT scan, or MRI. It includes the type of study performed, the findings, and the radiologist's interpretation.

6. Pathology Report: This report is created by a pathologist after analyzing a tissue sample (biopsy). It includes information about the type of tissue examined, the tests performed, the findings, and the pathologist's interpretation.

As a medical transcriptionist, it's important to understand these different types of reports and their typical formats.

Transcription Rules and Practices for Each Type of Report

Each type of medical report has specific transcription rules and practices. Here are some guidelines for the most common types:

1. History and Physical Examination (H&P): This report must accurately transcribe the patient's history, symptoms, and physician's findings during the physical examination. Use clear, concise language and follow the dictated format, which typically includes sections such as Chief Complaint, History of Present

Illness, Past Medical History, Family and Social History, Review of Systems, Physical Examination, and Assessment and Plan.

2. Consultation Report: Transcribe the reason for consultation, brief history, specialist's findings, and recommendations exactly as dictated. Pay close attention to any specific tests or treatments suggested by the consultant.

3. Operative Report: Transcribe the preoperative diagnosis, procedure, surgeon's name, findings, and postoperative diagnosis accurately. Include details of the operation such as type of anesthesia, description of the procedure, estimated blood loss, and any complications.

4. Discharge Summary: This summary must capture all essential information about the patient's hospital stay, including admission details, course in the hospital, treatment provided, final diagnosis, condition at discharge, and follow-up care instructions.

5. Radiology Report: Ensure you transcribe the name of the study, the findings, and the radiologist's impressions accurately. Misinterpretation or misrepresentation of findings can lead to incorrect treatment.

6. Pathology Report: Transcribe the type of specimen, macroscopic description, microscopic description, and diagnosis exactly as dictated. Again, any mistake could lead to misdiagnosis or incorrect treatment.

Remember to follow basic transcription guidelines for all types of reports: use correct spelling and punctuation, follow the dictated format, and ensure patient confidentiality at all times. If anything is unclear or sounds incorrect, flag it for review rather than guessing.

Common Challenges in Transcribing Different Reports

Transcribing medical reports can present several challenges:

1. Poor audio quality: This can be due to a bad phone line, background noise, or the speaker's voice being too quiet. This makes it difficult to understand what's being said and can lead to mistakes in transcription.

2. Accents and speech clarity: The physician dictating the report may have a strong accent, may speak too quickly, or may not enunciate clearly, which can make the dictation hard to understand.

3. Medical jargon and abbreviations: Medical reports are full of specialized terminology and abbreviations, which can be confusing if you're not familiar with them.

4. Similar sounding words: There are many medical terms that sound alike but have different meanings, like "hypertension" and "hypotension". Mishearing these can lead to serious errors in the transcription.

5. Formatting: Different types of reports have different formatting requirements, which can be difficult to remember and apply correctly.

6. Missing information: Sometimes, the speaker may leave out important information, or the dictation might be cut off. This requires the transcriptionist to be attentive and identify when something seems to be missing.

7. Keeping up with updates: Medical terminology and procedures are constantly evolving, so transcriptionists need to keep their knowledge up-to-date.

Despite these challenges, with the right training and practice, you can become proficient in transcribing a wide range of medical reports.

Practice Exercises and Examples

Practice is key in becoming proficient at medical transcription. Here are a few examples of practice exercises:

1. Transcription Practice: Try transcribing recorded medical dictations available online. Start with clear, slow-paced dictations and gradually move to ones with faster pace or thicker accents.

2. Terminology Quizzes: Regularly test your knowledge of medical terms. Try online quizzes or flashcards for different medical specialties.

3. Abbreviation Exercises: Write out common medical abbreviations and their full forms. Then, try writing out the full forms when you see the abbreviations.

4. Drug Name Drills: Practice spelling and pronouncing generic and brand names of common drugs.

5. Formatting Practice: Take a paragraph of medical text and practice formatting it as a different type of report (e.g., consultation report, operative report, discharge summary).

6. Listening Exercises: Improve your listening skills by watching medical lectures or seminars. This can help you become more accustomed to medical jargon and different accents.

7. Proofreading Exercises: Proofread transcribed medical reports to identify and correct errors. This can help you improve your accuracy and attention to detail.

8. Shadowing Exercises: Try to repeat what you hear in a dictation as closely as possible, mirroring the speaker's pace and intonation. This can help improve your listening skills and your understanding of how words and phrases are pronounced in different accents.

Remember, it's okay to make mistakes during practice. The goal is to learn from them and improve over time.

In the next chapter, we'll delve into the tools and technologies used in medical transcription. The right tools can make your work faster and more accurate, so let's explore them!

Hardware and Software Necessary for Transcription

Medical transcription requires a combination of hardware and software tools to perform the task efficiently. Here are some of the necessities:

Hardware:

1. Computer: A desktop or laptop computer with a good processor and enough memory to run transcription software efficiently.

2. Headphones: High-quality headphones are essential for clear audio playback. Some transcriptionists prefer noise-cancelling headphones to minimize distractions.

3. Foot Pedal: A transcription foot pedal allows you to control audio playback (play, pause, rewind, fast forward) with your foot, leaving your hands free to type.

4. Ergonomic Keyboard: An ergonomic keyboard can help prevent strain and injury from long hours of typing.

Software:

1. Transcription Software: There are many types of transcription software available, ranging from basic audio players to advanced programs that integrate with word processing software and provide tools for speeding up or slowing down playback, inserting timestamps, and more.

2. Word Processing Software: A good word processing program is essential for typing and formatting transcriptions. Microsoft Word is a commonly used option.

3. Medical Dictionary Software: A comprehensive medical dictionary software can be helpful for looking up unfamiliar terms quickly.

4. Spell Check and Grammar Software: Software like Grammarly can help ensure that your transcriptions are grammatically correct and free of typos.

5. Speech Recognition Software: While not necessary for all transcriptionists, speech recognition software like Dragon NaturallySpeaking can be a valuable tool, especially for those with fast typing speeds and a good understanding of how to use the software effectively.

Remember that while having the right tools is important, success in medical transcription ultimately comes down to your skills and knowledge. Practice regularly, stay updated with the latest medical terminology, and continuously strive to improve your typing speed and accuracy.

Speech recognition software, also known as speech-to-text or voice recognition software, converts spoken language into written text. It's becoming increasingly popular in various fields, including medical transcription. These tools can significantly speed up the transcription process, especially for individuals with fast and clear speech.

Here's a basic guide to understanding and using speech recognition software:

1. Selecting the Right Software: Different speech recognition programs have different strengths. Dragon NaturallySpeaking is a widely recognized program that many medical transcriptionists use due to its high accuracy and extensive customizability. Other options may include Google's speech-to-text capabilities or software like Express Scribe.

2. Training the Software: Most speech recognition software requires a training period to learn the specifics of your voice, including accent, speech patterns, and pacing. During this training period, you'll read specific texts aloud to allow the program to adjust to your voice. The more you use it, the better it becomes at understanding your speech.

3. Using a Good Quality Microphone: Speech recognition software relies heavily on the quality of the audio it receives. Therefore, using a good quality microphone can significantly improve the software's accuracy.

4. Correcting Mistakes: While speech recognition software has become quite accurate, it can still make mistakes. Always proofread the transcriptions and correct any errors. Over time, the software learns from these corrections and improves.

5. Using Commands: Many speech recognition programs include commands that you can use to control your computer or the software itself. For example, you might say "new paragraph" to start a new paragraph or "delete that" to erase the last thing you said.

6. Customizing the Software: Some advanced speech recognition software allows you to customize commands or add new vocabulary. This feature can be especially useful in medical transcription, where you frequently use specific medical terminology.

Keep in mind that while speech recognition software can be a valuable tool, it isn't a replacement for a skilled transcriptionist. It's best used as a tool to aid in your transcription efforts. You'll still need to proofread and edit the transcriptions to ensure accuracy.

Keeping up with Technological Advancements

In an industry as dynamic as healthcare, staying up-to-date with technological advancements is critical. These advancements could be in the form of new software tools, updated transcription guidelines, or innovative hardware equipment. Here are some strategies to keep up with technological advancements:

1. Attend Industry Conferences and Webinars: Conferences and webinars are great places to learn about new developments in medical transcription. They often feature industry experts who discuss recent trends, share their experiences, and demonstrate new tools or techniques.

2. Subscribe to Industry Publications: There are numerous industry-specific publications, both online and in print, which cover the latest advancements in medical transcription technology. Regularly reading these can provide you with valuable insights.

3. Join Online Communities: Online communities such as forums or social media groups provide platforms for people in the same field to share their experiences, ask questions, and discuss the latest trends. LinkedIn, for example, hosts several groups dedicated to medical transcription.

4. Take Continuing Education Courses: Many organizations offer courses on new technologies, transcription practices, and updates in the medical field. These can be great opportunities to learn new skills and stay current.

5. Experiment with New Tools: As new tools and software become available, try them out. Many companies offer free trials of their products. This hands-on experience can give you a better understanding of the tool's capabilities and whether it could be beneficial for your work.

6. Build a Network: Networking with other professionals in your field can provide you with insights into what tools they're using and how they're adapting to technological changes.

Remember, the goal of leveraging technology is to enhance efficiency, accuracy, and overall quality of work in medical transcription. While it's important to stay current with the latest technologies, it's equally important to master the tools you're using and understand their functionality thoroughly.

Troubleshooting Common Technical Issues

Technical issues are an inevitable part of working with computers and digital systems. Here are some common issues medical transcriptionists might encounter, along with suggested troubleshooting steps:

1. No Sound or Low Sound Quality in Dictation: Ensure your speakers or headphones are correctly plugged in and the volume is turned up. Check if the sound is muted on your computer or within the transcription software. If the problem persists, it could be an issue with the audio file itself, and you may need to request a better-quality version.

2. Slow or Unresponsive Software: This could be due to your computer's memory being overtaxed. Close any unnecessary applications. If the issue persists, you might need to restart your computer. If the problem continues even after rebooting, it could be a sign that your system lacks the resources to run the software efficiently, and you may need to upgrade your hardware or software.

3. Typing Lags or Errors: First, confirm that the issue is not physical, like a faulty keyboard. Then check if the problem occurs only with the transcription software or with other applications as well. If it's the latter, your computer could be low on resources. If it's the former, you might need to reinstall the transcription software or contact the software's support team.

4. Issues with Speech Recognition Software: If your speech recognition software is not transcribing accurately, make sure you're speaking clearly and at a moderate pace. It may require some training to adapt to your voice and speaking style. Also, ensure your microphone is working properly and is correctly configured with the software.

5. Trouble Connecting to the Internet: First, check to make sure your router is online and working properly. If it's not, you may need to reset it. If the problem persists, contact your internet service provider (ISP) for further assistance.

6. Software Updates Not Installing: This could be due to a lack of storage space on your device or a problem with your internet connection. Free up some space by deleting unnecessary files or applications and make sure your internet connection is stable before attempting to install updates again.

Remember, it's essential to regularly backup your work and files to prevent data loss in case of major technical issues. If you frequently encounter problems with your software or hardware, you may need to contact a professional for assistance.

Up next, we'll walk through the medical transcription process step by step. We'll cover everything from receiving the audio file to submitting the completed transcription. Stay tuned!

Step-by-Step Walkthrough of the Transcription Process

The transcription process involves several steps, each requiring attention to detail and accuracy. Here's a basic step-by-step guide:

1. Receiving and Reviewing the Dictation: The first step is to receive the audio file that you will transcribe. Review the file briefly to understand the subject matter, the speaker's accent and speaking speed, and the audio quality. You may also receive instructions or guidelines specific to the file.

2. Setting Up Your Workspace: Ensure your workspace is quiet and distraction-free. Prepare your transcription software, headset, and foot pedal, if you're using one. Open your word processing software and set it up according to your or your client's formatting requirements.

3. Transcribing the Audio: Start playing the audio file and begin transcribing. If you're using a foot pedal, you can use your foot to pause, play, rewind, or fast forward the recording, leaving your hands free to type. Try to transcribe verbatim (word for word) unless instructed otherwise.

4. Looking Up Unfamiliar Terms: If you come across any unfamiliar words or terms, pause the recording and look them up. This is particularly important in medical transcription, where accuracy can impact patient care.

5. Proofreading the Transcript: Once you've transcribed the entire audio file, review your work. Check for spelling, grammar, and punctuation errors. Also, make sure medical terms and drug names are spelled correctly.

6. Formatting the Transcript: Format the transcript according to the guidelines provided. This could include adding speaker labels, timestamps, or section headings.

7. Submitting the Transcript: Once you're satisfied with the accuracy and formatting of your transcript, save it in the required format (usually .doc or .txt) and submit it to your client or supervisor.

8. Handling Feedback and Revisions: Be prepared to receive feedback and make revisions if necessary. This is part of the learning process and helps you improve as a transcriptionist.

Remember, the goal of medical transcription is to create a clear, accurate written record of a spoken dictation. Quality is crucial. It's more important to take your time to produce an accurate transcript than to rush and make mistakes.

Importance of Accuracy and Techniques for Verification

Accuracy in medical transcription is of utmost importance as the transcribed documents are used for patient care, medical references, and legal purposes. Errors in medical transcription can lead to incorrect diagnosis, inappropriate treatment, and other potentially harmful consequences. Here are a few techniques to maintain and verify the accuracy of your transcriptions:

1. Know Your Subject: Have a good understanding of medical terminology, abbreviations, drug names, and procedures related to the specific medical specialty you are transcribing for.

2. Use Reliable References: Always keep a good medical dictionary, drug index, and reference books handy. Websites of professional medical organizations can also be a good source of information.

3. Listen Carefully: Pay close attention to the audio. If something doesn't sound right or make sense, it probably isn't. Listen to that part again. If still in doubt, mark the spot and move on. You can come back to it later.

4. Clarify Doubts: If you have a question about a dictation, don't hesitate to ask. Most organizations would prefer you ask questions rather than make an error in the transcript.

5. Proofread Your Work: Always proofread your work at least once. This helps you catch and correct any spelling, punctuation, grammar, or formatting errors.

6. Use Speech Recognition Software Sparingly: While speech recognition software can help increase productivity, they are not always accurate, especially with medical terms. Always review and edit the drafts produced by speech recognition software.

7. Continuous Learning: Medicine is a field that's always evolving. Make it a point to learn about new drugs, treatments, and medical procedures. This will help you stay updated and improve your accuracy.

Remember, the goal is to provide the most accurate transcription possible. Even small errors can have big consequences, so always prioritize accuracy over speed.

Confidentiality Laws and Ethical Practices in Medical Transcription

Medical transcriptionists play a crucial role in healthcare and have access to sensitive patient information. Thus, they are bound by strict laws and ethical guidelines to ensure patient confidentiality. Here are some important principles to understand:

1. Health Insurance Portability and Accountability Act (HIPAA): In the United States, HIPAA is the primary law governing patient privacy. It mandates that healthcare providers and their associates, including medical transcriptionists, must protect the privacy and security of a patient's health information. Violations can lead to significant penalties.

2. Confidentiality: As a medical transcriptionist, you must keep all patient information confidential. This includes not discussing patient information with friends, family, or anyone else who does not have a legitimate need to know.

3. Data Security: Medical transcription often involves digital data, which must be protected from unauthorized access. This involves using secure networks, strong passwords, and secure storage solutions for patient data.

4. Ethical Behavior: Beyond specific laws and regulations, medical transcriptionists are expected to behave ethically. This means being honest, accurate, and professional in all dealings. For instance, transcriptionists should not guess or make up information if they can't understand something in the audio file. Instead, they should seek clarification.

5. Continuous Learning: Laws, regulations, and best practices in healthcare often change. Therefore, medical transcriptionists need to engage in continuous learning to stay updated.

6. Reporting Violations: If a transcriptionist witnesses violations of these principles, such as unauthorized access or misuse of patient information, they have a duty to report these to the appropriate authority in their organization.

Overall, confidentiality and ethical practices are not just about legal compliance, but also about maintaining trust between patients and the healthcare system. Medical transcriptionists, like all healthcare professionals, play a crucial role in maintaining this trust.

Dealing with Difficult or Unclear Dictations

Transcribing unclear or difficult dictations can be challenging. Here are a few strategies to help handle such situations:

1. Slow Down Playback Speed: Most transcription software allows you to adjust the playback speed. Slowing down the dictation can help you understand unclear or fast speech.

2. Use Headphones: A good set of headphones can make it easier to hear and understand the dictation, especially if there's background noise.

3. Repeated Listening: Don't hesitate to replay difficult parts of the dictation. It's better to take your time to ensure accuracy than to rush and make mistakes.

4. Use Context Clues: If a particular word or phrase isn't clear, consider the context. What is the topic of the dictation? What words or phrases were used before and after the unclear section? This can often help you figure out the intended meaning.

5. Research: If you're unsure about a term, look it up. Use medical dictionaries, textbooks, or reputable online sources.

6. Flag for Review: If a portion of the dictation remains unclear despite your best efforts, flag it for review. Most transcription services have a process for reviewing and resolving unclear dictations.

7. Seek Help: If allowed by your organization's policies, ask a colleague or supervisor for help. They might be able to offer a different perspective or suggest something you hadn't considered.

Remember, the goal of medical transcription is accuracy. If you're unsure about something, it's better to seek clarification than to guess and risk making a mistake.

In the next chapter, we'll also discuss how to ensure the quality of your transcriptions and how to improve your skills over time. Keep reading!

CHAPTER 12: QUALITY CONTROL IN MEDICAL TRANSCRIPTION

Standards and Best Practices for Quality Control

Ensuring quality in medical transcription is essential due to the importance of accurate medical records in patient care. Here are some standards and best practices for quality control in medical transcription:

1. Accuracy: This is the most critical aspect of medical transcription. Transcripts must be accurate, with correct spelling of all terms and appropriate use of medical terminology.

2. Consistency: Consistency in the style and format of transcripts is also important. This includes consistent use of abbreviations, punctuation, and capitalization.

3. Proofreading: Every transcript should be thoroughly proofread to identify and correct any errors. This includes checking for omitted words or phrases, misheard words, typographical errors, and formatting issues.

4. Knowledge and Training: Transcriptionists should have a good understanding of medical terminology, anatomy and physiology, and the principles of health records management. They should also be well-versed in the specific documentation requirements and terminology of the medical specialty they are transcribing for.

5. Confidentiality and Security: Medical transcripts contain sensitive patient information, so transcriptionists must adhere to all applicable laws and regulations related to health information privacy and security, such as the Health Insurance Portability and Accountability Act (HIPAA) in the United States.

6. Audit and Feedback: Regular audits of transcripts, with feedback provided to transcriptionists, can help to identify common errors or areas for improvement. This can be part of a broader quality assurance process within a medical transcription service or healthcare organization.

7. Continuing Education: Medical terminology and technology are always evolving, so ongoing training and education are crucial for maintaining transcription quality.

Remember, the ultimate goal of these standards and best practices is to provide accurate and timely medical records that support high-quality patient care.

Techniques for Error Detection and Correction

Error detection and correction in medical transcription are critical to ensure the accuracy and reliability of medical records. Here are some techniques commonly used:

1. Proofreading: This is the process of carefully reading the transcribed document to identify and correct any errors. It's crucial to check for spelling mistakes, incorrect use of medical terminology, grammatical errors, and formatting issues.

2. Double-checking Unclear Parts: If parts of the dictation are unclear, it's important to replay and listen carefully to accurately transcribe the information. If it's still unclear, the transcriptionist should flag it for review or clarification from the person who dictated the report.

3. Software Tools: Some transcription software comes with built-in spelling and grammar checkers that can help identify errors. There are also specialized medical spell-checking tools that can catch misused or misspelled medical terms.

4. Cross-Referencing: Cross-referencing the transcription with any available related documents can help identify inconsistencies or errors.

5. Peer Review: Sometimes, another medical transcriptionist or a supervisor reviews the transcription for accuracy and provides feedback. This is particularly useful for complex or challenging transcriptions.

6. Continuing Education: Keeping up to date with medical terminology, drug names, and new medical procedures is crucial for accuracy in medical transcription. Regular training can help prevent errors due to outdated or incorrect knowledge.

7. Use of Templates and Standards: Using templates and adhering to established transcription standards can reduce the likelihood of errors related to formatting and structure.

8. Quality Control Processes: Implementing systematic quality control processes, including regular audits of transcriptions, can help identify common errors and patterns, leading to improvements in error detection and correction.

Remember, the goal of error detection and correction in medical transcription is to ensure the production of accurate and reliable medical records to support patient care.

Strategies for Continuous Improvement and Skill Enhancement

Continuous improvement and skill enhancement are essential for a successful career in medical transcription. Here are some strategies to consider:

1. Ongoing Education: The medical field is always evolving, with new procedures, drugs, and diseases. Staying up-to-date with the latest medical knowledge is crucial. You can do this through online courses, seminars, or medical journals.

2. Practice: The more you transcribe, the more proficient you'll become. Practice not only helps improve speed but also accuracy.

3. Feedback and Review: Regularly ask for feedback on your work from supervisors or experienced colleagues. Constructive criticism can be incredibly helpful for recognizing areas where you can improve.

4. Networking: Joining professional organizations or online communities for medical transcriptionists can provide valuable resources, advice, and opportunities to learn from others in your field.

5. Technology Training: As technology advances, new tools become available that can make transcription faster and more accurate. Stay current with these changes and be open to learning new software and technology.

6. Quality Control: Regularly check your work for errors and aim to continuously decrease them. Learning from mistakes is one of the best ways to improve your skills.

7. Set Personal Goals: Have clear, achievable goals in place to motivate your improvement. This could be improving your typing speed, reducing errors, or mastering transcription in a new medical specialty.

8. Health and Wellness: Transcription requires intense focus and can be mentally exhausting. Take care of your mental and physical health. Regular breaks, a comfortable workspace, and a healthy lifestyle can contribute to improved performance.

Remember, continuous improvement is a journey. Be patient with yourself and celebrate your achievements along the way.

Regular Audits and Feedback in Professional Settings

Regular audits and feedback are important components of professional growth in any field, including medical transcription. They ensure quality control and facilitate continuous improvement in your work. Here's how they typically operate in professional settings:

1. Audits: In a medical transcription context, audits involve a detailed review of your transcriptions by a supervisor or a quality assurance specialist. The auditor checks for errors in grammar, punctuation, terminology, formatting, and adherence to the transcription policies of the healthcare facility or transcription service. The frequency of audits can vary depending on the organization, but they're typically performed on a regular basis.

2. Feedback: After the audit, you should receive feedback on your performance. This feedback is a valuable tool for identifying areas of strength and areas that need improvement. Feedback may cover a range of areas such as accuracy, consistency, productivity, and adherence to deadlines.

3. Performance Appraisals: In addition to regular feedback, many organizations have formal performance appraisal systems where they evaluate your work over a longer period, typically annually. This appraisal may be used to determine promotions, salary increases, or bonuses.

4. Feedback and Learning: The goal of audits and feedback isn't to criticize, but to help you learn and grow as a professional. Take all feedback into consideration, and try to learn from any mistakes identified. If you disagree with feedback or don't understand it, don't hesitate to ask for clarification.

5. Continuous Improvement: Use the feedback to set personal goals and strive for continuous improvement. If specific issues are consistently appearing in audits, focus on those areas. For example, you could take a course or read up on a specific area of medical terminology that you find challenging.

Remember, the aim of regular audits and feedback in professional settings is to ensure the high quality of medical transcription, which ultimately contributes to quality patient care. They are essential tools for your professional development.

In the next chapter, we will discuss the legal and ethical aspects of medical transcription. This is a very important area that all medical transcriptionists need to be aware of.

CHAPTER 13: LEGAL AND ETHICAL ASPECTS OF MEDICAL TRANSCRIPTION

Legal Responsibilities of a Medical Transcriptionist

As a medical transcriptionist, you have several legal responsibilities tied to privacy, accuracy, and professionalism. Here are some key ones:

1. Patient Privacy: Probably the most important legal responsibility is adhering to patient privacy laws. In the U.S., the Health Insurance Portability and Accountability Act (HIPAA) is the main law protecting patient health information. You must ensure that all patient information you handle is kept confidential and is only shared with individuals authorized to see it.

2. Accuracy: Medical transcriptionists are legally responsible for providing accurate transcriptions. Errors in transcription can lead to misdiagnoses, improper treatment, and other medical mistakes. If it's found that negligence in transcription was the cause of a medical error, you could potentially be held liable.

3. Record Keeping: Transcriptionists might be responsible for managing and storing medical records. This can include ensuring records are properly filed and stored, ensuring they're accessible to authorized individuals, and destroying records when legally appropriate.

4. Professional Conduct: Medical transcriptionists are expected to conduct themselves professionally. This includes maintaining patient confidentiality, but also treating colleagues respectfully, adhering to workplace policies, and performing duties to the best of their ability.

5. Continuing Education: While not always legally mandated, ongoing education is crucial in a field that's constantly evolving due to medical advancements and changes in health laws and regulations. You may be required by your employer, or by a professional certification you hold, to undertake continuing education to ensure your knowledge stays current.

6. Copyright Laws: If you use any resources or reference materials in your work, you need to ensure you do so legally and within copyright laws.

Remember, these responsibilities exist to protect patients, medical professionals, and you as a medical transcriptionist. Violating these can lead to serious consequences, including loss of job, legal action, or fines.

Understanding HIPAA and Patient Confidentiality Laws

HIPAA, or the Health Insurance Portability and Accountability Act, is a U.S. law passed in 1996. One of its main components is to protect patient privacy and set guidelines for the use and disclosure of Protected Health Information (PHI).

HIPAA's Privacy Rule establishes national standards to protect individuals' medical records and other personal health information. It applies to health plans, healthcare clearinghouses, and healthcare providers who conduct specific healthcare transactions electronically.

Under HIPAA, patient confidentiality is of utmost importance. This means that any information about a patient's health status, provision of health care, or payment for health care that can be linked to a specific individual is considered protected. This includes any part of a patient's medical record or payment history.

Violating these rules can lead to significant fines and criminal charges. As a medical transcriptionist, it is your responsibility to ensure the confidentiality and security of all the medical records you handle. Here are some basic principles:

1. Only access and disclose patient information when necessary for your job.

2. Never share patient information with unauthorized individuals, including friends or family.

3. Use secure methods for storing and transmitting patient information. This could include encrypted emails or secure servers.

4. Dispose of patient information securely when it is no longer needed.

5. Follow all of your organization's privacy and security procedures.

Note that other countries have similar laws regarding patient confidentiality. For instance, in the EU, the General Data Protection Regulation (GDPR) is the relevant law. It's important to understand and adhere to the laws that apply in your location.

Remember, respecting patient privacy isn't just about legal compliance. It's also about building trust with patients and maintaining professional ethics.

Ethical Dilemmas in Medical Transcription

Ethical dilemmas in medical transcription may arise in various forms. Here are a few examples:

1. Accuracy vs. Speed: There can be pressure to transcribe reports quickly due to a high workload or tight deadlines. This can lead to a dilemma between maintaining accuracy and meeting the deadline. The ethical choice is always to prioritize accuracy to ensure patient safety.

2. Confidentiality: Sometimes, transcriptionists may handle sensitive information about someone they know. The ethical response is to respect confidentiality and not disclose or discuss this information, as per HIPAA guidelines and other confidentiality laws.

3. Correcting Errors: If a transcriptionist notices a potential error in the doctor's dictation, they might face a dilemma about whether to correct it. The right course of action is to flag it for review but not to make clinical changes on their own, as this would be outside the scope of their role.

4. Working Conditions: Transcriptionists may sometimes be asked to work long hours, leading to physical strain and fatigue, which could potentially affect their performance and the accuracy of their work. It's important to maintain a work-life balance and speak up about unreasonable conditions.

It's important to adhere to the code of ethics in medical transcription, which promotes respect for patient confidentiality, commitment to accuracy, and professional conduct.

Case Studies and Legal Precedents

While I can't provide specific case studies or legal precedents, I can tell you that there have been legal cases involving medical transcription. These typically involve issues like violations of patient confidentiality, errors in transcription leading to medical errors, and unfair labor practices. Here are some hypothetical examples:

1. Violations of Patient Confidentiality: A medical transcriptionist shares private patient information with someone else, either knowingly or unknowingly. This is a violation of the Health Insurance Portability and Accountability Act (HIPAA) and can lead to legal consequences. The transcriptionist and their employer could face hefty fines or other penalties.

2. Errors Leading to Medical Errors: A medical transcriptionist makes a mistake while transcribing a doctor's notes, which leads to a patient receiving the wrong treatment. If this error could have been reasonably avoided, the transcriptionist or their employer might be held liable for any harm caused to the patient.

3. Unfair Labor Practices: A medical transcription company requires its employees to work long hours without adequate breaks, leading to physical strain and potentially mistakes in their work. The employees could bring a case against the company for violating labor laws.

In any of these scenarios, the specific outcome would depend on the laws of the country or state, the details of the case, and the decision of the court.

In the next chapter, we will discuss the working environment and conditions for a medical transcriptionist. This will include a comparison of in-house and remote working, along with tips for maintaining health and wellness as a transcriptionist.

CHAPTER 14: WORKING ENVIRONMENT AND CONDITIONS

Comparison of In-house and Remote Working Conditions

In-house and remote working conditions each have their own advantages and disadvantages, particularly in the field of medical transcription. Here's a brief comparison:

In-house Medical Transcription:

Advantages:

1. Training and Support: Working in-house often provides more direct access to training resources and support from experienced colleagues. If you're just starting out or if you're dealing with complex medical records, this support can be invaluable.

2. Structured Environment: Working in-house often comes with a more structured work schedule and environment. This might help you stay focused and productive.

3. Access to Equipment: You'll have access to all the equipment you need, and the organization will take care of maintenance and upgrades.

Disadvantages:

1. Commute: You'll need to travel to and from work, which can take up a significant amount of time and money.

2. Less Flexibility: In-house jobs usually come with fixed hours, so you'll have less flexibility to manage your work schedule according to your personal needs.

Remote Medical Transcription:

Advantages:

1. Flexibility: Working remotely allows for a flexible schedule. You can adjust your working hours to fit around other commitments, and you can work from anywhere with a good internet connection.

2. No Commute: Since you're working from home, there's no need to travel. This can save a significant amount of time and reduce stress.

Disadvantages:

1. Self-Discipline Required: Working from home requires a great deal of self-discipline. It can be easy to get distracted or to overwork yourself without the structure of an office environment.

2. Limited Direct Support: While remote employers often provide virtual support and training, it might not be as readily available or comprehensive as in an office setting.

3. Equipment Maintenance: You're typically responsible for your own equipment, including maintenance and upgrades.

Choosing between in-house and remote medical transcription jobs often comes down to personal preference and lifestyle. You'll need to weigh these factors to decide which is the best fit for you.

Coping with Occupational Challenges such as Stress and Repetitive Strain Injuries

Working as a medical transcriptionist can be challenging at times. It requires high levels of concentration and involves repetitive tasks, which can lead to stress and physical strain. Here are some strategies to help cope with these occupational challenges:

Managing Stress:

1. Time Management: Plan your day and prioritize your tasks. Try to maintain a consistent work schedule to avoid rushing or working overtime. Breaks are crucial – take short breaks during your work day and ensure you take days off as well.

2. Self-Care: Ensure you're getting enough sleep, eating a healthy diet, and getting regular exercise. These can all help reduce stress and improve overall wellbeing.

3. Mindfulness and Relaxation Techniques: Consider incorporating mindfulness techniques, like meditation or deep breathing, into your routine to help manage stress.

4. Reach Out: Don't hesitate to reach out to others when you're feeling stressed. Talk to colleagues, supervisors, or consider seeking support from a mental health professional.

Avoiding Repetitive Strain Injuries (RSIs):

1. Ergonomics: Make sure your workspace is set up correctly. Your chair should support your lower back, and your keyboard and monitor should be at comfortable heights. Consider using an ergonomic keyboard or a standing desk.

2. Take Breaks: Take regular short breaks to stretch and rest your eyes. Even a few minutes every hour can make a difference.

3. Exercises: Regular physical exercise can help prevent RSIs. Consider exercises that strengthen your wrists and hands.

4. Posture: Maintain good posture while working. Keep your back straight and your feet flat on the floor.

Remember, everyone is different. What works for one person might not work for another. It may take some trial and error to find what strategies work best for you. It's also important to seek professional advice if you're experiencing significant stress or physical discomfort.

Tips for Maintaining Health and Wellness as a Transcriptionist

Maintaining health and wellness as a transcriptionist is critical since the job often involves long hours of sitting and focusing on a screen, which can lead to physical and mental health concerns. Here are some tips to maintain your health and wellness:

Physical Health:

1. Regular Exercise: Incorporate regular exercise into your routine. This could include walking, cycling, yoga, or any other form of physical activity that you enjoy.

2. Posture and Ergonomics: Ensure your workstation is set up properly to maintain good posture. An ergonomic chair, suitable desk height, and appropriate positioning of your keyboard and monitor can make a big difference.

3. Eye Health: Protect your eyes by taking regular breaks from the screen, adjusting your monitor's brightness, and considering using anti-glare screens or glasses.

4. Healthy Diet: Eat balanced meals and stay hydrated. Avoid excessive intake of caffeine or sugary snacks.

Mental Health:

1. Breaks: Regular breaks can help maintain focus and reduce stress. Even a five-minute break every hour can help recharge your mind.

2. Stress Management: Incorporate stress-reducing activities into your day, such as deep breathing exercises, meditation, or listening to calming music.

3. Social Interactions: Stay connected with friends, family, and colleagues. Social interactions, even if virtual, can help reduce feelings of isolation or burnout.

4. Professional Development: Regularly learning and developing your skills can help maintain your motivation and interest in your work.

5. Boundaries: Create clear boundaries between your work and personal life, especially if you are working from home. This might involve designating specific working hours and creating a separate workspace at home.

Remember, your health and wellbeing are crucial. If you're experiencing serious or prolonged physical discomfort, stress, or other health concerns, seek professional medical advice.

Balancing Work and Personal Life in a Transcription Career

Balancing work and personal life can be a challenge in any career, including medical transcription. Here are some tips for achieving a healthier work-life balance:

1. Set boundaries: It's important to designate specific working hours and stick to them. Avoid overworking by setting a firm end time each day. Make sure to communicate these boundaries to your employer or clients.

2. Take breaks: Regular breaks are essential to maintain focus and productivity, and to avoid burnout. This could be a short walk, a tea break, or a few minutes of stretching.

3. Create a dedicated workspace: Having a separate, designated workspace can help separate your work life from your personal life. This space should be comfortable, well-lit, and free from distractions.

4. Practice time management: Prioritize your tasks and manage your time effectively. This can help you complete your work within designated hours, leaving time for personal activities and relaxation.

5. Stay organized: Keeping your workspace tidy and your work organized can save time and reduce stress. This might involve organizing digital files, managing emails efficiently, or using a planner or digital tool to keep track of tasks.

6. Take care of your health: Regular exercise, a healthy diet, adequate sleep, and relaxation techniques can all contribute to better work-life balance by improving your physical health and stress levels.

7. Make time for leisure activities: Make sure you have time for hobbies, socializing, and relaxation. Leisure activities can provide a refreshing break from work and help reduce stress.

8. Use vacation time: Make sure to use your vacation time to take breaks from work, even if you don't go away. This time can be used for relaxation, spending time with family or friends, or pursuing hobbies.

Remember, achieving a healthy work-life balance is a continuous process, and it's important to regularly reassess your needs and make necessary adjustments.

In the next chapter, we will discuss the future of medical transcription. This will include the impact of technological advancements on the industry, emerging trends, and the changing role of a transcriptionist.

CHAPTER 15: THE FUTURE OF MEDICAL TRANSCRIPTION

Impact of Technological Advancements on Medical Transcription

Technological advancements have significantly impacted the field of medical transcription in various ways:

1. Speech Recognition Software: Automatic speech recognition software has greatly streamlined the transcription process. It converts spoken language into written text, which the transcriptionist can then edit for accuracy. This technology can increase productivity and reduce turnaround time.

2. Digital Dictation Devices: The shift from analog to digital dictation devices has improved sound quality, making it easier for transcriptionists to understand the dictation. Digital files can also be easily transferred over the internet, which is more efficient than handling physical tapes.

3. Electronic Health Records (EHRs): The adoption of EHRs allows medical transcriptionists to directly input transcribed reports into patients' digital records, making the information instantly available to healthcare providers. This has improved the efficiency of healthcare delivery and continuity of care.

4. Secure File Transfer Protocols: With the advent of secure file transfer protocols, physicians can safely and quickly send dictations to transcriptionists, and transcriptionists can securely send transcribed reports back. This ensures the confidentiality of patient information.

5. Transcription Software: There are now various software tools designed specifically for medical transcription, which include features like foot pedal control for playback, text expanders for common phrases, and automatic timestamping.

6. Artificial Intelligence (AI): AI and machine learning are being integrated into transcription services to further enhance speech recognition, improve accuracy, and predict common words or phrases, saving transcriptionists' time and effort.

7. Ergonomic Equipment: Technological advancements in ergonomic equipment, like keyboards, chairs, and foot pedals, help to reduce the risk of repetitive strain injuries, a common risk for transcriptionists.

However, it's also important to note that with these advancements come challenges, such as keeping up with rapidly changing technology, maintaining data security in digital platforms, and managing the potential loss of jobs due to automation. It's crucial for medical transcriptionists to stay updated with the latest technologies and adapt their skills accordingly.

Emerging Trends in Medical Transcription

Medical transcription, like many fields, is evolving in response to advancements in technology and changing needs within the healthcare industry. Some emerging trends in medical transcription include:

1. Voice Recognition Technology: With the growth of AI and machine learning, speech recognition technology is becoming increasingly sophisticated. Some organizations are moving towards systems where physicians' spoken words are directly transcribed into written documents, which are then edited by medical transcriptionists for accuracy. This trend may change the role of transcriptionists from typists to editors.

2. Integration with Electronic Health Records (EHRs): As EHRs become more prevalent, the need for seamless integration of transcribed reports into these systems is growing. Transcriptionists may need to become more familiar with various EHR systems and how to work with them effectively.

3. Outsourcing and Offshoring: In an effort to reduce costs, some healthcare organizations are outsourcing their transcription services to third-party companies, both domestically and overseas. This can change the job market for transcriptionists.

4. Data Security: With the increase in digital transcription and record keeping, there's an increasing focus on ensuring the privacy and security of patient data. Transcriptionists will need to be aware of and compliant with regulations like HIPAA in the United States, as well as best practices for data security.

5. Continuing Education: Given these changes and advancements, there's a growing emphasis on continuing education for medical transcriptionists. This may include staying up-to-date with changes in medical terminology, learning to use new technologies, and understanding new regulatory requirements.

6. Emerging Roles: As the healthcare documentation field evolves, new roles are emerging for professionals with transcription skills. For example, some are moving into roles as scribes, who directly document healthcare encounters in real time. Others are moving into roles focused on data quality management within EHRs.

These trends indicate a dynamic field that is continuing to evolve in response to technological advancements and changing healthcare needs.

The Changing Role and Skillset of a Transcriptionist

The role of a medical transcriptionist has been evolving over the years due to technological advancements and the shifting landscape of the healthcare industry. Here are some key ways the role and skillset of a transcriptionist are changing:

1. From Transcribers to Editors: With the advent of speech recognition technology, medical transcriptionists are increasingly taking on the role of editors. The software transcribes the doctor's spoken words into text, and the transcriptionist then edits and formats the document for clarity, coherence, and accuracy.

2. Technological Savviness: Familiarity with various transcription software, EHR systems, and speech recognition technology is becoming increasingly crucial for modern transcriptionists. They may also need to troubleshoot technical issues that arise.

3. Data Security Knowledge: As medical records are primarily digital now, transcriptionists need to understand and comply with data security protocols to protect patient information. Knowledge of legislation like HIPAA (Health Insurance Portability and Accountability Act) in the U.S. is crucial.

4. Expanded Medical Knowledge: The growing complexity of medical care requires transcriptionists to have a solid understanding of medical terminology, pharmacology, and the various medical specialties.

5. Quality Control and Management: Transcriptionists are playing a larger role in quality control and data management. This includes ensuring that transcribed reports are accurate and properly integrated into EHR systems.

6. Soft Skills: Good communication skills, attention to detail, and a strong command of grammar and punctuation remain as important as ever. With more transcriptionists now working remotely, skills in self-motivation, time management, and independent problem-solving are also increasingly valuable.

In short, the role of a medical transcriptionist is becoming more multifaceted. The ability to adapt to new technologies and the evolving needs of the healthcare industry is becoming increasingly important.

Opportunities and Challenges for Future Transcriptionists

As with any profession, the future of medical transcription presents both opportunities and challenges.

Opportunities:

1. Increased Demand for Healthcare Services: As the population ages, the demand for healthcare services is expected to increase. This, in turn, will generate more clinical documentation, creating a need for skilled medical transcriptionists.

2. Remote Work Opportunities: The nature of medical transcription work makes it well-suited to remote working arrangements. This can offer greater flexibility and work-life balance for transcriptionists.

3. Technological Advancements: Advances in speech recognition technology can streamline the transcription process, allowing transcriptionists to focus more on editing and quality control tasks.

4. Specialization: There may be opportunities for transcriptionists to specialize in specific areas of medicine, offering a chance to deepen their expertise and potentially earn higher rates.

Challenges:

1. Automation and AI: While technology can make transcription work more efficient, it also presents a potential threat. If speech recognition technology continues to improve, there may be less need for human transcriptionists in the future.

2. Data Security: As medical records are increasingly digitized, ensuring their security becomes more challenging. Transcriptionists will need to be vigilant in protecting sensitive patient information.

3. Workload and Stress: Medical transcription requires a high degree of concentration and accuracy, which can lead to stress and fatigue. Balancing productivity with health and well-being can be a challenge.

4. Continuous Learning: Medical knowledge and technology are constantly evolving. Transcriptionists must commit to ongoing learning to keep their skills up-to-date.

5. Compensation: The pay for medical transcription can vary widely, and in some cases may not be commensurate with the skill and precision the job requires.

In conclusion, the future for medical transcriptionists will likely be characterized by continuous adaptation to new technologies and trends in healthcare. The most successful transcriptionists will be those who can balance the demands of accuracy and efficiency, continually update their skills, and navigate the challenges of data security and work-life balance.

That wraps up our chapters in the comprehensive guide on medical transcription. In the next sections, you will find practical classroom modules and useful appendices with additional resources to help you on your journey.

MODULE I. WEEKLY TRANSCRIPTION MASTERCLASS: COMPREHENSIVE GUIDE TO MEDICAL TERMINOLOGY

By following this module, students will gain a solid foundation in medical terminology, including an extensive understanding of prefixes, root words, suffixes, and combining forms. They will develop the skills necessary for accurately interpreting and transcribing medical terms, enabling them to excel in their transcription career.

1. INTRODUCTION TO MEDICAL TERMINOLOGY

Medical Terminology: Medical terminology is the language used in the field of healthcare to describe medical conditions, procedures, and anatomy. It consists of various components such as prefixes, root words, suffixes, and combining forms that combine to form medical terms.

Importance and Benefits of Medical Terminology in Transcription:

- **Enhances understanding of medical reports and dictations:** Knowledge of medical terminology enables transcriptionists to better comprehend and accurately transcribe medical reports, including diagnoses, procedures, and treatment plans.

- **Facilitates accurate transcription and interpretation of medical terms:** Proficiency in medical terminology allows transcriptionists to transcribe medical terms precisely, ensuring the accuracy and integrity of medical records.

- **Improves communication among healthcare professionals:** Medical terminology provides a standardized language for healthcare professionals, facilitating effective communication and collaboration in patient care.

Basic Structure of Medical Terms: Prefixes, Root Words, Suffixes, and Combining Forms:

- **Prefixes:** These are word parts added at the beginning of a medical term to modify or specify its meaning. For example, the prefix "hypo-" means below normal or deficient, as in hypotension (low blood pressure).

- **Root Words:** Root words are the main component of a medical term that provides its core meaning. For example, the root word "cardi(o)-" refers to the heart, as in cardiology (the study of the heart).

- **Suffixes:** Suffixes are added at the end of a medical term to modify its meaning or indicate a specific action or condition. For example, the suffix "-itis" indicates inflammation, as in arthritis (inflammation of the joints).

- **Combining Forms:** Combining forms are created by adding a vowel, usually "o," to a root word, allowing for easier word construction and pronunciation. For example, the combining form "cardi(o)-" combined with the suffix "-logy" forms cardiology (the study of the heart).

Exercises and Practice Activities:

- Create a table listing common prefixes, root words, suffixes, and combining forms, along with their meanings and examples.

- Match medical terms with their corresponding components (prefix, root word, suffix).

- Analyze medical terms to understand the significance of each component in forming the overall meaning.

2. COMMONLY USED PREFIXES AND THEIR MEANINGS

Definition and Examples of Prefixes Used in Medical Terminology:

Prefixes are word parts that are attached to the beginning of a medical term to modify or change its meaning. They provide important context and information about the medical word. Here are some commonly used prefixes in medical terminology:

- "Hyper-" (excessive or above normal): Hyperactive, hypertension, hyperglycemia.

- "Hypo-" (below normal or deficient): Hypothyroidism, hypoglycemia, hypotension.

- "Dys-" (difficult or impaired): Dysphagia, dysfunction, dyspnea.

- "Poly-" (many or excessive): Polyuria, polydipsia, polyneuropathy.

- "Tachy-" (fast or rapid): Tachycardia, tachypnea, tachyphylaxis.

- "Brady-" (slow): Bradycardia, bradypnea, bradycardic.

- "Micro-" (small): Microscopic, microorganism, microcytic.

- "Macro-" (large): Macroscopic, macrophage, macrocytic.

- "A-/An-" (without or lack of): Aseptic, anemia, anorexia.

- "Mono-" (one): Mononucleosis, monotherapy, monosomy.

- "Multi-" (many or multiple): Multifocal, multitasking, multivitamin.

- "Pre-" (before): Preoperative, prenatal, preexisting.

- "Post-" (after): Postoperative, postnatal, postprandial.

- "Sub-" (below or under): Subcutaneous, sublingual, subnormal.

- "Super-" (above or excessive): Superficial, superinfection, superimpose.

- "Trans-" (across or through): Transplant, transdermal, transvaginal.

- "Re-" (again or back): Reassess, reevaluate, reoccur.

Understanding How Prefixes Modify the Meaning of Medical Words:

Prefixes provide additional information to medical terms, helping to modify or specify their meaning. By understanding the meanings of prefixes, you can decipher the significance of the medical word. For example, the prefix "hyper-" denotes excessive or above normal, so "hyperactive" means excessively active or overactive.

Additional Examples of Commonly Used Prefixes:

- "Anti-" (against): Antibiotic, antiviral, antihistamine.

- "Bi-" (two): Bicuspid, bilateral, bifocal.

- "Dis-" (apart or absence): Disinfect, dislocate, discontinue.

- "Ex-" (out of or former): Exhale, excrete, exfoliate.

- "In-/Im-" (not or into): Inactive, impossible, implant.

- "Inter-" (between or among): Interact, intervertebral, intercostal.

- "Intra-" (within): Intravenous, intramuscular, intracranial.

- "Mal-" (bad or abnormal): Malfunction, malnutrition, malformation.

- "Non-" (not): Noninvasive, nonreactive, noncompliant.

- "Peri-" (around or surrounding): Pericardium, perioral, perineal.

- "Pseudo-" (false or imitation): Pseudoscience, pseudonym, pseudocyst.

- "Semi-" (half or partial): Semiconscious, semicircle, semiformal.

- "Sub-" (under or below): Sublingual, subcutaneous, substandard.

- "Super-" (above or beyond): Supernatural, superimpose, superconductivity.

- "Sym-/Syn-" (together or with): Symbiotic, synthesis, syndrome.

- "Tri-" (three): Tricycle, tricuspid, trilingual.

- "Uni-" (one or single): Unilateral, unisex, unidirectional.

Exercises and Practice Activities:

1. Fill in the blanks with the correct prefix to complete the medical term:

   a. ___lingual (under the tongue)

   b. ___reactive (not reactive)

   c. ___cellular (within the cell)

   d. ___bacterial (against bacteria)

   e. ___partum (after childbirth)

2. Match the prefix with its correct definition or meaning:

   a. Anti-

b. Bi-

c. Dis-

d. Peri-

e. Sym-/Syn-

Definition/meaning:

i. Against

ii. Two

iii. Partial or incomplete

iv. Around or surrounding

v. Together or with

3. **Create three medical terms using the prefixes provided:**

a. Ex-

b. Intra-

c. Non-

[Note: Feel free to use Google for the answers or any other assistance. As a transcriptionist, you will always have access to the search engine.]

3. ESSENTIAL ROOT WORDS IN MEDICAL TERMINOLOGY

Medical terminology relies heavily on root words, which form the foundation of many medical terms. Understanding root words is crucial for deciphering the meaning of complex medical terms and enhancing your overall comprehension of medical terminology. In this chapter, we will explore the importance of root words and provide examples of commonly used root words and their meanings. Additionally, we will engage in exercises and practice activities to help you identify root words and understand their significance in medical terms.

Explanation of Root Words and Their Importance in Medical Terminology:

Root words are the core components of medical terms, derived from Greek or Latin origins. They convey the basic meaning or concept of a term and serve as the building blocks for creating new medical words. By understanding root words, you can break down complex medical terms into their components and gain insight into their meaning. This knowledge is essential for accurate transcription and interpretation of medical terminology.

Examples of Commonly Used Root Words and Their Meanings:

1. Cardi-: Pertaining to the heart

   - Cardiology: Study of the heart and its diseases

   - Cardiologist: Medical specialist who diagnoses and treats heart diseases

2. Derm-: Pertaining to the skin

   - Dermatology: Study of the skin and its diseases

   - Dermatitis: Inflammation of the skin

3. Neuro-: Pertaining to the nerves or nervous system

   - Neurology: Study of the nervous system and its disorders

   - Neurologist: Medical specialist who diagnoses and treats neurological disorders

4. Osteo-: Pertaining to the bones

   - Osteoporosis: Condition characterized by weak and brittle bones

   - Osteopath: Medical professional who uses manual techniques to treat musculoskeletal disorders

5. Gastro-: Pertaining to the stomach

   - Gastroenterology: Study of the digestive system and its disorders

   - Gastroscopy: Examination of the stomach using a flexible tube with a camera

6. Pulmo-: Pertaining to the lungs

   - Pulmonology: Study of the respiratory system and its disorders

   - Pulmonologist: Medical specialist who diagnoses and treats respiratory diseases

7. Nephro-: Pertaining to the kidneys

   - Nephrology: Study of the kidneys and their functions

   - Nephrologist: Medical specialist who diagnoses and treats kidney diseases

8. Hepato-: Pertaining to the liver

   - Hepatology: Study of the liver and its diseases

   - Hepatitis: Inflammation of the liver

9. Ortho-: Pertaining to the bones and joints

   - Orthopedics: Branch of medicine focused on the musculoskeletal system

   - Orthopedic surgeon: Medical specialist who performs surgical procedures on the musculoskeletal system

10. Hemato-: Pertaining to the blood

   - Hematology: Study of blood and blood disorders

   - Hemoglobin: Protein in red blood cells that carries oxygen

Additional Examples of Commonly Used Root Words:

1. acro-: extremity (acromegaly - enlargement of extremities)

2. aden-: gland (adenoma - tumor of a gland)

3. angi-: vessel (angiography - imaging of blood vessels)

4. arthr-: joint (arthritis - inflammation of joints)

5. audi-: hearing (audiology - study of hearing)

6. cardi-: heart (cardiology - study of the heart)

7. cephal-: head (cephalalgia - headache)

8. cerebr-: brain (cerebral - related to the brain)

9. dermat-: skin (dermatology - study of the skin)

10. gastr-: stomach (gastritis - inflammation of the stomach)

11. hemat-: blood (hematology - study of blood)

12. hepat-: liver (hepatitis - inflammation of the liver)

13. hyster-: uterus (hysterectomy - removal of the uterus)

14. laryng-: larynx (laryngitis - inflammation of the larynx)

15. leuk-: white (leukocyte - white blood cell)

16. mamm-: breast (mammogram - X-ray of the breast)

17. nephro-: kidney (nephrology - study of the kidneys)

18. neur-: nerve (neurology - study of the nerves)

19. ophthalm-: eye (ophthalmology - study of the eye)

20. oste-: bone (osteoporosis - decreased bone density)

21. ot-: ear (otitis - inflammation of the ear)

22. pulmon-: lung (pulmonology - study of the lungs)

23. ren-: kidney (renal - related to the kidneys)

24. rheum-: flow (rheumatoid arthritis - chronic inflammatory joint disease)

25. thromb-: clot (thrombosis - formation of a blood clot)

26. ur-: urine (urology - study of the urinary system)

27. vas-: vessel (vascular - related to blood vessels)

28. cyt-: cell (cytology - study of cells)

29. my-: muscle (myopathy - muscle disease)

30. osteo-: bone (osteoporosis - decreased bone density)

31. rhin-: nose (rhinitis - inflammation of the nose)

32. angi-: vessel (angioplasty - surgical repair of a blood vessel)

33. dent-: tooth (dentist - dental professional)

34. erythr-: red (erythrocyte - red blood cell)

35. hepat-: liver (hepatomegaly - enlarged liver)

36. mamm-: breast (mammography - imaging of the breast)

37. neuro-: nerve (neuropathy - nerve damage)

38. ot-: ear (otology - study of the ear)

39. pneum-: lung (pneumonia - inflammation of the lungs)

40. pod-: foot (podiatry - study of the feet)

41. somat-: body (somatology - study of the human body)

42. tox-: poison (toxicology - study of poisons)

43. cyst-: bladder (cystitis - inflammation of the bladder)

44. derm-: skin (dermatologist - skin specialist)

45. encephal-: brain (encephalitis - inflammation of the brain)

46. gastr-: stomach (gastroenterology - study of the stomach and intestines)

47. hem-: blood (hemorrhage - excessive bleeding)

48. mamm-: breast (mammoplasty - breast reconstruction)

49. nephro-: kidney (nephrectomy - surgical removal of a kidney)

50. neur-: nerve (neurologist - nerve specialist)

51. ot-: ear (otolaryngology - study of the ear, nose, and throat)

52. pneum-: lung (pneumothorax - collapsed lung)

53. pod-: foot (podiatrist - foot specialist)

54. somat-: body (somatotype - body type classification)

55. tox-: poison (toxicologist - specialist in poisons)

56. cyst-: bladder (cystoscopy - examination of the bladder)

57. derm-: skin (dermatitis - inflammation of the skin)

58. encephal-: brain (encephalopathy - brain disorder)

59. gastr-: stomach (gastroscopy - examination of the stomach)

60. hem-: blood (hematology - study of blood)

61. nephro-: kidney (nephropathy - kidney disease)

62. neur-: nerve (neuritis - inflammation of a nerve)

63. ot-: ear (otitis media - middle ear infection)

64. pneum-: lung (pneumonectomy - surgical removal of a lung)

65. pod-: foot (podiatry - medical care of the feet)

66. somat-: body (somatization - conversion of mental distress into physical symptoms)

67. tox-: poison (toxicity - degree of being poisonous)

68. cyst-: bladder (cystectomy - surgical removal of the bladder)

69. derm-: skin (dermatologist - specialist in skin diseases)

70. encephal-: brain (encephalogram - record of brain activity)

71. gastr-: stomach (gastric - related to the stomach)

72. hem-: blood (hemorrhoid - swollen blood vessel in the rectum)

73. nephro-: kidney (nephrolithiasis - kidney stone formation)

74. neur-: nerve (neurological - related to the nervous system)

75. ot-: ear (otoscopy - examination of the ear)

These are just a few examples of root words used in medical terminology. Familiarizing yourself with these root words will greatly enhance your understanding of medical terms and improve your overall proficiency in medical transcription. Practice identifying and analyzing root words to build a strong foundation in medical terminology.

Exercises and Practice Activities:

1. Identify the root word in the following medical terms and explain its meaning:

  - Cardiomyopathy

  - Nephrology

  - Dermatitis

  - Osteoporosis

  - Rhinoplasty

2. Create new medical terms by combining different root words. Provide the meaning of each new term.

1. Cardi-:

2. Derm-:

3. Neuro-:

4. Osteo-:

5. Gastro-:

3. Fill in the blanks with the appropriate root word to complete the medical term:

- ____________ectomy: Surgical removal

- ____________itis: Inflammation of

- ____________logy: Study of

- ____________ology: Science of

- ____________oma: Tumor of

[Note: Feel free to use Google for the answers or any other assistance. As a transcriptionist, you will always have access to the search engine.]

These exercises will help reinforce your understanding of root words and their significance in medical terminology. Practice regularly to enhance your knowledge and proficiency in deciphering medical terms. Remember, developing a solid understanding of root words is essential for successful medical transcription.

4. IMPORTANT SUFFIXES AND THEIR SIGNIFICANCE

Suffixes play a crucial role in medical terminology by modifying the meaning or function of medical words. Understanding the various suffixes used in medical terminology is essential for accurate transcription. Here are the key points to consider:

Definition and Examples of Suffixes:

In medical terminology, suffixes are word parts added to the end of a root word to modify its meaning or function. Suffixes can indicate a condition, a procedure, a diagnostic test, a symptom, or a specific body part, among other things. Here are some examples of commonly used suffixes in medical terminology:

  - "-itis": Denotes inflammation. For example, "gastritis" refers to inflammation of the stomach.

  - "-ectomy": Indicates surgical removal. For example, "appendectomy" is the surgical removal of the appendix.

  - "-osis": Suggests a condition or state. For example, "hypnosis" refers to a state of altered consciousness.

  - "-ology": Refers to the study or science of a particular subject. For example, "cardiology" is the study of the heart.

  - "-pathy": Denotes a disease or disorder. For example, "neuropathy" refers to a disorder affecting the nerves.

  - "-graphy": Indicates a technique or process of recording. For example, "mammography" is the imaging technique used for breast examination.

These examples represent just a few of the many suffixes used in medical terminology. Each suffix has a specific meaning and helps to convey important information about a medical term.

Understanding how suffixes change the meaning or function of medical words:

Here's an explanation of how suffixes can modify the meaning or function of medical terms:

1. Alteration of Meaning: Suffixes can modify the basic meaning of a root word by indicating a condition, a procedure, a state, or a specific body part. For example:

  - Adding the suffix "-itis" to the root word "derm" (skin) changes it to "dermatitis," which refers to inflammation of the skin.

- The suffix "-ectomy" added to the root word "append" (appendix) transforms it into "appendectomy," meaning the surgical removal of the appendix.

2. Change in Function: Suffixes can also indicate the function or purpose of a medical term. For example:

- The suffix "-gram" indicates a recording or image. When added to the root word "mamm" (breast), it becomes "mammogram," which refers to the imaging technique used for breast examination.

- The suffix "-scopy" suggests a procedure involving the use of an instrument for visual examination. When combined with the root word "colon" (large intestine), it forms "colonoscopy," which is the endoscopic examination of the colon.

Understanding how suffixes modify medical words allows you to interpret the precise meaning and function of terms within a medical context. It helps you accurately transcribe reports by recognizing the significance of each suffix and its impact on the overall meaning of the term.

By practicing exercises and activities focused on recognizing and applying suffixes, you will develop proficiency in understanding the role of suffixes in medical terminology. This skill is essential for producing high-quality transcriptions that accurately reflect the intended meaning of medical reports.

Remember, as a medical transcriptionist, developing proficiency in recognizing and understanding suffixes will greatly enhance your ability to accurately transcribe and interpret medical reports.

Additional Examples of Commonly Used Suffixes:

Here is a list of 75 common suffixes used in medical terminology along with their meanings and examples:

1. -algia: pain (Arthralgia - joint pain)

2. -cele: hernia or swelling (Cystocele - herniation of the bladder)

3. -centesis: surgical puncture (Thoracentesis - puncture of the chest wall to remove fluid)

4. -cide: killing or destruction (Bactericide - substance that kills bacteria)

5. -cyte: cell (Leukocyte - white blood cell)

6. -desis: fusion or fixation (Arthrodesis - surgical fusion of a joint)

7. -ectomy: surgical removal (Appendectomy - surgical removal of the appendix)

8. -emia: blood condition (Anemia - deficiency of red blood cells)

9. -gram: recording or image (Electrocardiogram - record of the electrical activity of the heart)

10. -graphy: process of recording or imaging (Mammography - imaging of the breast)

11. -ia: condition or state (Anemia - condition of low red blood cell count)

12. -iasis: abnormal condition or presence of (Nephrolithiasis - presence of kidney stones)

13. -itis: inflammation (Appendicitis - inflammation of the appendix)

14. -logy: study or science of (Cardiology - study of the heart)

15. -lysis: breakdown or destruction (Hemolysis - destruction of red blood cells)

16. -oma: tumor or mass (Sarcoma - cancerous tumor)

17. -opsy: examination or viewing (Biopsy - examination of tissue samples)

18. -osis: abnormal condition or increase (Osteoporosis - loss of bone density)

19. -otomy: surgical incision (Tracheotomy - surgical incision into the trachea)

20. -pathy: disease or disorder (Neuropathy - nerve disorder)

21. -plasty: surgical repair or reconstruction (Rhinoplasty - surgical repair of the nose)

22. -rrhage: excessive flow or bleeding (Hemorrhage - excessive bleeding)

23. -scopy: visual examination (Colonoscopy - visual examination of the colon)

24. -stomy: surgical creation of an opening (Colostomy - surgical creation of an artificial opening in the colon)

25. -therapy: treatment (Chemotherapy - treatment with drugs to kill cancer cells)

26. -uria: presence of a substance in the urine (Hematuria - presence of blood in the urine)

27. -y: condition or process (Cardiomyopathy - disease of the heart muscle)

28. -crit: to separate or choose (Hematocrit - percentage of red blood cells in the blood)

29. -esthesia: sensation or feeling (Anesthesia - loss of sensation)

30. -gen: substance or agent that produces (Carcinogen - substance that causes cancer)

31. -rrhexis: rupture or bursting (Arteriorrhexis - rupture of an artery)

32. -thorax: chest or pleural cavity (Pneumothorax - presence of air in the pleural cavity)

33. -plegia: paralysis or loss of movement (Hemiplegia - paralysis of one side of the body)

34. -pexy: surgical fixation or suspension (Nephropexy - surgical fixation of a floating kidney)

35. -phonia: voice or sound (Dysphonia - hoarseness or difficulty in producing sound)

36. -sclerosis: hardening or thickening (Arteriosclerosis - hardening of the arteries)

37. -stasis: stopping or controlling (Hemostasis - stopping of bleeding)

38. -tomy: incision or cutting (Phlebotomy - incision into a vein to withdraw blood)

39. -ac: pertaining to (Cardiac - pertaining to the heart)

40. -ation: process or action (Respiration - process of breathing)

41. -phagia: eating or swallowing (Dysphagia - difficulty in swallowing)

42. -ptosis: drooping or sagging (Blepharoptosis - drooping of the eyelid)

43. -tripsy: crushing or fragmentation (Lithotripsy - breakdown of kidney stones)

44. -drome: run or course (Syndrome - collection of symptoms that run together)

45. -dipsia: thirst or desire for (Polydipsia - excessive thirst)

46. -ectasis: dilation or expansion (Bronchiectasis - abnormal dilation of the bronchi)

47. -ptosis: drooping or sagging (Proptosis - protrusion of the eyeball)

48. -tocia: childbirth or labor (Dystocia - difficult or abnormal childbirth)

49. -plasia: growth or development (Hyperplasia - excessive growth of cells)

50. -rrhage: bleeding or abnormal discharge (Hemorrhage - excessive bleeding)

51. -aphy: recording or representation (Electroencephalography - recording of brain activity)

52. -dynia: pain (Myalgia - muscle pain)

53. -ectopia: displacement or abnormal position (Ectopia - abnormal positioning of an organ or body part)

54. -esthesia: sensation or feeling (Anesthesia - loss of sensation)

55. -genesis: origin or production (Carcinogenesis - development of cancer)

56. -genous: producing or originating from (Endogenous - originating from within the body)

57. -ia: condition or state (Anemia - condition of low red blood cell count)

58. -itis: inflammation (Gastritis - inflammation of the stomach)

59. -logist: specialist or expert (Cardiologist - specialist in the field of cardiology)

60. -malacia: softening (Osteomalacia - softening of the bones)

61. -megaly: enlargement or abnormal growth (Hepatomegaly - enlargement of the liver)

62. -oid: resembling or similar to (Carcinoid - tumor resembling cancer)

63. -oma: tumor or mass (Melanoma - malignant tumor of melanocytes)

64. -opsy: examination or viewing (Biopsy - examination of tissue samples)

65. -osis: abnormal condition or increase (Hypertension - high blood pressure)

66. -ous: pertaining to or characterized by (Nervous - pertaining to the nerves)

67. -plasia: formation or growth (Hyperplasia - excessive growth of cells)

68. -rrhaphy: suturing or stitching (Herniorrhaphy - surgical repair of a hernia)

69. -sis: process or condition (Diagnosis - process of identifying a disease)

70. -stasis: stopping or controlling (Homeostasis - maintaining a stable internal environment)

71. -tomy: incision or cutting (Laparotomy - surgical incision into the abdomen)

72. -uria: presence of a substance in the urine (Proteinuria - presence of protein in the urine)

73. -xerosis: abnormal dryness (Xerosis - abnormal dryness of the skin)

74. -blast: immature or embryonic cell (Osteoblast - bone-forming cell)

75. -cele: hernia or swelling (Rectocele - herniation of the rectum)

Remember that this is not an exhaustive list of suffixes, but it includes many commonly used ones in medical terminology. The meanings provided are general and may vary depending on the specific medical context.

Exercises and Practice Activities:

To reinforce the learning, this section includes exercises and practice activities. These exercises involve identifying the correct suffixes for given medical terms, constructing new medical terms using specific suffixes, and completing sentences by adding appropriate suffixes. For example:

Exercise 1: Identify the correct suffix for the following medical terms:

- Hypertension:

- Arthritis:

- Cardiologist:

Exercise 2: Construct new medical terms by adding the correct suffix to the given root words:

- Neuro:

- Dermato:

- Cardi:

Exercise 3: Complete the sentences by adding the appropriate suffix:

- The ___________ refers to the study of cells.

- ___________ refers to the condition of high blood pressure.

- Osteo___________ refers to the inflammation of bones.

[Note: Feel free to use Google for the answers or any other assistance. As a transcriptionist, you will always have access to the search engine.]

By engaging in these exercises and practice activities, you will develop a solid understanding of suffixes and their significance in medical terminology. This will enhance your ability to accurately interpret and transcribe medical terms.

Remember, practicing and familiarizing yourself with suffixes is crucial for mastering medical terminology.

5. COMBINING FORMS IN MEDICAL TERMINOLOGY

Combining forms are linguistic elements derived from Greek and Latin roots that are used to create medical terms. They serve as a foundation upon which prefixes and suffixes are added to form complete medical words. Combining forms are typically word roots that have been modified by adding a vowel, such as 'o' or 'i', to make them easier to pronounce and connect to other word parts.

The purpose of combining forms is to provide a consistent and standardized way of representing specific anatomical structures, organs, diseases, and medical concepts. They allow for the precise description and communication of medical information across healthcare professionals.

Combining forms are often derived from Greek or Latin words that describe anatomical features or medical conditions. For example:

- Cardi/o: Pertaining to the heart

  Example: Cardiology (study of the heart)

- Derm/o: Pertaining to the skin

  Example: Dermatology (study of the skin)

- Gastr/o: Pertaining to the stomach

  Example: Gastroenteritis (inflammation of the stomach and intestines)

- Hepat/o: Pertaining to the liver

  Example: Hepatitis (inflammation of the liver)

- Nephro/o: Pertaining to the kidney

  Example: Nephrology (study of the kidneys)

- Oste/o: Pertaining to bone

  Example: Osteoporosis (loss of bone density)

- Pulmon/o: Pertaining to the lungs

  Example: Pulmonology (study of the lungs)

By combining these combining forms with appropriate prefixes and suffixes, medical terms can be created to describe specific medical conditions, procedures, or anatomical structures.

Understanding combining forms is essential in medical transcription as it allows transcriptionists to accurately interpret and transcribe medical terms. Mastery of combining forms enables transcriptionists to decipher the meaning of complex medical words and effectively communicate medical information in the written format.

Examples of commonly used combining forms and their meanings:

- Cardi/o: Pertaining to the heart

- Derm/o: Pertaining to the skin

- Gastr/o: Pertaining to the stomach

- Hepat/o: Pertaining to the liver

- Nephro/o: Pertaining to the kidney

- Oste/o: Pertaining to bone

- Pulmon/o: Pertaining to the lungs

- Neuro/o: Pertaining to the nervous system

- Ophthalm/o: Pertaining to the eye

- Ot/o: Pertaining to the ear

- Arthr/o: Pertaining to the joints

- Gynec/o: Pertaining to the female reproductive system

- Uro/o: Pertaining to the urinary system

- Hemat/o: Pertaining to blood

- My/o: Pertaining to muscle

- Cerebr/o: Pertaining to the brain

- Psych/o: Pertaining to the mind or mental processes

- Pod/o: Pertaining to the foot

- Dent/o: Pertaining to teeth

- Laryng/o: Pertaining to the larynx (voice box)

These are just a few examples of commonly used combining forms in medical terminology. There are many more combining forms that represent different anatomical structures, diseases, and medical concepts. By understanding the meanings of these combining forms, you can decipher the meaning of complex medical terms and accurately transcribe them in your work as a medical transcriptionist.

Combining forms in medical terminology serve as the foundation upon which medical words are built. They are typically derived from Greek or Latin roots and carry a specific meaning related to a body part, condition, or medical concept. Combining forms can be combined with prefixes, suffixes, and other combining forms to create complex medical terms.

When combining forms are combined with prefixes, they usually appear at the beginning of a word. For example:

- Cardi/o (combining form for heart) + Megaly (suffix meaning enlargement) = Cardiomegaly (enlargement of the heart)

When combining forms are combined with suffixes, they usually appear at the end of a word. For example:

- Nephro (combining form for kidney) + Itis (suffix meaning inflammation) = Nephritis (inflammation of the kidney)

Combining forms can also combine with other combining forms to create compound words. For example:

- Osteo (combining form for bone) + Arthritis (suffix meaning inflammation of a joint) = Osteoarthritis (inflammation of the joints involving bone)

Understanding how combining forms combine with other components is crucial for deciphering the meaning of complex medical terms. It allows medical transcriptionists to accurately transcribe and interpret medical reports and dictations. Through practice and familiarity with commonly used combining forms, you will develop the skills to break down and understand the structure of medical words effectively.

Additional Examples of Commonly Used Combining Forms:

Here's a list of 100 commonly used combining forms in medical terminology, along with their meanings and examples:

1. Abdomin/o - abdomen (abdominal pain)

2. Aden/o - gland (adenoma)

3. Angi/o - vessel (angiogram)

4. Arthr/o - joint (arthritis)

5. Audi/o - hearing (audiology)

6. Bio - life (biology)

7. Bronch/o - bronchus (bronchoscopy)

8. Cardi/o - heart (cardiology)

9. Cephal/o - head (cephalalgia)

10. Cerebr/o - brain (cerebrovascular)

11. Chem/o - chemical (chemotherapy)

12. Cholecyst/o - gallbladder (cholecystectomy)

13. Col/o - colon (colonoscopy)

14. Derm/o - skin (dermatology)

15. Enter/o - intestine (enteritis)

16. Gastr/o - stomach (gastritis)

17. Gynec/o - female (gynecology)

18. Hemat/o - blood (hematology)

19. Hepat/o - liver (hepatitis)

20. Immun/o - immune (immunology)

21. Lith/o - stone (lithotripsy)

22. Mamm/o - breast (mammogram)

23. Nephr/o - kidney (nephrology)

24. Neuro/o - nerve (neurology)

25. Ophthalm/o - eye (ophthalmology)

26. Oste/o - bone (osteoporosis)

27. Ot/o - ear (otitis)

28. Path/o - disease (pathology)

29. Pulmon/o - lung (pulmonology)

30. Ren/o - kidney (renal)

31. Rhin/o - nose (rhinoplasty)

32. Scler/o - hardening (sclerosis)

33. Thromb/o - clot (thrombosis)

34. Ureter/o - ureter (ureterolithiasis)

35. Vas/o - vessel (vasodilation)

36. Angi/o - vessel (angioplasty)

37. Erythr/o - red (erythrocyte)

38. Lymph/o - lymph (lymphoma)

39. My/o - muscle (myopathy)

40. Oss/e, Oss/i, Oste/o - bone (osteomyelitis)

41. Phleb/o - vein (phlebitis)

42. Pneum/o - lung (pneumonia)

43. Rhiz/o - root (rhizotomy)

44. Splen/o - spleen (splenomegaly)

45. Thyr/o, Thyroid/o - thyroid (hyperthyroidism)

46. Urethr/o - urethra (urethritis)

47. Ven/o - vein (venipuncture)

48. Adrenal/o - adrenal gland (adrenaline)

49. Aur/o - ear (auricle)

50. Bronchi/o - bronchus (bronchiectasis)

51. Angi/o - vessel (angioplasty)

52. Arteri/o - artery (arteriosclerosis)

53. Chondr/o - cartilage (chondritis)

54. Chron/o - time (chronic)

55. Cyt/o - cell (cytology)

56. Encephal/o - brain (encephalitis)

57. Hem/o, Hemat/o - blood (hemorrhage, hematoma)

58. Immun/o - immune (immunotherapy)

59. Leuk/o - white (leukemia)

60. Mening/o - meninges (meningitis)

61. Myel/o - bone marrow (myeloma)

62. Necr/o - death (necrosis)

63. Onco/o - tumor (oncology)

64. Ophthalm/o - eye (ophthalmoscope)

65. Oste/o - bone (osteotomy)

66. Ot/o - ear (otology)

67. Pancreat/o - pancreas (pancreatitis)

68. Phag/o - eat, swallow (phagocytosis)

69. Psych/o - mind (psychology)

70. Radi/o - radiation (radiology)

71. Ren/o - kidney (renogram)

72. Retin/o - retina (retinopathy)

73. Sarc/o - flesh (sarcoidosis)

74. Splen/o - spleen (splenectomy)

75. Thromb/o - clot (thrombolysis)

76. Thyroid/o - thyroid (hypothyroidism)

77. Vascul/o - blood vessel (vasculitis)

78. Bi/o - life (biology)

79. Carcin/o - cancer (carcinoma)

80. Dent/o, Odont/o - tooth (dentistry, odontoma)

81. Erythr/o - red (erythrocyte)

82. Gastro/o - stomach (gastroenterology)

83. Hyster/o - uterus (hysterectomy)

84. Laryng/o - larynx (laryngoscopy)

85. Mast/o - breast (mastectomy)

86. My/o - muscle (myalgia)

87. Nephr/o - kidney (nephrolithiasis)

88. Ocul/o - eye (oculomotor)

89. Pneum/o, Pneumat/o - air, lung (pneumonia, pneumothorax)

90. Proct/o - rectum (proctoscopy)

91. Psych/o - mind (psychiatry)

92. Radi/o - radiation (radiography)

93. Spondyl/o - vertebrae (spondylitis)

94. Thyr/o - thyroid (thyroidectomy)

95. Trache/o - trachea (tracheostomy)

96. Ureter/o - ureter (ureteroscopy)

97. Viscer/o - internal organs (visceral)

98. Glyc/o - sugar (glycosuria)

99. Lith/o - stone (lithotripsy)

100. Oss/e, Oss/i, Oste/o - bone (osteoporosis)

This comprehensive list provides additional combining forms commonly used in medical terminology. Please note that this is not an exhaustive list, but it covers a wide range of commonly used combining forms in medical terminology.

Exercises and Practice Activities:

Exercise 1: Fill in the Blanks

Fill in the blanks with the appropriate combining form to complete the medical terms:

1. ________ + gastr + itis = Inflammation of the stomach

2. Nephro + ________ + itis = Inflammation of the kidneys

3. ________ + dermat + ology = Study of the skin

4. ________ + hepat + itis = Inflammation of the liver

5. ________ + osteo + arthr + itis = Inflammation of the joints and bones

Exercise 2: Matching Game

Match the combining forms with their corresponding meanings:

1. Cardi/o   a. Kidney

2. Derm/a   b. Heart

3. Nephro   c. Skin

4. Hepat/o   d. Bone

5. Oste/o   e. Liver

Exercise 3: Create New Medical Terms

Combine the given combining forms to create new medical terms:

1. Hepat + _________ = Pertaining to the liver

2. Derm + ________ = Pertaining to the skin

3. Nephro + ________ = Pertaining to the kidneys

4. Osteo + ________ = Pertaining to the bones

5. Cardi + ________ = Pertaining to the heart

Exercise 4: Break It Down

Break down the following medical terms into their combining forms:

1. Gastroenterology

2. Dermatologist

3. Nephrology

4. Cardiology

5. Osteoporosis

Exercise 5: Medical Term Transformation

Transform the following medical terms by replacing the combining form with the appropriate root word or suffix:

1. Cardiologist = ________ + logist

2. Dermatitis = derm + _________

3. Nephropathy = nephro + _________

4. Osteotomy = osteo + _________

5. Cardiomyopathy = _________ + myopathy

Exercise 6: Medical Term Scramble

Unscramble the letters to form medical terms using the given combining forms:

1. gast + ropy

2. derm + logo

3. nephro + loyg

4. osteo + thaomy

5. cardi + tlogiso

[Note: Feel free to use Google for the answers or any other assistance. As a transcriptionist, you will always have access to the search engine.]

Remember, practicing these exercises and activities regularly will enhance your proficiency in utilizing combining forms effectively in medical terminology.

In the world of medical transcription, it is essential to have a comprehensive understanding of how prefixes, root words, and suffixes combine to form medical terms. This knowledge allows you to accurately interpret and transcribe medical reports, ensuring clear communication between healthcare professionals.

Within this chapter, we will explore the intricacies of building medical terms by examining the individual roles and functions of prefixes, root words, and suffixes. By understanding these components and their specific contributions to medical terminology, you will gain the necessary skills to construct and interpret medical terms effectively.

To develop a strong foundation in word building, we will discuss the rules and guidelines that govern the combination of prefixes, root words, and suffixes. By adhering to these guidelines, you can construct medical terms with precision and accuracy, ensuring that the intended meaning is conveyed accurately in your transcription work.

Throughout the chapter, you will encounter various exercises and practice activities designed to reinforce your understanding of combining components to form medical terms. These exercises will provide you with hands-on experience in constructing medical terms, enabling you to apply your knowledge in a practical and meaningful way.

By mastering the art of building medical terms, you will enhance your transcription skills and expand your ability to accurately interpret and transcribe medical reports. This chapter serves as a valuable resource in your journey towards becoming a proficient medical transcriptionist, equipping you with the tools necessary to navigate the complex world of medical terminology with confidence and precision.

Rules and guidelines for word building and combining components correctly:

In order to build medical terms effectively, it is important to follow certain rules and guidelines to ensure that the components - prefixes, root words, and suffixes - are combined correctly. These rules help maintain consistency and accuracy in medical terminology. Here are some key rules and guidelines to consider:

1. Maintain the correct order: When constructing a medical term, it is important to follow the proper order of components. Generally, the prefix comes before the root word, and the suffix comes after the root word. This order ensures that the term is structured correctly and conveys the intended meaning.

2. Understand the meaning of each component: It is crucial to have a thorough understanding of the meanings of prefixes, root words, and suffixes. This knowledge allows you to combine the components in a way that accurately represents the medical concept being described. For example, the prefix "hyper-" denotes excessive or above normal, while the suffix "-itis" indicates inflammation.

3. Consider the combining vowel: In some cases, a combining vowel is used to connect the components in a medical term. The most common combining vowel is "o." It is added between the root word and the suffix to improve pronunciation and maintain clarity. For example, in the term "cardiologist," the combining vowel "o" is used to connect the root word "cardio" and the suffix "-logist."

4. Recognize variations in spelling: Depending on the combination of components, there may be changes in spelling or alterations in the components themselves. For example, when the suffix "-al" is added to the root word "digest," the final term becomes "digestive," with the letter "e" added before the suffix.

5. Pay attention to combining form changes: Some root words undergo changes when combined with certain prefixes or suffixes. These changes are known as combining form changes and are necessary to maintain proper pronunciation and word flow. For example, the root word "dermato" changes to "dermat" when combined with the suffix "-logy" to form "dermatology."

Understanding and following these rules and guidelines ensures that you can effectively build medical terms and create accurate transcriptions. By adhering to these principles, you will develop a solid foundation in constructing medical terms and enhance your overall proficiency as a medical transcriptionist.

Examples of Commonly Used Medical Terms broken in Prefix, Root Words, and Suffix:

Here are 100 medical terms broken down into their respective prefix, suffix, and root words:

1. Anemia: Without blood (prefix: An-; suffix: -emia)

2. Bradycardia: Slow heart rate (prefix: Brady-; root word: Cardi/o)

3. Dermatitis: Inflammation of the skin (root word: Dermat/o; suffix: -itis)

4. Gastrectomy: Surgical removal of the stomach (root word: Gastr/o; suffix: -ectomy)

5. Hematology: Study of blood (root word: Hem/o; suffix: -logy)

6. Neurology: Study of the nervous system (root word: Neur/o; suffix: -logy)

7. Osteoporosis: Abnormal condition of weak bones (root word: Oste/o; suffix: -osis)

8. Pulmonology: Study of the lungs (root word: Pulmon/o; suffix: -logy)

9. Renalgia: Pain in the kidney (root word: Ren/o; suffix: -algia)

10. Thermography: Recording of heat patterns (root word: Therm/o; suffix: -graphy)

11. Abdominoplasty: Surgical repair of the abdomen (root word: Abdomin/o; suffix: -plasty)

12. Cephalalgia: Headache (root word: Cephal/o; suffix: -algia)

13. Dermatologist: Medical professional specializing in skin conditions (root word: Dermat/o; suffix: -logist)

14. Gastroenteritis: Inflammation of the stomach and intestines (root word: Gastroenter/o; suffix: -itis)

15. Hemorrhage: Excessive bleeding (root word: Hemorrh/o; suffix: -age)

16. Nephrology: Study of the kidneys (root word: Nephro/o; suffix: -logy)

17. Orthopedic: Relating to the correction of deformities of the musculoskeletal system (root word: Orth/o; suffix: -edic)

18. Pneumonia: Infection of the lungs (root word: Pneumon/o; suffix: -ia)

19. Rhinoplasty: Surgical repair of the nose (root word: Rhin/o; suffix: -plasty)

20. Thrombosis: Formation of a blood clot (root word: Thromb/o; suffix: -osis)

21. Acromegaly: Excessive growth of the extremities (root word: Acro/o; suffix: -megaly)

22. Bronchitis: Inflammation of the bronchial tubes (root word: Bronch/o; suffix: -itis)

23. Cardiovascular: Relating to the heart and blood vessels (root word: Cardi/o; suffix: -vascular)

24. Dermatology: Study of the skin (root word: Dermat/o; suffix: -logy)

25. Gastroscope: Instrument used for visual examination of the stomach (root word: Gastro/o; suffix: -scope)

26. Hepatitis: Inflammation of the liver (root word: Hepat/o; suffix: -itis)

27. Neurologist: Medical professional specializing in the nervous system (root word: Neur/o; suffix: -logist)

28. Ophthalmology: Study of the eyes and eye diseases (root word: Ophthalm/o; suffix: -logy)

29. Podiatrist: Medical professional specializing in foot care (root word: Pod/o; suffix: -iatrist)

30. Urology: Study of the urinary system (root word: Ur/o; suffix: -logy)

31. Adenoma: Benign tumor of glandular tissue (root word: Aden/o; suffix: -oma)

32. Cystoscopy: Visual examination of the bladder (root word: Cyst/o; suffix: -scopy)

33. Endoscopy: Visual examination of internal organs or cavities (root word: End/o; suffix: -scopy)

34. Hemoglobin: Protein in red blood cells that carries oxygen (root word: Hem/o; suffix: -globin)

35. Nephrectomy: Surgical removal of a kidney (root word: Nephr/o; suffix: -ectomy)

36. Orthodontist: Dental specialist who corrects irregularities of the teeth (root word: Orth/o; suffix: -odontist)

37. Phlebotomy: Process of drawing blood (root word: Phleb/o; suffix: -tomy)

38. Radiology: Study of medical imaging (root word: Radi/o; suffix: -logy)

39. Tracheotomy: Surgical procedure to create an opening in the windpipe (root word: Trache/o; suffix: -tomy)

40. Vasectomy: Surgical sterilization procedure for males (root word: Vas/o; suffix: -ectomy)

41. Allergy: Hypersensitivity to a substance (root word: All/o; suffix: -ergy)

42. Cardiologist: Medical professional specializing in heart conditions (root word: Cardi/o; suffix: -logist)

43. Dermatopathy: Disease of the skin (root word: Dermat/o; suffix: -pathy)

44. Gastroscopy: Visual examination of the stomach (root word: Gastro/o; suffix: -scopy)

45. Hematology: Study of blood and blood disorders (root word: Hem/o; suffix: -logy)

46. Neurologist: Medical professional specializing in neurological disorders (root word: Neur/o; suffix: -logist)

47. Osteotomy: Surgical cutting of bone (root word: Oste/o; suffix: -tomy)

48. Pulmonologist: Medical professional specializing in lung diseases (root word: Pulmon/o; suffix: -logist)

49. Renal: Relating to the kidneys (root word: Ren/o; suffix: -al)

50. Thermometer: Instrument used to measure temperature (root word: Therm/o; suffix: -meter)

51. Adrenal: Relating to the adrenal glands (root word: Adren/o; suffix: -al)

52. Bronchoscopy: Visual examination of the bronchial tubes (root word: Bronch/o; suffix: -scopy)

53. Cardioversion: Restoring normal heart rhythm through electrical shock (root word: Cardi/o; suffix: -version)

54. Dermatology: Study and treatment of skin diseases (root word: Dermat/o; suffix: -logy)

55. Gastrotomy: Surgical incision into the stomach (root word: Gastro/o; suffix: -tomy)

56. Hepatologist: Medical professional specializing in liver diseases (root word: Hepat/o; suffix: -logist)

57. Nephropathy: Disease of the kidneys (root word: Nephr/o; suffix: -pathy)

58. Orthopedics: Branch of medicine dealing with the musculoskeletal system (root word: Orth/o; suffix: -pedics)

59. Phlebotomist: Medical professional trained to draw blood (root word: Phleb/o; suffix: -tomist)

60. Radiography: Technique of producing images using X-rays (root word: Radi/o; suffix: -graphy)

61. Urologist: Medical professional specializing in the urinary system (root word: Ur/o; suffix: -logist)

62. Adenitis: Inflammation of a gland (root word: Aden/o; suffix: -itis)

63. Cystectomy: Surgical removal of the bladder (root word: Cyst/o; suffix: -ectomy)

64. Endocrinology: Study of hormones and the endocrine system (root word: Endocrin/o; suffix: -logy)

65. Hematoma: Collection of blood outside of blood vessels (root word: Hem/o; suffix: -toma)

66. Nephrologist: Medical professional specializing in kidney diseases (root word: Nephr/o; suffix: -logist)

67. Orthotic: Device used to support or correct a part of the body (root word: Orth/o; suffix: -otic)

68. Phlebitis: Inflammation of a vein (root word: Phleb/o; suffix: -itis)

69. Radiologist: Medical professional who interprets medical images (root word: Radi/o; suffix: -logist)

70. Uroscopy: Examination of the urine (root word: Ur/o; suffix: -scopy)

71. Allergist: Medical professional specializing in allergies (root word: All/o; suffix: -gist)

72. Cardiology: Study of the heart and its diseases (root word: Cardi/o; suffix: -logy)

73. Dermatologist: Medical professional specializing in skin disorders (root word: Dermat/o; suffix: -logist)

74. Gastroenterology: Study of the digestive system and its diseases (root word: Gastroenter/o; suffix: -logy)

75. Hematology: Study of blood and blood disorders (root word: Hem/o; suffix: -logy)

76. Neurologist: Medical professional specializing in neurological disorders (root word: Neur/o; suffix: -logist)

77. Osteoarthritis: Degenerative joint disease (root word: Oste/o; suffix: -arthritis)

78. Pulmonary: Relating to the lungs (root word: Pulmon/o; suffix: -ary)

79. Renovascular: Relating to blood vessels of the kidneys (root word: Ren/o; suffix: -vascular)

80. Thermoregulation: Maintenance of internal body temperature (root word: Therm/o; suffix: -regulation)

81. Adenopathy: Enlargement or disease of a gland (root word: Aden/o; suffix: -opathy)

82. Cystolithiasis: Presence of stones in the urinary bladder (root word: Cyst/o; suffix: -lithiasis)

83. Endoscope: Instrument used for visual examination inside the body (root word: End/o; suffix: -scope)

84. Hematologist: Medical professional specializing in the study of blood (root word: Hem/o; suffix: -logist)

85. Nephrology: Study of the kidneys and their diseases (root word: Nephr/o; suffix: -logy)

86. Orthopedic: Relating to the correction of deformities of the musculoskeletal system (root word: Orth/o; suffix: -pedic)

87. Phlebotomy: Procedure of drawing blood for diagnostic or therapeutic purposes (root word: Phleb/o; suffix: -tomy)

88. Radiologist: Medical professional specializing in medical imaging and interpretation (root word: Radi/o; suffix: -logist)

89. Urologist: Medical professional specializing in the urinary system (root word: Ur/o; suffix: -logist)

90. Adrenaline: Hormone released in response to stress, also known as epinephrine (root word: Adren/o; suffix: -ine)

91. Bronchoscope: Instrument used for visual examination of the bronchial tubes (root word: Bronch/o; suffix: -scope)

92. Cardiovascular: Pertaining to the heart and blood vessels (root word: Cardi/o; suffix: -vascular)

93. Dermatology: Branch of medicine dealing with the skin and its diseases (root word: Dermat/o; suffix: -logy)

94. Gastroenteritis: Inflammation of the stomach and intestines (root word: Gastroenter/o; suffix: -itis)

95. Hemorrhage: Abnormal bleeding (root word: Hemorrh/o; suffix: -age)

96. Nephropathy: Disease or disorder of the kidneys (root word: Nephr/o; suffix: -pathy)

97. Orthodontics: Branch of dentistry concerned with the alignment of teeth (root word: Orth/o; suffix: -odontics)

98. Phlebitis: Inflammation of a vein (root word: Phleb/o; suffix: -itis)

99. Radiography: Imaging technique using X-rays (root word: Radi/o; suffix: -graphy)

100. Uroscopy: Examination of the urine (root word: Ur/o; suffix: -scopy)

Exercise and Practice Activities:

Exercise 1: Prefixes, Root Words, and Suffixes Matching

Match the correct prefix, root word, and suffix to form a complete medical term.

Example:

Prefix: Pre-

Root Word: Cardi

Suffix: -ology

Medical Term: Precardiology

1. Prefix: Sub-

   Root Word: Dermat

   Suffix: -itis

Medical Term: ___________

2. Prefix: Hypo-

   Root Word: Glyc

   Suffix: -emia

   Medical Term: ___________

3. Prefix: Poly-

   Root Word: Neur

   Suffix: -pathy

   Medical Term: ___________

4. Prefix: Dys-

   Root Word: Pnea

   Suffix: -ia

   Medical Term: ___________

5. Prefix: Peri-

   Root Word: Oste

   Suffix: -itis

   Medical Term: ___________

Exercise 2: Building Medical Terms

Construct medical terms by combining the given prefix, root word, and suffix.

Example:

Prefix: Hypo-

Root Word: Thyroid

Suffix: -ism

Medical Term: Hypothyroidism

1. Prefix: Macro-

   Root Word: Vascular

   Suffix: -ectomy

   Medical Term: ___________

2. Prefix: Bradycardio-

   Root Word: Graphy

   Suffix: -gram

   Medical Term: ___________

3. Prefix: Hyper-

   Root Word: Tension

   Suffix: -ectomy

   Medical Term: ___________

4. Prefix: Sub-

   Root Word: Gastr

   Suffix: -itis

   Medical Term: ___________

5. Prefix: Anti-

   Root Word: Inflammatory

   Suffix: -otic

   Medical Term: ___________

Exercise 3: Fill in the Blanks

Complete the following sentences by filling in the blanks with the appropriate prefix, root word, or suffix.

1. The study of the nervous system is known as ____________.

2. Inflammation of the liver is called ___________.

3. The process of recording the electrical activity of the heart is called ___________.

4. The medical term for the surgical removal of the appendix is ___________.

5. The condition of excessive thirst is known as ___________.

[Note: Feel free to use Google for the answers or any other assistance. As a transcriptionist, you will always have access to the search engine.]

7. MEDICAL TERMINOLOGY AND WORD ANALYSIS

In this section, we will delve into the strategies for analyzing complex medical terms and deciphering their meaning. Understanding how medical terms are constructed and being able to break them down into their component parts will greatly enhance your ability to comprehend and interpret medical documentation accurately. Here are some key points to explore:

1. Breaking Down Medical Terms:

  - Learn to identify and separate prefixes, root words, and suffixes in a medical term.

  - Understand the role of each component in modifying the meaning or function of the term.

  - Practice dissecting medical terms into their component parts to better understand their overall meaning.

2. Analyzing Medical Terms:

  - Examine the meaning of individual prefixes, root words, and suffixes to determine their significance.

  - Understand common combining forms and their meanings.

  - Recognize how the combination of different components influences the overall meaning of the term.

3. Deciphering Medical Terminology:

  - Develop strategies for determining the meaning of unfamiliar medical terms by analyzing their components.

  - Utilize resources such as medical dictionaries, online databases, and reference materials to assist in deciphering complex terms.

  - Practice breaking down and interpreting medical terms through exercises and real-world examples.

4. Contextual Analysis:

  - Understand the importance of considering the context in which a medical term is used.

  - Consider the patient's medical condition, symptoms, and other relevant factors to aid in understanding the intended meaning of a term.

  - Analyze the entire medical report or documentation to gather additional information that may provide insights into the intended meaning of specific terms.

By developing effective strategies for analyzing medical terms and applying word analysis techniques, you will be better equipped to navigate the vast array of medical terminology encountered in transcription. This skill will contribute to your overall proficiency in accurately transcribing and understanding medical documentation.

Exercise:

Analyze the following medical terms by breaking them down into their component parts (prefixes, root words, and suffixes) and provide a brief explanation of their meaning:

1. Hyperthyroidism:

   Components: _______________

   Meaning: _______________

2. Dermatologist:

   Components: _______________

   Meaning: _______________

3. Gastroenteritis:

   Components: _______________

   Meaning: _______________

4. Ophthalmology:

   Components: _______________

   Meaning: _______________

5. Hemorrhage:

   Components: _______________

   Meaning: _______________

[Note: Feel free to use Google for the answers or any other assistance. As a transcriptionist, you will always have access to the search engine.]

Breaking down medical terms into their component parts for better comprehension

Here is a list of 25 medical terms broken down into their component parts for better comprehension:

1. Cardiologist:

   - Cardio: Relating to the heart

   - Logist: Specialist or expert

   Meaning: A cardiologist is a specialist who deals with the study and treatment of heart-related conditions.

2. Hepatitis:

   - Hepat: Pertaining to the liver

   - Itis: Inflammation

   Meaning: Hepatitis is the inflammation of the liver.

3. Ophthalmology:

   - Ophthalm: Relating to the eye

   - Logy: Study or science of

   Meaning: Ophthalmology is the study and treatment of eye-related conditions.

4. Gastroenteritis:

   - Gastro: Pertaining to the stomach or gastrointestinal tract

   - Enter: Relating to the intestines

   - Itis: Inflammation

   Meaning: Gastroenteritis is the inflammation of the stomach and intestines, usually resulting in symptoms like vomiting and diarrhea.

5. Dermatologist:

   - Dermat: Referring to the skin

   - Logist: Specialist or expert

   Meaning: A dermatologist is a specialist who deals with the study and treatment of skin-related conditions.

6. Nephrology:

   - Nephro: Relating to the kidney

   - Logy: Study or science of

   Meaning: Nephrology is the study and treatment of kidney-related conditions.

7. Neurologist:

   - Neuro: Relating to the nervous system

   - Logist: Specialist or expert

   Meaning: A neurologist is a specialist who deals with the study and treatment of nervous system disorders.

8. Orthopedics:

   - Ortho: Correct or straight

   - Ped: Relating to the foot or child

   - Ics: Study or science of

   Meaning: Orthopedics is the study and treatment of conditions related to the musculoskeletal system, particularly the bones and joints.

9. Hematology:

   - Hema: Pertaining to blood

   - Logy: Study or science of

   Meaning: Hematology is the study and treatment of blood-related conditions.

10. Urology:

- Uro: Relating to the urinary system

- Logy: Study or science of

Meaning: Urology is the study and treatment of urinary system disorders.

11. Cardiology:

 - Cardio: Relating to the heart

 - Logy: Study or science of

Meaning: Cardiology is the study of the heart and its disorders.

12. Endoscopy:

 - Endo: Inside or within

 - Scopy: Examination or visualization

Meaning: Endoscopy is a medical procedure used to examine the internal organs or cavities of the body using an endoscope.

13. Dermatology:

 - Dermat: Referring to the skin

 - Logy: Study or science of

Meaning: Dermatology is the study and treatment of diseases and conditions related to the skin.

14. Osteoporosis:

 - Osteo: Relating to the bones

 - Porosis: Porous or brittle condition

Meaning: Osteoporosis is a condition characterized by weak and brittle bones.

15. Gastroscopy:

 - Gastro: Pertaining to the stomach or gastrointestinal tract

 - Scopy: Examination or visualization

Meaning: Gastroscopy is a medical procedure used to visually examine the interior of the stomach using a flexible tube with a camera.

16. Nephropathy:

- Nephro: Relating to the kidney

- Pathy: Disease or disorder

Meaning: Nephropathy refers to any disease or disorder affecting the kidneys.

17. Neurology:

- Neuro: Relating to the nervous system

- Logy: Study or science of

Meaning: Neurology is the branch of medicine that deals with the study and treatment of disorders of the nervous system.

18. Orthodontics:

- Ortho: Correct or straight

- Dont: Referring to teeth

- Ics: Study or science of

Meaning: Orthodontics is the branch of dentistry that focuses on the correction of irregularities in teeth and jaw alignment.

19. Hemoglobin:

- Hemo: Relating to blood

- Globin: Protein

Meaning: Hemoglobin is the protein in red blood cells that carries oxygen throughout the body.

20. Urologist:

- Uro: Relating to the urinary system

- Logist: Specialist or expert

Meaning: A urologist is a specialist who deals with the study and treatment of diseases and disorders of the urinary system.

21. Gynecology:

   - Gyneco: Relating to women or female reproductive system

   - Logy: Study or science of

Meaning: Gynecology is the branch of medicine that focuses on the health and diseases of the female reproductive system.

22. Oncology:

   - Onco: Relating to tumors or cancer

   - Logy: Study or science of

Meaning: Oncology is the branch of medicine that deals with the prevention, diagnosis, and treatment of cancer.

23. Ophthalmologist:

   - Ophthalm: Relating to the eye

   - Logist: Specialist or expert

Meaning: An ophthalmologist is a medical doctor specializing in the diagnosis and treatment of eye disorders.

24. Podiatry:

   - Pod: Referring to the foot

   - Iatry: Medical treatment or specialty

Meaning: Podiatry is a branch of medicine that focuses on the study and treatment of disorders of the foot and ankle.

25. Radiology:

   - Radi: Relating to radiation or X-rays

   - Logy: Study or science of

Meaning: Radiology is the branch of medicine that deals with the use of medical imaging technologies, such as X-rays, to diagnose and treat

Remember, breaking down medical terms into their component parts can help in understanding their meaning and context. This knowledge is valuable for accurate transcription and effective communication within the medical field.

Techniques for identifying and understanding unfamiliar medical terms

Here are some examples of techniques for identifying and understanding unfamiliar medical terms:

1. Breaking down the word: Break the medical term into its component parts—prefix, root word, and suffix. Analyze each part to understand its meaning and how it contributes to the overall term. For example, in the word "gastroenteritis," "gastro" refers to the stomach, "enter" refers to the intestines, and "itis" indicates inflammation.

2. Using a medical dictionary or online resources: Look up unfamiliar medical terms in a medical dictionary or reliable online resources. These resources provide definitions, pronunciations, and explanations of medical terms, helping you understand their meaning and usage.

3. Analyzing the word roots: Familiarize yourself with common word roots used in medical terminology. Understanding the meanings of these roots will help you decipher the meaning of new medical terms. For example, "derm" refers to the skin, "cardi" refers to the heart, and "neuro" refers to the nervous system.

4. Identifying prefixes and suffixes: Pay attention to the prefixes and suffixes in medical terms as they provide clues about the term's meaning. For instance, the prefix "hypo-" indicates something is below normal or deficient, while the suffix "-ectomy" refers to the surgical removal of a specific organ or tissue.

5. Contextual understanding: Consider the context in which the medical term is used. Look for clues in the surrounding information, such as symptoms, body parts, or medical procedures, to help you deduce the meaning of the term.

6. Utilizing mnemonic devices: Mnemonic devices can be helpful for remembering complex medical terms. Create associations or memorable phrases using the first letters of the word parts to aid in recall and understanding. For example, "BRAT" can be used as a mnemonic for "Bananas, Rice, Applesauce, Toast" to remember the dietary recommendations for gastrointestinal upset.

7. Practice with flashcards: Create flashcards with unfamiliar medical terms, their meanings, and any relevant components. Quiz yourself regularly to reinforce your understanding and memorization of the terms.

8. Engaging in hands-on practice: Apply your knowledge by transcribing medical reports, listening to dictations, or participating in medical case studies. Hands-on practice helps you become familiar with different medical terms and their usage in real-world scenarios.

Remember, building a strong foundation in medical terminology takes time and practice. Consistent exposure to medical terms, active learning techniques, and ongoing reinforcement will enhance your ability to identify and understand unfamiliar medical terms.

8. PRACTICAL APPLICATIONS OF MEDICAL TERMINOLOGY

Applying medical terminology knowledge in transcription practice

Here are some practical applications of medical terminology in transcription practice:

1. Transcribing Medical Reports: Put your medical terminology knowledge into practice by transcribing various types of medical reports, such as discharge summaries, progress notes, or operative reports. Pay attention to the accurate spelling and usage of medical terms within the context of the report.

2. Identifying Medical Terminology in Dictations: Listen to medical dictations and practice identifying and understanding the medical terms used by healthcare professionals. Enhance your listening skills and develop the ability to recognize and interpret medical terminology accurately.

3. Researching Unfamiliar Medical Terms: Encounter unfamiliar medical terms during transcription? Use your knowledge of medical terminology to research and understand their meaning. Utilize reputable medical dictionaries, online resources, or consult with colleagues to ensure accurate interpretation and transcription.

4. Contextual Understanding: Develop the ability to comprehend medical terminology within the context of the patient's condition, diagnosis, treatment, and medical procedures. Apply critical thinking skills to ensure accurate transcription and convey the intended meaning of the medical terms in the reports.

5. Creating a Personal Medical Terminology Glossary: As you encounter new medical terms during transcription, maintain a personal glossary to record their meanings, context, and usage. Regularly review and update this glossary to expand your knowledge and enhance accuracy in future transcriptions.

6. Continuing Education and Professional Development: Stay updated with advancements in medical terminology and transcription practices by participating in workshops, webinars, or courses. Continuously expand your knowledge base and keep abreast of changes in medical terminology to provide accurate and quality transcription services.

7. Collaborating with Healthcare Professionals: Maintain open communication with healthcare professionals to clarify any doubts or seek clarification regarding medical terminology. Develop a collaborative relationship to ensure accurate transcription and to contribute effectively to the healthcare team.

By actively applying your medical terminology knowledge in transcription practice, you will enhance your transcription skills, accuracy, and efficiency. Continuously seek opportunities to practice, learn, and refine your understanding of medical terminology in the context of transcription, thus ensuring high-quality transcription services.

Certainly! Here are some exercises and practice activities for transcribing medical reports using correct terminology:

1. Dictation Transcription: Listen to a recorded medical dictation and transcribe it accurately, focusing on using the correct medical terminology. Pay attention to the context of the dictation, identify medical terms, and ensure their correct spelling, capitalization, and usage.

2. Case Study Transcription: Obtain a case study or patient scenario, and transcribe the relevant medical information, such as the patient's medical history, symptoms, diagnosis, treatment, and progress. Use appropriate medical terminology specific to the case study and maintain consistency throughout the transcription.

3. Verbatim Transcription: Practice transcribing medical dictations verbatim, including all the spoken words, including fillers (such as "um" or "uh") and non-verbal sounds. This exercise helps you accurately capture the details of the dictation, including specific medical terms used by healthcare professionals.

4. Practice with Medical Journals or Textbooks: Select a medical journal article or textbook chapter, and transcribe relevant sections, focusing on incorporating the correct medical terminology used in the text. Pay attention to the context and use accurate terminology to convey the intended meaning.

5. Transcription Review and Editing: Obtain previously transcribed medical reports, and review them for accuracy, particularly in terms of medical terminology usage. Identify any errors or inconsistencies and edit the reports to ensure correct terminology is used throughout.

6. Team-based Transcription Exercises: Collaborate with other transcriptionists or healthcare professionals to simulate real-life transcription scenarios. Each participant can transcribe different sections of a medical report, and then come together to compare and discuss their transcriptions, focusing on accuracy and correct terminology usage.

7. Continuing Education Courses: Enroll in medical transcription courses or workshops that provide specific exercises and practice activities for transcribing medical reports using correct terminology. These courses often include case studies, role-playing exercises, and quizzes to reinforce learning and application of medical terminology.

Remember, practice is key in developing proficiency in transcribing medical reports with correct terminology. Regularly engage in these exercises and seek opportunities to transcribe a variety of medical reports to enhance your skills and confidence in using accurate medical terminology.

Real-world examples and case studies demonstrating the practical use of medical terminology

Here are some real-world examples and case studies demonstrating the practical use of medical terminology:

1. Case Study: Patient Diagnosis and Treatment

- Scenario: A 45-year-old patient presents with severe abdominal pain and vomiting. After a thorough examination, the patient is diagnosed with acute appendicitis.

- Practical Use of Medical Terminology: In this case, medical terminology is used to document the patient's symptoms, perform relevant diagnostic tests (e.g., abdominal ultrasound), and describe the surgical procedure (e.g., appendectomy). Accurate and precise medical terminology is essential for clear communication among healthcare professionals involved in the patient's care.

2. Radiology Report: Interpretation of Imaging Studies

- Scenario: A patient undergoes a chest X-ray to evaluate persistent cough and shortness of breath. The radiologist examines the images and prepares a report.

- Practical Use of Medical Terminology: The radiology report uses medical terminology to describe the findings, such as "pulmonary infiltrates," "pleural effusion," or "mediastinal widening." Accurate medical terminology is crucial for conveying the radiologist's observations and assisting other healthcare providers in making informed treatment decisions.

3. Laboratory Report: Analysis of Blood Tests

- Scenario: A patient has routine blood work done, including a complete blood count (CBC) and liver function tests (LFTs). The laboratory technician analyzes the blood samples and generates a report.

- Practical Use of Medical Terminology: The laboratory report utilizes medical terminology to report the results, such as "hemoglobin," "platelet count," "alanine aminotransferase (ALT)," or "total bilirubin." Precise and standardized medical terminology ensures accurate interpretation of the test results by healthcare professionals.

4. Clinical Note: Documentation of Patient Progress

- Scenario: A physician sees a patient with diabetes who has been recently started on a new medication regimen. The physician documents the patient's progress during follow-up visits.

- Practical Use of Medical Terminology: The clinical note employs medical terminology to describe the patient's glycemic control, medication adjustments, and the management of complications related to diabetes. Consistent use of medical terminology helps healthcare providers accurately communicate and track the patient's progress over time.

These examples highlight how medical terminology is applied in various medical contexts, including patient diagnosis, imaging and laboratory analysis, and documentation of patient progress. Understanding and using accurate medical terminology enables effective communication, proper documentation, and optimal patient care.

9. TEST MODULE: ASSESSING MEDICAL TERMINOLOGY SKILLS

Comprehensive test module to assess the understanding and application of medical terminology

The Test Module is designed to provide a comprehensive assessment of your medical terminology skills and ensure that you have a solid understanding of the concepts and their practical application. It allows you to apply your knowledge, test your proficiency, and identify areas for improvement.

Multiple-choice questions, fill-in-the-blanks, and matching exercises

Here are some examples of multiple-choice questions, fill-in-the-blanks, and matching exercises in the Test Module for assessing medical terminology skills:

Multiple-Choice Questions:

1. Which of the following suffixes means "inflammation"?

a) -ectomy

b) -osis

c) -itis

d) -algia

2. What does the prefix "poly-" mean?

a) Above

b) Below

c) Many

d) Within

Fill-in-the-Blanks:

1. The medical term for "study of the ear" is ___________.

2. "Dyspnea" is a term that describes ___________.

Matching Exercises:

Match the following medical terms with their meanings:

1. Erythrocyte

2. Gastroenteritis

3. Osteoporosis

a) Inflammation of the stomach and intestines

b) Abnormal condition of weak bones

c) Red blood cell

Answers:

Multiple-Choice Questions:

1. c) -itis

2. c) Many

Fill-in-the-Blanks:

1. Otology

2. Difficulty breathing

Matching Exercises:

1. c) Red blood cell

2. a) Inflammation of the stomach and intestines

3. b) Abnormal condition of weak bones

These types of questions and exercises provide a comprehensive assessment of your knowledge and understanding of medical terminology. They require you to apply your knowledge of prefixes, suffixes, root words, and combining forms to determine the correct answers. By including a variety of question formats, the Test Module ensures that you have a well-rounded understanding of medical terminology and can effectively use it in a transcription context.

Here are some realistic transcription exercises involving medical terms:

Exercise 1: "The patient presented with symptoms of dyspnea, cough, and wheezing. Upon examination, the physician noted decreased breath sounds in the lower lobes and diagnosed the patient with pneumonia. The treatment plan includes antibiotics, bronchodilators, and rest."

Exercise 2:

Consultation Report:

Chief Complaint: Abdominal pain and bloating.

History of Present Illness: The patient reports intermittent sharp pain in the lower abdomen for the past week. The pain is aggravated by eating and relieved by rest. She also complains of bloating and occasional diarrhea. No significant weight loss or fever noted.

Physical Examination: Abdomen is tender upon palpation in the lower quadrants. No signs of peritonitis. Bowel sounds are normal. No palpable masses or organomegaly.

Assessment and Plan: Suspected irritable bowel syndrome. Recommended dietary modifications and symptom management with antispasmodics. Follow-up in 4 weeks.

Exercise 3:

Operative Report:

Preoperative Diagnosis: Cholecystitis with cholelithiasis.

Postoperative Diagnosis: Cholecystitis with cholelithiasis.

Procedure: Laparoscopic cholecystectomy.

Operative Findings: Inflamed gallbladder with multiple gallstones.

Description of Procedure: The patient was placed under general anesthesia. Four incisions were made in the abdomen for the laparoscopic instruments. The gallbladder was dissected and removed using electrocautery and a retrieval bag. Hemostasis was achieved, and the incisions were closed with absorbable sutures.

Postoperative Care: The patient tolerated the procedure well and was transferred to the recovery room in stable condition.

These transcription exercises simulate real-life scenarios and require you to accurately transcribe medical dictation and reports using appropriate medical terminology. By practicing these exercises, you can enhance your transcription skills and familiarity with medical terms in different clinical contexts.

Feedback and explanations for correct answers to enhance learning

Providing feedback and explanations for correct answers can greatly enhance learning. Here's an example of feedback and explanations for the transcription exercises mentioned earlier:

Exercise 1: Transcription Feedback and Explanations

Question: The patient presented with symptoms of dyspnea, cough, and wheezing. Upon examination, the physician noted decreased breath sounds in the lower lobes and diagnosed the patient with pneumonia. The treatment plan includes antibiotics, bronchodilators, and rest.

Feedback: Great job transcribing the dictation! You accurately captured the patient's symptoms, examination findings, and the diagnosis of pneumonia. The treatment plan includes antibiotics to treat the infection, bronchodilators to relieve wheezing, and rest to aid in recovery.

Explanation: Dyspnea refers to difficulty in breathing, cough is the act of expelling air from the lungs to clear the airways, and wheezing is a high-pitched whistling sound during breathing. Decreased breath sounds in the lower lobes can indicate a localized lung infection like pneumonia. Antibiotics are prescribed to target the specific pathogen causing the infection, bronchodilators help relax and open up the airways, and rest allows the body to recover and heal.

Exercise 2: Transcription Feedback and Explanations

Question: Chief Complaint: Abdominal pain and bloating. History of Present Illness: The patient reports intermittent sharp pain in the lower abdomen for the past week. The pain is aggravated by eating and relieved by rest. She also complains of bloating and occasional diarrhea. No significant weight loss or fever noted. Physical Examination: Abdomen is tender upon palpation in the lower quadrants. No signs of peritonitis. Bowel sounds are normal. No palpable masses or organomegaly. Assessment and Plan: Suspected irritable bowel syndrome. Recommended dietary modifications and symptom management with antispasmodics. Follow-up in 4 weeks.

Feedback: Excellent job transcribing the consultation report! You accurately captured the patient's chief complaint, history of present illness, physical examination findings, and the assessment and plan. The patient is suspected to have irritable bowel syndrome, and the recommended management includes dietary modifications and antispasmodics to alleviate symptoms.

Explanation: The chief complaint refers to the main reason for the patient's visit, which in this case is abdominal pain and bloating. The history of present illness provides details about the patient's symptoms, such as intermittent sharp pain in the lower abdomen aggravated by eating and relieved by rest, along with bloating and occasional diarrhea. The physical examination findings indicate tenderness in the lower quadrants of the abdomen but no signs of peritonitis (inflammation of the abdominal lining). Normal bowel sounds and the absence of palpable masses or organomegaly (enlarged organs) are also noted. The assessment is a suspected diagnosis of irritable bowel syndrome, a common gastrointestinal disorder. The plan involves dietary modifications and the use of antispasmodics to manage symptoms, with a follow-up appointment in 4 weeks for further evaluation.

Exercise 3: Transcription Feedback and Explanations

Question: Preoperative Diagnosis: Cholecystitis with cholelithiasis. Postoperative Diagnosis: Cholecystitis with cholelithiasis. Procedure: Laparoscopic cholecystectomy. Operative Findings: Inflamed gallbladder with multiple gallstones. Description of Procedure: The patient was placed under general anesthesia. Four incisions were made in the abdomen for the laparoscopic instruments. The gallbladder was dissected and removed using electrocautery and a retrieval bag. Hemostasis was achieved, and the incisions were closed with absorbable sutures. Postoperative Care: The patient tolerated the procedure well and was transferred to the recovery room in stable condition.

Feedback: Well done transcribing the operative report! You accurately captured the preoperative and postoperative diagnoses, the procedure performed, the operative findings, the description of the procedure, and the postoperative care. The patient underwent a laparoscopic cholecystectomy to remove an inflamed gallbladder with multiple gallstones. The procedure was successful, and the patient was transferred to the recovery room.

Explanation: Cholecystitis refers to inflammation of the gallbladder, and cholelithiasis refers to the presence of gallstones. A laparoscopic cholecystectomy is a minimally invasive surgical procedure to remove the gallbladder. The operative findings indicate an inflamed gallbladder with multiple gallstones. The description of the procedure mentions the use of general anesthesia, the creation of four incisions in the abdomen for the laparoscopic instruments, dissection and removal of the gallbladder using electrocautery and a retrieval bag, achievement of hemostasis (control of bleeding), and closure of the incisions with absorbable sutures. The postoperative care statement indicates that the patient tolerated the procedure well and was transferred to the recovery room in stable condition.

By providing detailed feedback and explanations for correct answers, learners can understand the rationale behind their responses, reinforce their knowledge, and improve their transcription skills and understanding of medical terminology.

MODULE II. WEEKLY TRANSCRIPTION MASTERCLASS: DEEP DIVE INTO DIFFERENT MEDICAL SPECIALTIES

1. INTRODUCTION TO MEDICAL SPECIALTIES

In the field of medicine, there are numerous specialized areas known as medical specialties. Each specialty focuses on a specific aspect of healthcare, targeting particular organs, systems, age groups, or conditions. Understanding medical specialties is crucial for transcriptionists to accurately transcribe medical reports and documents. Here are key points covered in the introduction to medical specialties:

1. Overview of Various Medical Specialties: This section provides a broad overview of different medical specialties, highlighting their distinct focus areas and the types of patients they serve. It includes specialties such as cardiology, dermatology, endocrinology, gastroenterology, hematology, oncology, neurology, obstetrics, gynecology, orthopedics, and more. The aim is to familiarize transcriptionists with the breadth and diversity of medical specialties.

2. Unique Focus Areas: Each medical specialty has its own unique focus, addressing specific organs, systems, or medical conditions. For example, cardiology deals with the heart and circulatory system, dermatology focuses on skin disorders, and neurology specializes in the nervous system. Transcriptionists need to grasp the core areas of each specialty to accurately transcribe medical reports in those fields.

3. Importance of Understanding Medical Specialties in Transcription: Transcriptionists play a crucial role in accurately documenting medical information. Understanding medical specialties is essential for them to comprehend the context, terminology, and specific requirements of each specialty. By having a good grasp of medical specialties, transcriptionists can ensure precise transcription, effective communication, and quality documentation.

Transcriptionists should familiarize themselves with the different medical specialties, their focus areas, and the types of patients they serve. This understanding will enable them to accurately transcribe medical reports, ensuring that the appropriate terminology, context, and nuances are captured in the documentation process.

2. TRANSCRIPTION CONSIDERATIONS FOR MEDICAL SPECIALTIES

Transcribing medical reports across different specialties requires a deep understanding of the specific terminology and language used in each specialty. Here are key points covered in the transcription considerations for medical specialties:

1. Understanding Specialty-Specific Terminology: Each medical specialty has its own set of unique terms, abbreviations, acronyms, and jargon. Transcriptionists must familiarize themselves with the terminology used in different specialties to ensure accurate transcription. For example, cardiology may include terms like angioplasty, arrhythmia, and stenosis, while dermatology may involve terms such as eczema, psoriasis, and biopsy.

2. Guidelines for Accurate Transcription: Transcriptionists should follow guidelines specific to each medical specialty to ensure accurate transcription. These guidelines may include formatting preferences, preferred abbreviations, usage of specialty-specific symbols or notations, and documentation requirements. Adhering to these guidelines helps maintain consistency and clarity in the transcribed reports.

3. Practice Activities for Familiarizing with Specialty-Specific Terms: To enhance their familiarity with specialty-specific terms, transcriptionists can engage in practice activities. These activities may involve reviewing sample reports from various specialties, listening to audio recordings, and transcribing reports with a focus on specific specialties. By actively engaging with specialty-specific terms, transcriptionists can improve their accuracy and confidence in transcribing reports in different medical specialties.

By understanding the specific terminology and language used in different medical specialties, following specialty-specific transcription guidelines, and actively practicing with specialty-specific terms, transcriptionists can ensure accurate and reliable transcriptions. This attention to detail and specialty-specific knowledge contributes to effective communication and documentation within each medical specialty.

Human heart anatomy

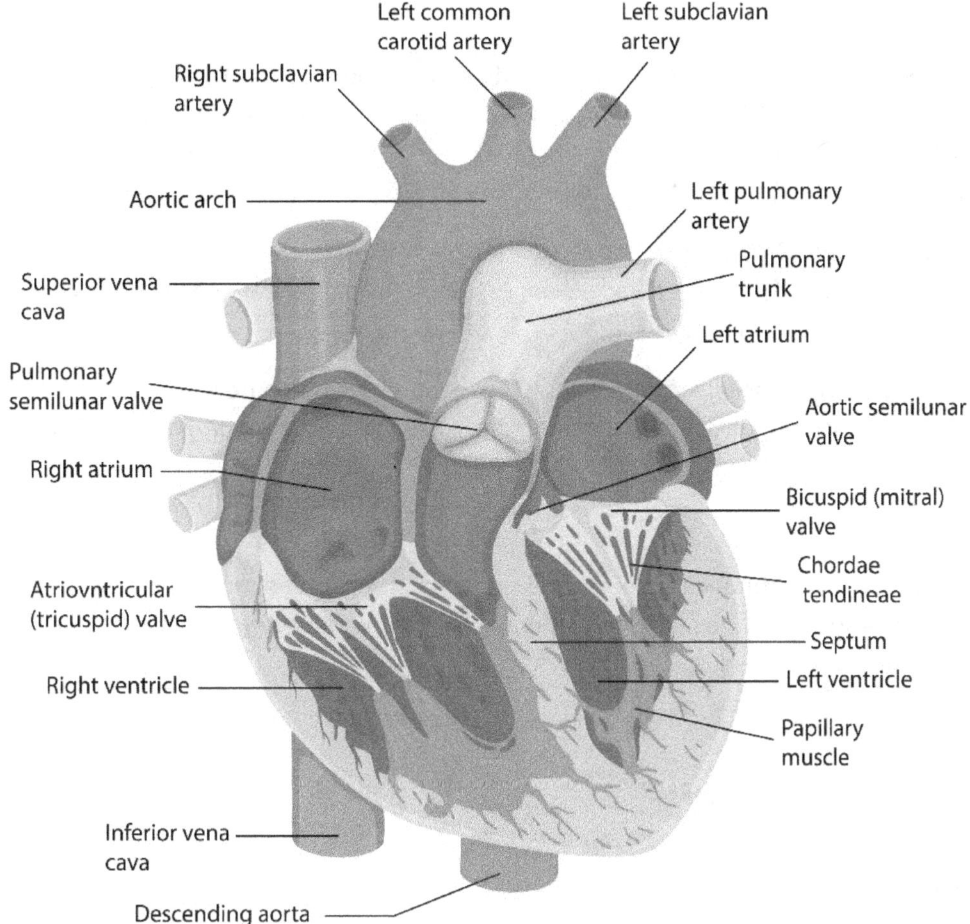

Overview of the field of cardiology and its key terminology

Cardiology is a branch of medicine that deals with disorders of the heart and certain parts of the cardiovascular system. The cardiovascular system includes the heart, the blood vessels, and the blood itself. If you're new to this field, here are some key concepts that you'll want to understand:

1. The Heart: The heart is a muscular organ that pumps blood throughout the body. It has four chambers - two atria (right and left) and two ventricles (right and left). Each chamber has a specific role in pumping blood. The right side of the heart pumps blood to the lungs for oxygenation, while the left side pumps oxygen-rich blood to the rest of the body.

2. Cardiovascular Diseases: These are conditions that involve narrowed or blocked blood vessels that can lead to a heart attack, chest pain (angina), or stroke. Other heart conditions, such as those that affect your heart's muscle, valves or rhythm, also are considered forms of heart disease.

3. Common Conditions: Some of the common conditions a cardiologist might treat include coronary artery disease, heart failure, valvular heart disease, heart rhythm disorders (arrhythmias), and congenital heart defects.

4. Diagnostic Tools: Cardiologists use a range of diagnostic tools to identify heart conditions. These include electrocardiograms (EKG/ECG), which record the electrical activity of the heart; echocardiograms, which use ultrasound to create images of the heart; and catheterization procedures, which involve threading a small tube into the heart through a blood vessel to perform diagnostic tests.

5. Treatment Approaches: Cardiologists can recommend a range of treatments, depending on the specific heart condition. These might include lifestyle changes, medications, cardiac procedures (such as stents or angioplasty), or surgery (such as bypass surgery or valve replacement).

6. Preventive Cardiology: This area of cardiology focuses on preventing heart disease in the first place. This often involves helping patients manage risk factors like high blood pressure, high cholesterol, obesity, smoking, and diabetes.

Remember, cardiology is a complex field that requires a strong foundation in biology, anatomy, and physiology. It's a rewarding field where you can make a profound difference in people's lives by helping them prevent, manage, and overcome heart disease.

Common cardiac conditions, diagnostic tests, and procedures

I. Cardiac Conditions:

1. Atrial fibrillation: A common cardiac arrhythmia characterized by rapid and irregular heartbeat originating in the atria.

2. Mitral valve prolapse: A condition where the valve between the left atrium and left ventricle doesn't close properly, causing blood to leak backward.

3. Ventricular septal defect: A congenital heart defect characterized by a hole in the wall (septum) separating the heart's lower chambers (ventricles).

4. Aortic stenosis: The narrowing of the aortic valve, restricting blood flow from the left ventricle to the aorta.

5. Hypertrophic cardiomyopathy: A genetic condition causing the thickening of the heart muscle, leading to impaired heart function.

6. Pulmonary embolism: A blockage of the pulmonary artery or its branches by a blood clot, typically originating from a deep vein thrombosis.

7. Bradycardia: An abnormally slow heart rate, usually defined as fewer than 60 beats per minute.

8. Myocarditis: Inflammation of the heart muscle often caused by a viral infection or autoimmune response.

9. Tetralogy of Fallot: A congenital heart defect consisting of four abnormalities in the structure of the heart, leading to oxygen deprivation in the body.

10. Endocarditis: Infection or inflammation of the inner lining of the heart, usually involving the heart valves.

11. Pulmonary hypertension: High blood pressure in the pulmonary arteries, which carry blood from the heart to the lungs.

12. Dilated cardiomyopathy: A condition characterized by the enlargement of the heart chambers, leading to weakened heart muscle and impaired pumping ability.

13. Supraventricular tachycardia: A rapid heart rate originating above the ventricles, often causing palpitations and shortness of breath.

14. Ventricular fibrillation: A life-threatening arrhythmia characterized by irregular and chaotic contractions of the ventricles.

15. Rheumatic heart disease: Heart damage resulting from rheumatic fever, an inflammatory condition caused by untreated streptococcal infection.

16. Mitral regurgitation: A condition where the mitral valve doesn't close properly, causing blood to leak back into the left atrium.

17. Wolff-Parkinson-White syndrome: A congenital condition characterized by an abnormal electrical pathway in the heart, leading to rapid heart rates.

18. Long QT syndrome: A disorder of the heart's electrical system, causing an increased risk of arrhythmias and sudden cardiac arrest.

19. Aortic dissection: A tear in the inner layer of the aorta, causing blood to flow between the layers and potentially leading to life-threatening complications.

20. Ischemic heart disease: A condition where there is reduced blood flow to the heart muscle due to narrowed or blocked coronary arteries.

21. Cardiac tamponade: The accumulation of fluid or blood in the pericardial sac, compressing the heart and impairing its function.

22. Pulmonary valve stenosis: The narrowing of the pulmonary valve, restricting blood flow from the right ventricle to the pulmonary artery.

23. Coarctation of the aorta: A congenital heart defect characterized by a narrowing of the aorta, leading to reduced blood flow to the body.

24. Arrhythmogenic right ventricular dysplasia: A condition where the muscle tissue in the right ventricle is replaced by fatty or fibrous tissue, increasing the risk of arrhythmias.

25. Restrictive cardiomyopathy: A rare condition where the heart muscle becomes stiff and less able to fill with blood properly.

II. Diagnostic Tests:

1. Electrocardiogram (ECG/EKG): A non-invasive test that records the electrical activity of the heart to evaluate its rhythm and detect abnormalities.

2. Echocardiogram: A test that uses sound waves (ultrasound) to create images of the heart's structure and assess its function.

3. Stress test: A test that measures the heart's response to physical activity or induced stress to evaluate its performance and detect potential abnormalities.

4. Holter monitor: A portable device that records the heart's electrical activity over a 24-hour period to assess for any irregularities or symptoms.

5. Cardiac catheterization: A procedure where a thin tube (catheter) is inserted into a blood vessel and threaded to the heart to diagnose and treat various cardiac conditions.

6. Coronary angiogram: A type of cardiac catheterization that uses contrast dye to visualize the coronary arteries and detect blockages or narrowing.

7. Nuclear stress test: A stress test that involves injecting a small amount of radioactive material to evaluate blood flow to the heart muscle.

8. Cardiac MRI (Magnetic Resonance Imaging): A non-invasive imaging technique that uses magnetic fields and radio waves to create detailed images of the heart's structure and function.

9. CT angiogram: A computed tomography (CT) scan that provides detailed images of the blood vessels, including the coronary arteries, to assess for blockages.

10. Blood tests: Various blood tests can be performed to assess cardiac markers, cholesterol levels, electrolyte imbalances, and other factors related to heart health.

11. Tilt table test: A test used to assess the cause of fainting episodes by tilting the patient on a table to monitor changes in blood pressure and heart rate.

12. Event monitor: A portable device worn by the patient to record heart rhythm irregularities when symptoms occur intermittently.

13. Transesophageal echocardiogram (TEE): A specialized echocardiogram where a small probe is inserted into the esophagus to obtain clearer images of the heart.

14. Exercise stress echocardiogram: A stress test combined with an echocardiogram to assess the heart's function during physical activity.

15. Genetic testing: Testing for specific genetic mutations or variations that may be associated with certain cardiac conditions or predisposition to cardiovascular diseases.

16. Ambulatory blood pressure monitoring (ABPM): A device worn by the patient to monitor blood pressure at regular intervals over a 24-hour period.

17. Electrophysiology study (EPS): A procedure where catheters are used to evaluate the heart's electrical system and identify abnormal rhythms.

18. Cardiac event monitor: A device worn by the patient to record heart rhythm irregularities for an extended period.

19. Myocardial perfusion imaging: A nuclear medicine imaging test that evaluates blood flow to the heart muscle during rest and stress conditions.

20. Chest X-ray: A radiographic imaging test that provides a visual representation of the heart and lungs.

21. Carotid ultrasound: A test that uses sound waves to evaluate the structure and blood flow in the carotid arteries in the neck.

22. Coronary calcium scan: A specialized CT scan that measures the amount of calcium in the coronary arteries, which can indicate the presence of plaque buildup.

23. Ambulatory electrocardiogram (AECG): A portable device that records the heart's electrical activity over an extended period, typically 24 to 48 hours.

24. Exercise stress test: A test that monitors the heart's electrical activity and blood pressure while the patient exercises on a treadmill or stationary bike.

25. Transcutaneous echocardiogram (TTE): A standard echocardiogram performed by placing an ultrasound probe on

III. Procedures:

1. Coronary angioplasty: A minimally invasive procedure that uses a balloon-tipped catheter to open blocked or narrowed coronary arteries and restore blood flow to the heart muscle.

2. Coronary artery bypass grafting (CABG): A surgical procedure in which a healthy blood vessel is harvested from another part of the body and used to bypass blocked or narrowed coronary arteries, improving blood flow to the heart.

3. Pacemaker implantation: A procedure in which a small electronic device (pacemaker) is implanted under the skin to regulate the heart's rhythm and treat abnormal heart rhythms.

4. Implantable cardioverter-defibrillator (ICD) insertion: A surgical procedure in which a device is implanted to monitor the heart's rhythm and deliver electric shocks to restore normal rhythm in the event of a life-threatening arrhythmia.

5. Cardiac ablation: A procedure that uses heat or cold energy to destroy or scar tissue in the heart that is causing abnormal heart rhythms.

6. Transcatheter aortic valve replacement (TAVR): A minimally invasive procedure in which a new artificial valve is implanted within the existing diseased aortic valve, typically used for patients with severe aortic stenosis.

7. Transcatheter mitral valve repair or replacement: Minimally invasive procedures to repair or replace the mitral valve using catheter-based techniques.

8. Heart transplant: A surgical procedure in which a diseased heart is replaced with a healthy heart from a donor.

9. Left ventricular assist device (LVAD) implantation: A procedure in which a mechanical pump is implanted to assist the left ventricle in pumping blood, typically used as a bridge to heart transplantation or as destination therapy for end-stage heart failure.

10. Percutaneous coronary intervention (PCI): A minimally invasive procedure that combines coronary angioplasty with the insertion of stents to treat blocked or narrowed coronary arteries.

11. Electrophysiology study (EPS): A procedure used to diagnose and treat abnormal heart rhythms by mapping the electrical pathways and using catheter-based techniques to correct them.

12. Radiofrequency ablation: A procedure that uses high-frequency electrical currents to destroy abnormal tissue responsible for causing arrhythmias.

13. Atherectomy: A procedure to remove plaque buildup within the blood vessels using specialized devices, improving blood flow.

14. Thoracic aortic aneurysm repair: A surgical procedure to repair an enlarged or weakened section of the aorta in the chest.

15. Percutaneous valve repair or replacement: Minimally invasive procedures to repair or replace heart valves using catheter-based techniques.

16. Heart valve repair or replacement surgery: A surgical procedure to repair or replace damaged or diseased heart valves with artificial or biological valves.

17. Ventricular assist device (VAD) implantation: A mechanical device implanted to assist the pumping function of the heart's ventricles in patients with advanced heart failure.

18. Patent foramen ovale (PFO) closure: A procedure to close a small hole between the heart's chambers that is present since birth.

19. Aortic aneurysm repair: A surgical procedure to repair an enlarged or weakened section of the aorta, the body's main artery.

20. Septal defect closure: A procedure to close abnormal openings between the heart's chambers, such as atrial septal defects or ventricular septal defects.

21. Maze procedure: A surgical procedure to treat atrial fibrillation by creating scar tissue in the heart to redirect the electrical impulses.

22. Cardiac resynchronization therapy (CRT): A procedure in which a special pacemaker with three leads is implanted to help synchronize the heart's contractions in patients with heart failure.

23. Pulmonary valve repair or replacement: A surgical procedure to repair or replace the pulmonary valve, which regulates blood flow from the heart to the lungs.

24. Endovascular aneurysm repair (EVAR): A minimally invasive procedure to repair abdominal aortic aneurysms using stent grafts.

25. Thrombectomy: A procedure to remove blood clots from blood vessels, restoring normal blood flow.

Exercises for transcribing cardiology reports accurately

Exercise 1: Fill in the blanks

Transcribe the following sentence:

The patient's ______ shows an irregular ______ rhythm with ______ intervals, indicative of atrial fibrillation.

Answer:

The patient's EKG shows an irregular cardiac rhythm with irregular intervals, indicative of atrial fibrillation.

Exercise 2: True or False

Indicate whether the following statement is true or false:

In coronary artery disease, there is a narrowing or blockage of the arteries that supply blood to the heart muscle.

Answer:

True

Exercise 3: Fill in the blanks

Transcribe the following sentence:

The patient's ______ levels are elevated, suggesting cardiac muscle damage.

Answer:

The patient's troponin levels are elevated, suggesting cardiac muscle damage.

Exercise 4: Matching

Match the diagnostic test with its description:

1. Echocardiography

2. Cardiac catheterization

3. Holter monitoring

4. Stress test

A. Measures the electrical activity of the heart

B. Uses sound waves to visualize the heart's structure and function

C. Evaluates the heart's electrical conduction system

D. Measures the heart's response to physical activity or medication

Answer:

1. Echocardiography

B. Uses sound waves to visualize the heart's structure and function

2. Cardiac catheterization

C. Evaluates the heart's electrical conduction system

3. Holter monitoring

A. Measures the electrical activity of the heart

4. Stress test

D. Measures the heart's response to physical activity or medication

Exercise 5: Fill in the blanks

Transcribe the following sentence:

The patient has a history of _____, _____, and _____, which are significant risk factors for cardiovascular disease.

Answer:

The patient has a history of hypertension, diabetes, and smoking, which are significant risk factors for cardiovascular disease.

Exercise 6: True or False

Indicate whether the following statement is true or false:

A myocardial infarction is commonly known as a heart attack and occurs when blood flow to the heart is blocked, leading to damage of the heart muscle.

Answer:

True

Exercise 7: Fill in the blanks

Transcribe the following sentence:

The patient is scheduled for _____, a procedure that uses a balloon-tipped catheter to open blocked coronary arteries.

Answer:

The patient is scheduled for percutaneous coronary intervention (PCI), a procedure that uses a balloon-tipped catheter to open blocked coronary arteries.

Exercise 8: Matching

Match the procedure with its description:

1. Angioplasty

2. Coronary artery bypass surgery

3. Stent placement

4. Endarterectomy

A. Surgical removal of atherosclerotic plaque from a blood vessel

B. Use of a balloon-tipped catheter to open narrowed or blocked blood vessels

C. Creation of a bypass around a blocked coronary artery using a blood vessel graft

D. Placement of a mesh-like device to keep a blood vessel open

Answer:

1. Angioplasty

B. Use of a balloon-tipped catheter to open narrowed or blocked blood vessels

2. Coronary artery bypass surgery

C. Creation of a bypass around a blocked coronary artery using a blood vessel graft

3. Stent placement

D. Placement of a mesh-like device to keep a blood vessel open

4. Endarterectomy

A. Surgical removal of atherosclerotic plaque from a blood vessel

Exercise 9: True or False

Indicate whether the following statement is true or false:

An echocardiogram is a non-invasive imaging test that uses sound waves to create pictures of the heart's structure and function.

Answer:

True

Exercise 10: Fill in the blanks

Transcribe the following sentence:

The patient's ______ is prescribed to help control blood pressure and reduce the risk of future cardiac events.

Answer:

The patient's antihypertensive medication is prescribed to help control blood pressure and reduce the risk of future cardiac events.

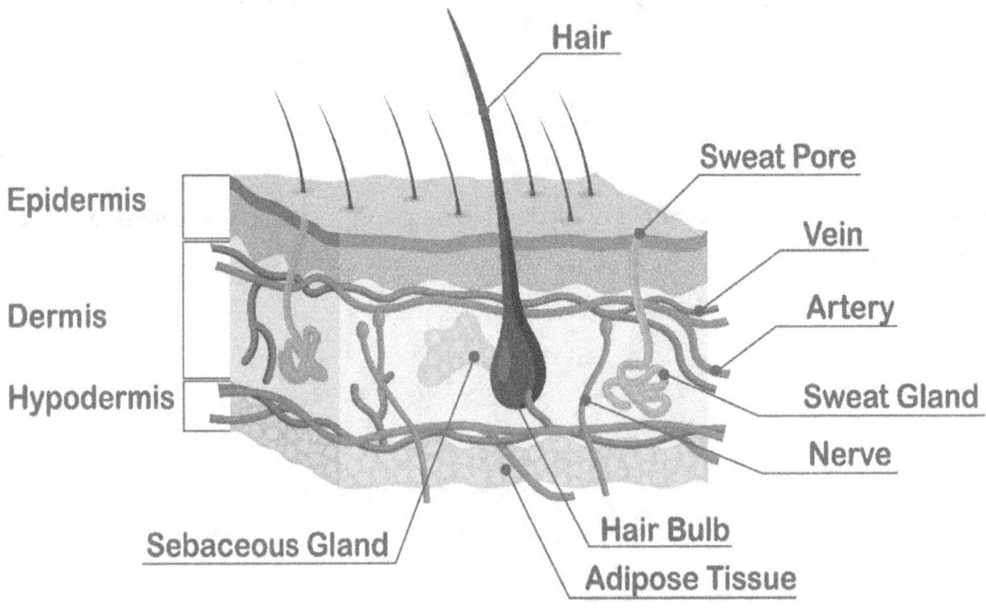

Introduction to dermatology and its specialized terminology

Dermatology is a branch of medicine that focuses on the health and diseases of the skin, hair, nails, and mucous membranes (like the lining inside the mouth, nose, and eyelids). If you're new to this field, here are some key concepts to understand:

1. The Skin: The skin is the largest organ of the body. It acts as a barrier protecting the body from environmental factors, helps regulate body temperature, allows sensation of touch, heat, and cold, and aids in vitamin D synthesis. It has three main layers: the epidermis (outermost layer), dermis (middle layer), and subcutaneous layer (innermost layer).

2. Common Conditions: Dermatologists diagnose and treat more than 3,000 different diseases. Some common conditions include acne, eczema, psoriasis, skin cancer, fungal infections, vitiligo, rosacea, warts, and alopecia (hair loss).

3. Diagnostic Tools: Dermatologists use various diagnostic tools like dermoscopy (handheld microscope to examine skin), patch testing (to find allergens causing skin reactions), skin biopsies (taking a small sample of skin for testing), and laboratory tests.

4. Treatment Approaches: Treatment in dermatology varies widely depending on the condition. It can involve topical medications (like creams or ointments), systemic medications (pills or injections that affect the whole body), minor surgical procedures, or more complex surgeries. Other treatment modalities include phototherapy (use of UV light), laser therapy, and cosmetic procedures like botox or fillers.

5. Dermatopathology and Mohs Surgery: Dermatopathology is a subspecialty focusing on the study of cutaneous diseases at a microscopic level. Mohs surgery is a precise surgical technique used to treat skin cancer, where layers of cancer-containing skin are progressively removed and examined until only cancer-free tissue remains.

6. Cosmetic Dermatology: This is a subfield that provides services designed to enhance appearance. These include procedures to improve skin tone and texture, reduce wrinkles, remove hair, and even alter the shape of certain features.

Skin conditions, diagnostic procedures, and treatments

I. Skin Conditions:

1. Acne: Common skin condition characterized by the formation of pimples, blackheads, and whiteheads.

2. Eczema: Chronic inflammatory condition causing red, itchy, and dry skin patches.

3. Psoriasis: Chronic autoimmune condition leading to thick, scaly patches on the skin.

4. Rosacea: Chronic inflammatory condition causing redness and flushing on the face.

5. Dermatitis: Inflammation of the skin caused by allergies, irritants, or infections.

6. Urticaria (Hives): Allergic reaction resulting in raised, itchy, and red welts on the skin.

7. Melanoma: Type of skin cancer developing in melanocytes, the pigment-producing cells.

8. Basal cell carcinoma: Most common type of skin cancer characterized by small, shiny bumps.

9. Squamous cell carcinoma: Skin cancer appearing as red nodules or scaly lesions.

10. Vitiligo: Condition causing loss of skin pigmentation and the appearance of white patches.

11. Impetigo: Contagious bacterial skin infection resulting in blisters and crusty sores.

12. Herpes simplex: Viral infection causing painful cold sores or blisters on the lips, mouth, or genitals.

13. Hives: Allergic reaction causing itchy, raised welts on the skin.

14. Ringworm: Fungal infection causing red, circular rashes on the skin.

15. Warts: Viral infection leading to the formation of rough, raised bumps on the skin.

16. Athlete's foot: Fungal infection causing itchy, peeling skin between the toes.

17. Cellulitis: Bacterial skin infection causing redness, warmth, and swelling.

18. Shingles: Viral infection causing painful, blistering rash along nerve pathways.

19. Moles: Common skin growths usually brown or black in color.

20. Hidradenitis suppurativa: Chronic skin condition characterized by painful, recurrent abscesses in the armpits, groin, or buttocks.

21. Actinic keratosis: Rough, scaly patches on the skin caused by long-term sun exposure.

22. Allergic contact dermatitis: Skin inflammation caused by an allergic reaction to a specific substance.

23. Pruritus: Persistent itching sensation of the skin.

24. Xerosis: Dry skin condition characterized by itching and scaling.

25. Stevens-Johnson syndrome: Severe allergic reaction causing widespread blistering and skin detachment.

II. Diagnostic Procedures:

1. Biopsy: Removal of a small sample of skin tissue for microscopic examination.

2. Patch testing: Application of patches with potential allergens to identify allergic contact dermatitis.

3. Skin scraping: Collection of skin cells for microscopic examination to diagnose fungal infections.

4. Skin prick test: Introduction of small amounts of allergens into the skin to identify specific allergies.

5. Wood's lamp examination: Use of ultraviolet light to detect certain skin conditions or infections.

6. Skin biopsy: Removal of a sample of skin tissue for laboratory analysis.

7. Dermoscopy: Examination of skin lesions using a dermatoscope to assess for signs of skin cancer.

8. Patch testing: Application of patches containing potential allergens to identify allergic reactions.

9. Skin allergy testing: Testing to identify specific allergens causing allergic reactions on the skin.

10. Skin culture: Collection of a skin sample to culture and identify bacterial, fungal, or viral infections.

11. Tzanck smear: Microscopic examination of cells from skin lesions to diagnose viral infections.

12. Skin prick test: Pricking the skin with potential allergens to observe allergic reactions.

13. Skin scraping: Collecting skin cells or scrapings to examine for the presence of parasites or fungal infections.

14. Skin punch biopsy: Removal of a small, circular piece of skin tissue for examination under a microscope.

15. Skin patch test: Application of patches with potential allergens to assess allergic reactions.

16. Skin cytology: Examination of skin cells to detect abnormalities or cancerous cells.

17. Skin prick allergy test: Introduction of potential allergens into the skin to identify allergic reactions.

18. Dermatopathology: Study of skin tissue samples to diagnose skin diseases and conditions.

19. Skin imaging (e.g., dermoscopy, reflectance confocal microscopy): Non-invasive imaging techniques used to assess skin lesions and identify potential abnormalities.

20. Skin scraping and potassium hydroxide (KOH) test: Microscopic examination of skin scrapings treated with KOH to detect fungal infections.

21. Skin biopsy with immunofluorescence: Removal of skin tissue for examination under a microscope, using immunofluorescent staining to identify specific proteins or antibodies.

22. Skin lesion aspiration: Use of a needle and syringe to extract fluid from skin lesions for laboratory analysis.

23. Skin allergy patch test: Application of patches containing potential allergens to identify delayed allergic reactions.

24. Skin perfusion pressure measurement: Non-invasive test to assess blood flow and tissue perfusion in the skin.

25. Reflectance confocal microscopy: Non-invasive imaging technique that allows for the visualization of cellular structures in the skin.

III. Treatments:

1. Topical corticosteroids: Anti-inflammatory medications applied to the skin to reduce itching and inflammation.

2. Topical retinoids: Medications derived from vitamin A used to treat acne, psoriasis, and other skin conditions.

3. Antibiotics: Medications used to treat bacterial skin infections such as cellulitis or impetigo.

4. Antifungal creams: Topical medications used to treat fungal skin infections such as athlete's foot or ringworm.

5. Antihistamines: Medications that block the effects of histamine and relieve itching in allergic skin conditions.

6. Moisturizers: Products used to hydrate and soothe dry skin, reducing itching and scaling.

7. Topical immunomodulators: Medications that modify the immune response to manage inflammatory skin conditions such as eczema.

8. Phototherapy: Treatment with ultraviolet light to reduce inflammation and symptoms in certain skin conditions.

9. Systemic corticosteroids: Oral or injectable medications used to manage severe inflammatory skin conditions.

10. Systemic immunosuppressants: Medications that suppress the immune system to manage autoimmune skin conditions.

11. Antiviral medications: Medications used to treat viral skin infections such as herpes or shingles.

12. Cryosurgery: Treatment method that uses extreme cold to freeze and destroy abnormal skin cells, such as warts or precancerous lesions.

13. Laser therapy: Use of lasers to target and treat specific skin conditions, including hair removal, scar reduction, or tattoo removal.

14. Chemical peels: Procedure involving the application of a chemical solution to the skin to exfoliate and improve its appearance.

15. Microdermabrasion: Exfoliation technique that removes dead skin cells and improves the texture and appearance of the skin.

16. Electrosurgery: Use of electrical current to cut, coagulate, or remove tissue, commonly used for the removal of skin lesions or the treatment of certain skin conditions.

17. Skin grafting: Surgical procedure that involves transplanting healthy skin to replace damaged or lost skin.

18. Cryotherapy: Treatment method that uses extreme cold to freeze and destroy abnormal skin cells, commonly used for warts or precancerous skin lesions.

19. Mohs surgery: Specialized surgical technique for the removal of skin cancers, layer by layer, to minimize damage to healthy tissue.

20. Excisional biopsy: Surgical removal of a skin lesion or abnormal tissue for further examination.

21. Microdermabrasion: A procedure that uses a handheld device to exfoliate the outer layer of skin, improving its texture and appearance.

22. Chemical peels: Application of a chemical solution to the skin to remove damaged outer layers and promote the growth of new, healthier skin.

23. Laser resurfacing: The use of laser technology to remove damaged skin layers and stimulate collagen production, reducing wrinkles, scars, and other skin imperfections.

24. Hair transplant: Surgical procedure that involves moving hair follicles from a donor area to areas of the scalp affected by hair loss or thinning.

25. Photodynamic therapy: A treatment that combines a light-activated photosensitizing agent with a specific wavelength of light to target and destroy abnormal cells or treat certain skin conditions.

Practice activities for transcribing dermatology reports effectively

Exercise 1: Fill in the blanks

Transcribe the following sentence:

The patient presented with a ______ rash characterized by ______, ______, and ______.

Answer:

The patient presented with a maculopapular rash characterized by redness, itching, and raised bumps.

Exercise 2: True or False

Indicate whether the following statement is true or false:

Psoriasis is an autoimmune skin condition characterized by red, scaly patches on the skin.

Answer:

True

Exercise 3: Fill in the blanks

Transcribe the following sentence:

The patient has a history of ______, ______, and ______, which are known risk factors for developing skin cancer.

Answer:

The patient has a history of sun exposure, fair skin, and a family history of skin cancer, which are known risk factors for developing skin cancer.

Exercise 4: Matching

Match the skin condition with its description:

1. Acne

2. Eczema

3. Rosacea

4. Psoriasis

A. Chronic skin condition characterized by redness and visible blood vessels on the face

B. Skin condition characterized by raised, red plaques covered with silver scales

C. Common skin condition characterized by clogged pores, pimples, and blackheads

D. Inflammatory skin condition characterized by dry, itchy, and inflamed patches

Answer:

1. Acne

C. Common skin condition characterized by clogged pores, pimples, and blackheads

2. Eczema

D. Inflammatory skin condition characterized by dry, itchy, and inflamed patches

3. Rosacea

A. Chronic skin condition characterized by redness and visible blood vessels on the face

4. Psoriasis

B. Skin condition characterized by raised, red plaques covered with silver scales

Exercise 5: Fill in the blanks

Transcribe the following sentence:

The patient's skin biopsy revealed the presence of ______, confirming the diagnosis of ______.

Answer:

The patient's skin biopsy revealed the presence of melanoma cells, confirming the diagnosis of melanoma.

Exercise 6: True or False

Indicate whether the following statement is true or false:

A dermatologist is a medical specialist who diagnoses and treats conditions related to the skin, hair, and nails.

Answer:

True

Exercise 7: Fill in the blanks

Transcribe the following sentence:

The patient was prescribed a _____ cream to alleviate the symptoms of _____.

Answer:

The patient was prescribed a corticosteroid cream to alleviate the symptoms of eczema.

Exercise 8: Matching

Match the diagnostic procedure with its description:

1. Patch testing

2. Wood's lamp examination

3. Skin biopsy

4. Dermoscopy

A. Procedure to examine the skin's reaction to various substances to identify allergies

B. Use of a special light to examine the skin for certain conditions, such as fungal infections

C. Surgical procedure to remove a sample of skin tissue for laboratory analysis

D. Examination of skin lesions using a handheld magnifying device to assess their characteristics

Answer:

1. Patch testing

A. Procedure to examine the skin's reaction to various substances to identify allergies

2. Wood's lamp examination

B. Use of a special light to examine the skin for certain conditions, such as fungal infections

3. Skin biopsy

C. Surgical procedure to remove a sample of skin tissue for laboratory analysis

4. Dermoscopy

D. Examination of skin lesions using a handheld magnifying device to assess their characteristics

Exercise 9: True or False

Indicate whether the following statement is true or false:

Contact dermatitis is a skin condition that occurs when the skin comes into contact with an irritant or allergen, leading to redness, itching, and rash.

Answer:

True

Exercise 10: Fill in the blanks

Transcribe the following sentence:

The patient's skin examination revealed the presence of ______, which required further evaluation for ______.

Answer:

The patient's skin examination revealed the presence of a suspicious mole, which required further evaluation for possible skin cancer.

ENDOCRINE SYSTEM

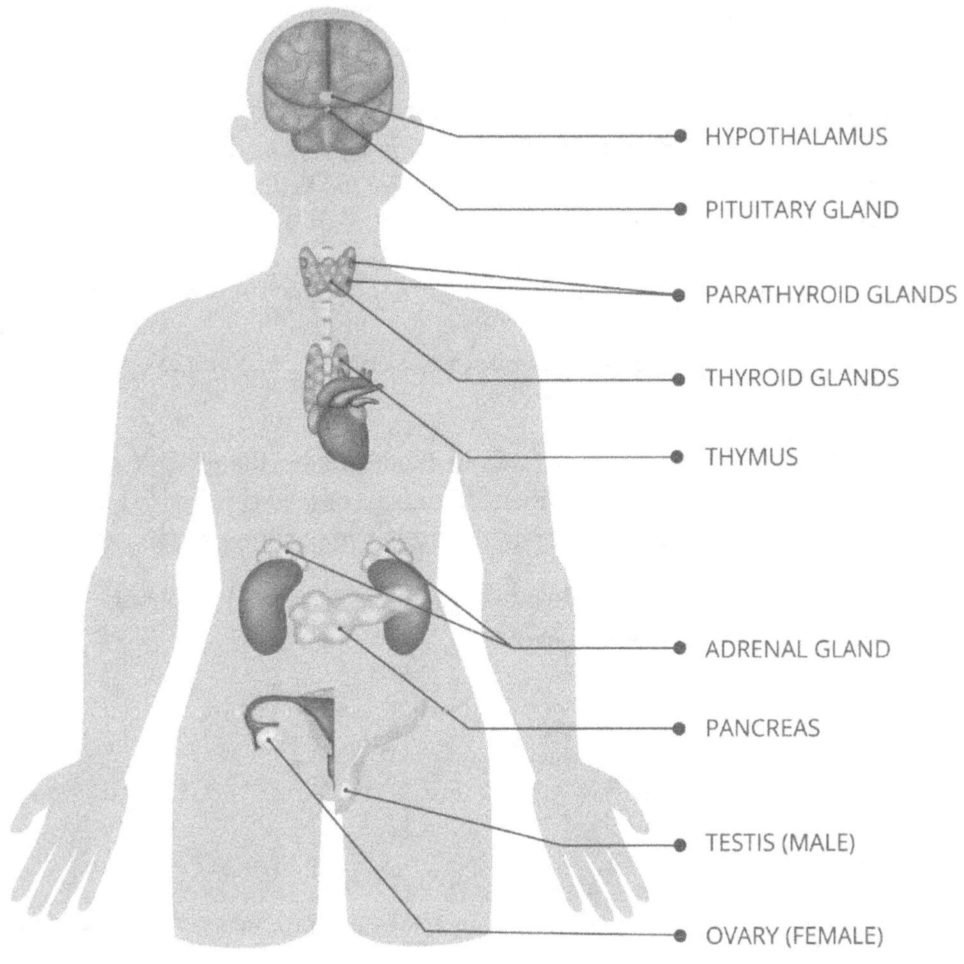

Understanding the field of endocrinology and its terminology

Endocrinology is a branch of medicine that focuses on the endocrine system and the hormones it produces. The endocrine system is a network of glands that produce and release hormones that help control many important body functions, especially the body's ability to change calories into energy that powers cells and organs.

If you're a beginner in this field, here are some fundamental concepts to comprehend:

1. Endocrine Glands: These are specialized organs and tissues that produce and secrete hormones. They include the pituitary gland, thyroid gland, adrenal glands, pancreas, ovaries in women, and testes in men. Each gland produces specific hormones that have specific roles.

2. Hormones: Hormones are chemical messengers that travel throughout the body coordinating complex processes like growth, metabolism, and fertility. They can influence the function of the immune system, and even alter behavior.

3. Common Conditions: Endocrinologists diagnose and treat conditions related to problems with the endocrine system. These can include diabetes (type 1 and type 2), thyroid diseases, metabolic disorders, lack of growth (short stature), over- or underproduction of hormones, menopause, osteoporosis, hypertension, and cancers of the endocrine glands.

4. Diagnostic Tools: Endocrinologists use a variety of diagnostic tools including blood and urine tests to measure hormone levels. They also use imaging studies like ultrasound, CT scans, MRIs, and nuclear medicine scans for diagnosis and management of endocrine disorders. In some cases, they may perform a biopsy.

5. Treatment Approaches: Treatment can vary widely depending on the specific condition. It often involves managing hormone imbalances with synthetic hormones or medications. In some cases, surgical intervention may be necessary to remove a tumor or a part of an endocrine gland.

6. Reproductive Endocrinology: This is a subfield that addresses hormonal functioning as it pertains to reproduction and infertility in both men and women.

Hormonal disorders, diagnostic tests, and treatment options

I. Hormonal Disorders:

1. Hypothyroidism: A condition where the thyroid gland does not produce enough thyroid hormones, leading to symptoms such as fatigue, weight gain, and depression.

2. Hyperthyroidism: A condition characterized by excessive production of thyroid hormones, resulting in symptoms like weight loss, rapid heartbeat, and irritability.

3. Diabetes mellitus: A metabolic disorder characterized by high blood sugar levels due to insufficient production or utilization of insulin.

4. Polycystic ovary syndrome (PCOS): A hormonal disorder affecting women that can cause irregular menstrual periods, excess hair growth, and fertility issues.

5. Cushing's syndrome: A disorder caused by excessive production of cortisol hormone, leading to symptoms like weight gain, high blood pressure, and fragile skin.

6. Addison's disease: A condition where the adrenal glands do not produce enough cortisol and aldosterone, resulting in fatigue, muscle weakness, and low blood pressure.

7. Growth hormone deficiency: A disorder characterized by inadequate production of growth hormone, leading to short stature in children and fatigue in adults.

8. Hyperparathyroidism: A condition in which the parathyroid glands produce too much parathyroid hormone, causing elevated calcium levels in the blood.

9. Hypoparathyroidism: A disorder where the parathyroid glands produce insufficient parathyroid hormone, leading to low calcium levels in the blood.

10. Pituitary adenomas: Benign tumors that develop in the pituitary gland and can affect hormone production, leading to various hormonal imbalances.

11. Polycystic kidney disease: A genetic disorder characterized by the formation of fluid-filled cysts in the kidneys, often associated with hormonal abnormalities.

12. Acromegaly: A hormonal disorder resulting from excessive growth hormone production in adults, leading to enlarged hands, feet, and facial features.

13. Hyperaldosteronism: A condition in which the adrenal glands produce too much aldosterone hormone, causing sodium retention and potassium loss.

14. Hypogonadism: A condition characterized by inadequate production of sex hormones, leading to reproductive and sexual dysfunction.

15. Pheochromocytoma: A tumor in the adrenal glands that can cause excessive production of adrenaline and noradrenaline, resulting in high blood pressure and other symptoms.

16. Congenital adrenal hyperplasia: A group of genetic disorders affecting the adrenal glands' hormone production, leading to various hormonal imbalances.

17. Hypopituitarism: A condition where the pituitary gland does not produce enough hormones, causing deficiencies in multiple hormonal pathways.

18. Parathyroid disorders: Conditions involving abnormal functioning of the parathyroid glands, leading to imbalances in calcium and phosphorus levels.

19. Hypothalamic disorders: Conditions affecting the hypothalamus, a region in the brain that plays a crucial role in hormone regulation.

20. Multiple endocrine neoplasia (MEN): A group of genetic disorders characterized by the development of tumors in multiple endocrine glands, leading to hormonal imbalances.

21. Adrenal insufficiency: A condition where the adrenal glands do not produce enough cortisol and sometimes aldosterone, resulting in fatigue and electrolyte imbalances.

22. Thyroid nodules: Abnormal growths or lumps in the thyroid gland, which can lead to hormone imbalances and may require further investigation.

23. Syndrome of inappropriate antidiuretic hormone secretion (SIADH): A condition where the body produces too much antidiuretic hormone, leading to water retention and dilutional hyponatremia.

24. Hyperprolactinemia: A condition characterized by high levels of prolactin hormone, leading to irregular menstrual periods, breast milk production in non-lactating individuals, and fertility issues.

25. Hypopituitarism: A condition where the pituitary gland does not produce enough hormones, causing deficiencies in multiple hormonal pathways.

II. Diagnostic Tests for Hormonal Disorders:

1. Blood tests: Measures hormone levels in the blood, such as thyroid-stimulating hormone (TSH), cortisol, insulin, growth hormone, and sex hormones.

2. Thyroid function tests: Evaluate the thyroid gland's activity by measuring levels of TSH, free T3, free T4, and sometimes thyroid antibodies.

3. Glucose tolerance test: Assesses how the body processes glucose and helps diagnose diabetes or impaired glucose tolerance.

4. Insulin tolerance test: Measures the body's response to insulin to evaluate insulin production and insulin sensitivity.

5. Oral glucose tolerance test: Involves consuming a glucose solution to assess how the body regulates blood sugar levels over time.

6. Adrenal function tests: Measure cortisol and aldosterone levels to evaluate adrenal gland function.

7. Growth hormone stimulation test: Determines the pituitary gland's ability to produce growth hormone by stimulating its release.

8. ACTH stimulation test: Evaluates the adrenal glands' response to adrenocorticotropic hormone (ACTH) to assess adrenal function.

9. Dexamethasone suppression test: Determines the body's cortisol response to dexamethasone, helping diagnose Cushing's syndrome.

10. Gonadotropin-releasing hormone (GnRH) stimulation test: Evaluates the pituitary gland's response to GnRH to assess reproductive hormone production.

11. Bone density scan (DXA scan): Measures bone mineral density to assess the risk of osteoporosis, often related to hormonal changes.

12. Ultrasonography: Uses sound waves to visualize the size and structure of organs, including the thyroid, adrenal glands, and ovaries.

13. Magnetic resonance imaging (MRI): Provides detailed images of the brain, pituitary gland, and other structures to detect abnormalities.

14. Computed tomography (CT) scan: Uses X-rays and computer processing to generate cross-sectional images for evaluating the adrenal glands, pituitary gland, and other structures.

15. Genetic testing: Identifies genetic mutations or abnormalities associated with specific hormonal disorders, such as multiple endocrine neoplasia.

16. Fine needle aspiration (FNA) biopsy: Involves extracting cells or tissue samples from nodules or tumors for microscopic examination and diagnosis.

17. Radioiodine uptake test: Measures the amount of radioactive iodine absorbed by the thyroid gland to evaluate its activity.

18. ACTH and cortisol rhythm assessment: Involves collecting multiple blood or saliva samples throughout the day to assess the diurnal cortisol rhythm.

19. Bone age assessment: Radiographic evaluation of skeletal development to determine growth abnormalities or hormone-related growth delays.

20. Serum calcium and phosphorus levels: Measure blood levels of calcium and phosphorus, which can provide insight into parathyroid function and disorders.

21. Genetic screening: Identifies inherited genetic mutations or abnormalities associated with specific hormonal disorders.

22. Pelvic ultrasound: Uses sound waves to visualize the reproductive organs, such as the ovaries and uterus, for assessing hormonal conditions like polycystic ovary syndrome.

23. Dynamic function tests: Evaluate hormonal responses to specific stimuli, such as insulin, GnRH, or corticotropin-releasing hormone (CRH).

24. Hormone suppression or stimulation tests: Assess hormone production and regulation by administering substances that suppress or stimulate specific hormone pathways.

25. Electrolyte panel: Measures blood levels of electrolytes such as sodium, potassium, and calcium, which can be affected by hormonal imbalances.

III. Treatment Options for Hormonal Disorders:

1. Hormone replacement therapy (HRT): Involves administering synthetic or bio-identical hormones to restore hormonal balance.

2. Thyroid hormone replacement: Prescribes synthetic thyroid hormones, such as levothyroxine, to supplement low thyroid hormone levels.

3. Insulin therapy: Administers insulin via injections or insulin pumps to regulate blood sugar levels in diabetes mellitus.

4. Antithyroid medications: Prescribed to treat hyperthyroidism by reducing the production of thyroid hormones.

5. Anti-androgen medications: Block the effects of androgen hormones, commonly used in the treatment of hormonal conditions like hirsutism or acne.

6. Oral contraceptives: Contain synthetic hormones to regulate menstrual cycles, treat hormonal conditions like PCOS, and provide contraception.

7. Growth hormone therapy: Administers synthetic growth hormone to individuals with growth hormone deficiency or certain growth disorders.

8. Adrenal hormone replacement: Prescribes synthetic corticosteroids, such as hydrocortisone or prednisone, to replace deficient cortisol or aldosterone.

9. Medications for pituitary disorders: Target specific hormone deficiencies or excesses caused by pituitary gland dysfunction.

10. Surgery: Removes tumors or abnormal glands affecting hormone production, such as pituitary adenomas or adrenal tumors.

11. Radioactive iodine therapy: Uses radioactive iodine to destroy thyroid tissue in cases of hyperthyroidism or thyroid cancer.

12. Androgen replacement therapy: Administers synthetic androgens to individuals with hormone deficiencies or certain conditions like hypogonadism.

13. Desmopressin therapy: Provides synthetic desmopressin to replace antidiuretic hormone in cases of diabetes insipidus or nocturnal enuresis.

14. Parathyroid hormone therapy: Administers synthetic parathyroid hormone to individuals with hypoparathyroidism to regulate calcium levels.

15. Gonadotropin therapy: Uses synthetic gonadotropins to stimulate ovulation in fertility treatments or hormone replacement in menopause.

16. Thyroidectomy: Surgical removal of the thyroid gland, usually performed in cases of thyroid cancer or severe hyperthyroidism.

17. Adrenalectomy: Removes one or both adrenal glands in cases of adrenal tumors, hyperplasia, or hormone overproduction.

18. Radiation therapy: Uses high-energy radiation to target and destroy tumors or abnormal tissue affecting hormone production.

19. Lifestyle modifications: Includes dietary changes, exercise, stress management, and weight management to support hormone balance.

20. Supportive care: Provides symptomatic relief and counseling to individuals with chronic or life-altering hormonal disorders.

21. Fertility treatments: Assists individuals with hormone-related fertility issues through techniques like in vitro fertilization (IVF) or hormonal stimulation.

22. Calcium and vitamin D supplementation: Prescribes these supplements to support bone health in conditions like hypoparathyroidism or osteoporosis.

23. Counseling and support groups: Offer emotional support and education to individuals living with hormonal disorders and their caregivers.

24. Immunomodulatory therapies: Used in certain autoimmune-related hormonal disorders to modulate the immune system's response.

25. Targeted therapy: Utilizes medications that specifically target the underlying cause or mechanism of certain hormonal disorders.

Exercises for transcribing endocrinology reports accurately

Exercise 1: Fill in the blanks

Transcribe the following sentence:

The patient's thyroid function test results showed elevated levels of ______ and decreased levels of ______.

Answer:

The patient's thyroid function test results showed elevated levels of TSH (thyroid-stimulating hormone) and decreased levels of free T4 (thyroxine).

Exercise 2: True or False

Indicate whether the following statement is true or false:

Type 2 diabetes is characterized by insulin resistance and high blood sugar levels.

Answer:

True

Exercise 3: Fill in the blanks

Transcribe the following sentence:

The patient was diagnosed with _____, a condition characterized by excess production of cortisol by the adrenal glands.

Answer:

The patient was diagnosed with Cushing's syndrome, a condition characterized by excess production of cortisol by the adrenal glands.

Exercise 4: Matching

Match the endocrine disorder with its description:

1. Hyperthyroidism

2. Hypothyroidism

3. Diabetes mellitus

4. Acromegaly

A. Insufficient production of insulin or inability of the body to properly use insulin

B. Excess production of growth hormone leading to enlarged body parts

C. Overactivity of the thyroid gland resulting in increased metabolism

D. Underactivity of the thyroid gland leading to decreased metabolism

Answer:

1. Hyperthyroidism

C. Overactivity of the thyroid gland resulting in increased metabolism

2. Hypothyroidism

D. Underactivity of the thyroid gland leading to decreased metabolism

3. Diabetes mellitus

A. Insufficient production of insulin or inability of the body to properly use insulin

4. Acromegaly

B. Excess production of growth hormone leading to enlarged body parts

Exercise 5: Fill in the blanks

Transcribe the following sentence:

The patient's adrenal function tests revealed normal levels of ______ and ______.

Answer:

The patient's adrenal function tests revealed normal levels of cortisol and aldosterone.

Exercise 6: True or False

Indicate whether the following statement is true or false:

Gestational diabetes is a type of diabetes that occurs during pregnancy and usually resolves after delivery.

Answer:

True

Exercise 7: Fill in the blanks

Transcribe the following sentence:

The patient's lab results showed low levels of ______, indicating ______.

Answer:

The patient's lab results showed low levels of parathyroid hormone (PTH), indicating hypoparathyroidism.

Exercise 8: Matching

Match the diagnostic test with its description:

1. Hemoglobin A1c

2. Glucose tolerance test

3. ACTH stimulation test

4. Thyroid ultrasound

A. Blood test to measure the average blood sugar levels over a period of 2-3 months

B. Test to evaluate the body's response to a glucose load, commonly used to diagnose gestational diabetes

C. Test to assess the functioning of the adrenal glands by measuring cortisol levels before and after administration of synthetic ACTH

D. Imaging test using sound waves to visualize the structure of the thyroid gland and detect any abnormalities

Answer:

1. Hemoglobin A1c

A. Blood test to measure the average blood sugar levels over a period of 2-3 months

2. Glucose tolerance test

B. Test to evaluate the body's response to a glucose load, commonly used to diagnose gestational diabetes

3. ACTH stimulation test

C. Test to assess the functioning of the adrenal glands by measuring cortisol levels before and after administration of synthetic ACTH

4. Thyroid ultrasound

D. Imaging test using sound waves to visualize the structure of the thyroid gland and detect any abnormalities

Exercise 9: True or False

Indicate whether the following statement is true or false:

Hypercalcemia is a condition characterized by high levels of calcium in the blood and can be associated with certain endocrine disorders.

Answer:

True

Exercise 10: Fill in the blanks

Transcribe the following sentence:

The patient's lab results showed elevated levels of ______, indicating ______.

Answer:

The patient's lab results showed elevated levels of prolactin, indicating hyperprolactinemia.

HUMAN DIGESTIVE SYSTEM

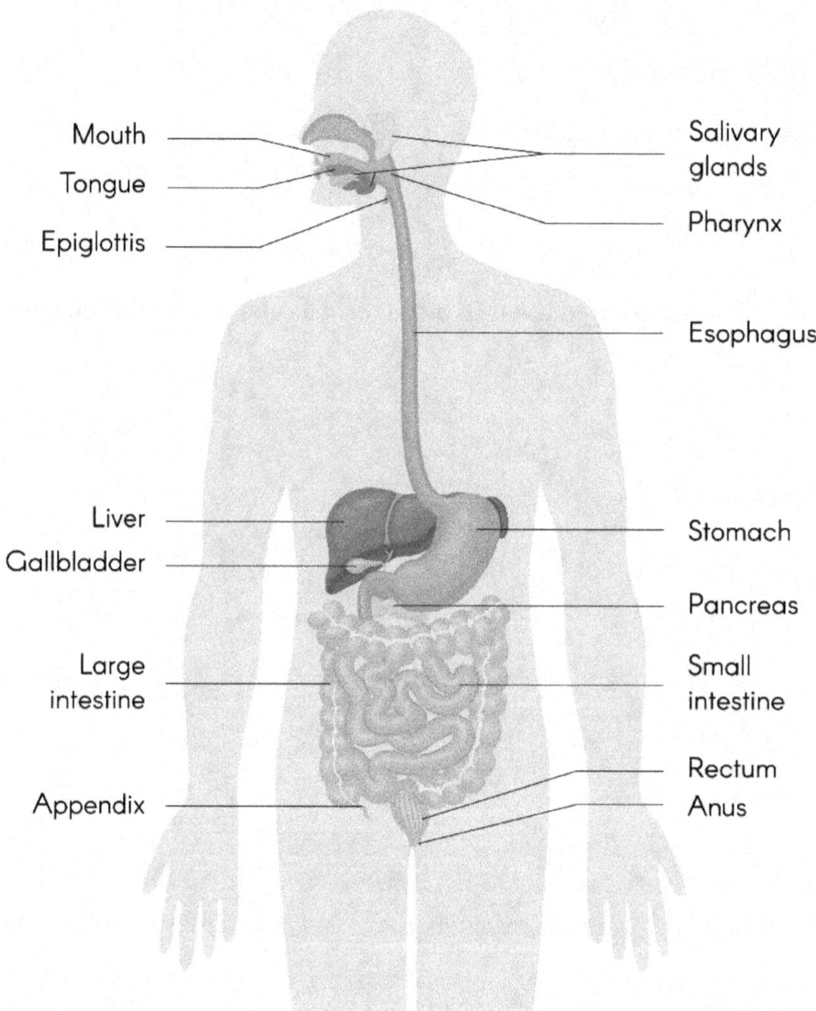

Overview of gastroenterology and its specialized vocabulary

Gastroenterology is the branch of medicine focused on the digestive system and its disorders. This includes organs from mouth to anus, along the alimentary canal, including the esophagus, stomach, small intestine, large intestine (colon), rectum, liver, gallbladder, and pancreas.

If you're new to this field, here are some important concepts to understand:

1. Digestive System: This system is responsible for breaking down food, absorbing nutrients, and removing waste from the body. Each part of the system has a specific role in this process, from initial intake and breakdown in the mouth and stomach, to nutrient absorption in the intestines, and waste excretion through the rectum.

2. Common Conditions: Gastroenterologists diagnose and treat many conditions. These include acid reflux (GERD), peptic ulcers, gallstones, liver diseases (such as hepatitis or cirrhosis), pancreatitis, inflammatory bowel diseases (like Crohn's disease and ulcerative colitis), irritable bowel syndrome (IBS), hemorrhoids, colorectal cancer, and many others.

3. Diagnostic Tools: Gastroenterologists use a variety of diagnostic tools. These include blood tests, stool tests, imaging studies (like CT scans or MRI), and endoscopic procedures. Endoscopies allow the doctor to visualize the inside of the gastrointestinal tract, and they include procedures like colonoscopy, upper endoscopy (also known as EGD), capsule endoscopy, and ERCP.

4. Treatment Approaches: Treatment in gastroenterology can involve dietary modifications, lifestyle changes, medication, and in some cases, endoscopic procedures or surgery. For example, a gastroenterologist might recommend a high-fiber diet and lifestyle changes for someone with IBS, prescribe medication for acid reflux or inflammatory bowel disease, or perform an endoscopic procedure to remove polyps or treat bleeding in the gastrointestinal tract.

5. Hepatology and Gastrointestinal Oncology: Hepatology is a sub-specialty of gastroenterology focusing on the liver, gallbladder, biliary tree, and pancreas. Gastrointestinal oncology focuses on cancers of the gastrointestinal system.

Digestive system disorders, diagnostic procedures, and interventions

I. Digestive System Disorders:

1. Gastroesophageal Reflux Disease (GERD): A condition in which stomach acid flows back into the esophagus, causing heartburn and acid reflux symptoms.

2. Peptic Ulcer Disease: Open sores that develop on the lining of the stomach, small intestine, or esophagus due to erosion by stomach acid and Helicobacter pylori infection.

3. Inflammatory Bowel Disease (IBD): A group of chronic conditions that cause inflammation in the digestive tract, including Crohn's disease and ulcerative colitis.

4. Irritable Bowel Syndrome (IBS): A common gastrointestinal disorder characterized by abdominal pain, bloating, and changes in bowel habits without any structural damage.

5. Gallstones: Hardened deposits that form in the gallbladder, causing pain and discomfort, often requiring surgical removal.

6. Pancreatitis: Inflammation of the pancreas, which can be acute or chronic and is often associated with alcohol consumption, gallstones, or certain medications.

7. Diverticulitis: Inflammation or infection of small pouches (diverticula) that develop in the lining of the colon, leading to abdominal pain and changes in bowel habits.

8. Celiac Disease: An autoimmune disorder triggered by the consumption of gluten, causing damage to the small intestine and difficulty absorbing nutrients.

9. Hepatitis: Inflammation of the liver, usually caused by viral infections (such as hepatitis A, B, or C), alcohol abuse, or autoimmune diseases.

10. Crohn's Disease: A chronic inflammatory bowel disease that primarily affects the lining of the digestive tract, causing abdominal pain, diarrhea, and weight loss.

11. Ulcerative Colitis: A chronic inflammatory bowel disease characterized by inflammation and ulcers in the colon and rectum, leading to symptoms like diarrhea, rectal bleeding, and abdominal cramps.

12. Gastroenteritis: Inflammation of the stomach and intestines caused by viral, bacterial, or parasitic infections, leading to diarrhea, vomiting, and abdominal pain.

13. Cirrhosis: A late stage of scarring (fibrosis) of the liver caused by various liver diseases and conditions, leading to liver dysfunction.

14. Gastritis: Inflammation of the stomach lining, which can be acute or chronic and may result from infection, certain medications, or autoimmune disorders.

15. Pancreatic Cancer: Malignant tumors that develop in the pancreas, often with symptoms such as abdominal pain, weight loss, and jaundice.

16. Hemorrhoids: Swollen blood vessels in the rectum or anus, causing discomfort, itching, and bleeding.

17. Gastrointestinal Bleeding: Any bleeding that occurs in the digestive tract, often resulting from ulcers, tumors, or vascular abnormalities.

18. Gastrointestinal Obstruction: Partial or complete blockage of the normal flow of food, fluids, or waste through the digestive tract, leading to symptoms like abdominal pain and vomiting.

19. Colorectal Cancer: Cancer that develops in the colon or rectum, usually starting as small polyps and progressing to malignant tumors.

20. Pancreatic Insufficiency: Impaired secretion of pancreatic enzymes, leading to poor digestion and malabsorption of nutrients.

21. Gastric Ulcers: Ulcers that develop in the lining of the stomach, often associated with Helicobacter pylori infection or long-term use of nonsteroidal anti-inflammatory drugs (NSAIDs).

22. Gastrointestinal Reflux Disease: A condition in which the contents of the stomach, including stomach acid, flow back into the esophagus, causing symptoms such as heartburn and regurgitation.

23. Gastroparesis: Delayed emptying of the stomach, resulting in symptoms like nausea, vomiting, and bloating.

24. Biliary Colic: Severe pain caused by the obstruction of the bile ducts due to gallstones or other conditions affecting the gallbladder or biliary system.

25. Esophageal Cancer: Cancer that develops in the lining of the esophagus, often associated with long-term exposure to factors like tobacco smoke or chronic acid reflux.

II. Diagnostic Procedures for Digestive System Disorders:

1. Upper Endoscopy (Esophagogastroduodenoscopy): A procedure that involves inserting a flexible tube with a camera into the esophagus, stomach, and upper small intestine to visualize the digestive tract and collect tissue samples for biopsy.

2. Colonoscopy: A procedure that examines the rectum and entire colon using a colonoscope to detect abnormalities, such as polyps or cancer, and remove them if necessary.

3. Endoscopic Retrograde Cholangiopancreatography (ERCP): A procedure that combines endoscopy and fluoroscopy to diagnose and treat conditions affecting the bile ducts and pancreatic ducts, such as gallstones or strictures.

4. Abdominal Ultrasound: An imaging test that uses sound waves to create images of the abdomen, helping to diagnose conditions like gallstones, liver disease, or abdominal masses.

5. Computerized Tomography (CT) Scan: A specialized X-ray technique that produces detailed cross-sectional images of the abdomen, providing valuable information about the digestive organs, blood vessels, and surrounding structures.

6. Magnetic Resonance Imaging (MRI): A non-invasive imaging technique that uses magnetic fields and radio waves to generate detailed images of the digestive system, assisting in the diagnosis of conditions like liver disease or tumors.

7. Barium Swallow/Upper Gastrointestinal (GI) Series: A series of X-ray images taken after drinking a barium solution to visualize the esophagus, stomach, and small intestine, aiding in the detection of abnormalities or structural issues.

8. Fecal Occult Blood Test (FOBT): A screening test to detect the presence of hidden blood in the stool, indicating possible gastrointestinal bleeding or colorectal cancer.

9. Esophageal Manometry: A diagnostic test that measures the pressure and coordination of the muscles in the esophagus to evaluate swallowing function and diagnose conditions like esophageal motility disorders or gastroesophageal reflux disease (GERD).

10. H. pylori Breath Test: A non-invasive test to detect the presence of Helicobacter pylori bacteria in the stomach, which can cause peptic ulcers and gastritis.

11. Liver Function Tests (LFTs): Blood tests that assess liver function and measure the levels of liver enzymes, bilirubin, and other substances to evaluate liver health and diagnose liver diseases.

12. Stool Culture: Laboratory testing of a stool sample to identify the presence of bacteria, parasites, or viruses that may cause gastrointestinal infections or diarrhea.

13. Sigmoidoscopy: A procedure that uses a flexible tube with a camera to examine the rectum and sigmoid colon, helping to diagnose conditions like colitis or colorectal cancer.

14. Gastric Emptying Study: A test that evaluates the rate at which the stomach empties its contents, helping to diagnose conditions like gastroparesis or delayed gastric emptying.

15. Anorectal Manometry: A test that measures the pressure and coordination of the muscles in the rectum and anus to evaluate conditions like fecal incontinence or pelvic floor dysfunction.

16. Capsule Endoscopy: A procedure in which a small capsule with a camera is swallowed, allowing for visualization of the small intestine to detect conditions like Crohn's disease or small bowel tumors.

17. Hydrogen Breath Test: A diagnostic test used to detect conditions like lactose intolerance or bacterial overgrowth in the small intestine by measuring the levels of hydrogen gas in breath samples.

18. Endoscopic Ultrasound (EUS): A procedure that combines endoscopy with ultrasound imaging to obtain detailed images of the gastrointestinal tract and adjacent organs, aiding in the diagnosis and staging of GI cancers.

19. Liver Biopsy: A procedure that involves the removal of a small tissue sample from the liver for microscopic examination, assisting in the diagnosis and staging of liver diseases.

20. ERCP (Endoscopic Retrograde Cholangiopancreatography): A procedure that combines endoscopy and X-ray imaging to visualize the bile ducts and pancreatic ducts, helping to diagnose and treat conditions such as gallstones or strictures.

21. Breath Tests: These tests measure the levels of certain gases in the breath to diagnose conditions like lactose intolerance or bacterial overgrowth in the digestive system.

22. Motility Studies: These tests evaluate the movement and function of the digestive tract, such as esophageal motility studies to diagnose disorders like achalasia or high-resolution anorectal manometry to assess anorectal function.

23. Endoscopic Mucosal Resection (EMR): A procedure used to remove abnormal tissue, such as polyps or early-stage cancers, from the digestive tract using an endoscope.

24. Chromoendoscopy: A technique that involves applying special stains or dyes during endoscopy to enhance the visualization and detection of abnormalities in the digestive tract.

25. Impedance pH Monitoring: A test that measures the reflux of stomach contents and the acidity levels in the esophagus, helping to diagnose and evaluate conditions like gastroesophageal reflux disease (GERD).

III. Interventions for Digestive System Disorders:

1. Medications: Prescribing and managing medications to treat specific digestive system disorders, such as proton pump inhibitors for GERD, anti-inflammatory drugs for inflammatory bowel disease, or antiviral drugs for hepatitis.

2. Dietary Modifications: Recommending specific dietary changes or restrictions to manage digestive system disorders, such as a low-FODMAP diet for irritable bowel syndrome or a gluten-free diet for celiac disease.

3. Lifestyle Modifications: Advising patients on lifestyle changes, such as quitting smoking, reducing alcohol consumption, managing stress, or regular physical exercise, to improve digestive health and prevent complications.

4. Endoscopic Procedures: Performing minimally invasive endoscopic procedures, such as polyp removal, stricture dilation, or stent placement, to treat conditions like gastrointestinal bleeding or strictures.

5. Surgical Interventions: Recommending and performing surgical procedures when necessary, such as gallbladder removal for gallstones, bowel resection for Crohn's disease, or liver transplantation for end-stage liver disease.

6. Endoscopic Retrograde Cholangiopancreatography (ERCP): A procedure that combines endoscopy and X-ray imaging to diagnose and treat conditions affecting the bile ducts and pancreatic ducts, such as removing gallstones or placing stents.

7. Radiofrequency Ablation: A technique that uses heat energy to destroy abnormal tissue, such as precancerous cells or small tumors, in the digestive system.

8. Transjugular Intrahepatic Portosystemic Shunt (TIPS): A procedure that creates a shunt between the portal vein and hepatic vein to relieve portal hypertension in conditions like cirrhosis.

9. Bowel Resection: Surgical removal of a portion of the intestine affected by conditions like diverticulitis, Crohn's disease, or colorectal cancer.

10. Hemorrhoidectomy: Surgical removal of hemorrhoids that are causing significant symptoms and not responding to conservative treatments.

11. Bariatric Surgery: Surgical procedures, such as gastric bypass or sleeve gastrectomy, performed to treat obesity and associated digestive disorders.

12. Colostomy/Ileostomy: Surgical creation of an opening in the abdominal wall to divert the passage of stool or digestive waste in conditions like colorectal cancer or inflammatory bowel disease.

13. Enteral Nutrition: Providing nutrition through a feeding tube directly into the gastrointestinal tract for patients who are unable to eat or digest food normally.

14. Percutaneous Endoscopic Gastrostomy (PEG): A procedure that involves the insertion of a feeding tube directly into the stomach through the abdominal wall to provide nutrition and fluids.

15. Liver Transplantation: A surgical procedure in which a diseased liver is replaced with a healthy liver from a donor, typically reserved for end-stage liver disease or liver cancer.

16. Colonic Stent Placement: A minimally invasive procedure in which a stent is placed in the colon to relieve bowel obstruction caused by tumors or strictures.

17. Percutaneous Transhepatic Cholangiography (PTC): A procedure that involves the insertion of a catheter into the liver to visualize and treat conditions affecting the bile ducts.

18. Sphincterotomy: A surgical procedure to cut the sphincter muscles in the digestive tract, such as the anal sphincter or the sphincter of Oddi, to relieve blockages or improve the flow of fluids.

19. Colectomy: Surgical removal of all or part of the colon, often performed for conditions like colon cancer, ulcerative colitis, or diverticulitis.

20. Gastric Bypass Surgery: A surgical procedure that involves rerouting the digestive tract to bypass a portion of the stomach, promoting weight loss and improved metabolic function in patients with severe obesity.

21. Colonic Resection: Surgical removal of a portion of the colon affected by conditions like colorectal cancer, diverticulitis, or inflammatory bowel disease.

22. Esophageal Dilation: A procedure to widen a narrowed or strictured esophagus using dilators or balloons, helping to relieve swallowing difficulties caused by conditions like esophageal strictures or eosinophilic esophagitis.

23. Gastric Balloon: A non-surgical intervention in which a deflated balloon is placed in the stomach and then filled with saline to create a feeling of fullness and promote weight loss.

24. Colonic Polypectomy: The removal of polyps from the colon during a colonoscopy to prevent the development of colorectal cancer.

25. Percutaneous Endoscopic Jejunostomy (PEJ): A procedure that involves the placement of a feeding tube directly into the jejunum (part of the small intestine) for long-term enteral feeding when the stomach is not accessible or functional.

Practice activities for transcribing gastroenterology reports effectively

Exercise 1: Fill in the blanks

Transcribe the following sentence:

The patient presented with abdominal pain, bloating, and ______.

Answer:

The patient presented with abdominal pain, bloating, and diarrhea.

Exercise 2: True or False

Indicate whether the following statement is true or false:

Gastroesophageal reflux disease (GERD) is characterized by the backward flow of stomach acid into the esophagus.

Answer:

True

Exercise 3: Fill in the blanks

Transcribe the following sentence:

The patient's colonoscopy revealed the presence of multiple _____ throughout the colon.

Answer:

The patient's colonoscopy revealed the presence of multiple polyps throughout the colon.

Exercise 4: Matching

Match the gastrointestinal disorder with its description:

1. Gastritis

2. Hepatitis

3. Cholecystitis

4. Pancreatitis

A. Inflammation of the liver

B. Inflammation of the stomach lining

C. Inflammation of the gallbladder

D. Inflammation of the pancreas

Answer:

1. Gastritis

B. Inflammation of the stomach lining

2. Hepatitis

A. Inflammation of the liver

3. Cholecystitis

C. Inflammation of the gallbladder

4. Pancreatitis

D. Inflammation of the pancreas

Exercise 5: Fill in the blanks

Transcribe the following sentence:

The patient's stool sample tested positive for the presence of ______.

Answer:

The patient's stool sample tested positive for the presence of blood.

Exercise 6: True or False

Indicate whether the following statement is true or false:

Crohn's disease and ulcerative colitis are types of inflammatory bowel disease (IBD).

Answer:

True

Exercise 7: Fill in the blanks

Transcribe the following sentence:

The patient's liver function tests showed elevated levels of ______, indicating ______.

Answer:

The patient's liver function tests showed elevated levels of bilirubin, indicating possible liver dysfunction.

Exercise 8: Matching

Match the diagnostic test with its description:

1. Upper gastrointestinal (GI) endoscopy

2. Abdominal ultrasound

3. Colonoscopy

4. Magnetic resonance cholangiopancreatography (MRCP)

A. Imaging test using sound waves to visualize the liver, gallbladder, and bile ducts

B. Endoscopic procedure to examine the esophagus, stomach, and upper part of the small intestine

C. Endoscopic examination of the large intestine and rectum

D. Imaging technique that uses magnetic fields and radio waves to visualize the biliary and pancreatic ducts

Answer:

1. Upper gastrointestinal (GI) endoscopy   B. Endoscopic procedure to examine the esophagus, stomach, and upper part of the small intestine

2. Abdominal ultrasound   A. Imaging test using sound waves to visualize the liver, gallbladder, and bile ducts

3. Colonoscopy   C. Endoscopic examination of the large intestine and rectum

4. Magnetic resonance cholangiopancreatography (MRCP)   D. Imaging technique that uses magnetic fields and radio waves to visualize the biliary and pancreatic ducts

Exercise 9: True or False

Indicate whether the following statement is true or false:

Celiac disease is an autoimmune disorder characterized by the inability to tolerate gluten.

Answer:

True

Exercise 10: Fill in the blanks

Transcribe the following sentence:

The patient's endoscopy revealed the presence of an _____ in the stomach.

Answer:

The patient's endoscopy revealed the presence of an ulcer in the stomach.

THE COMPOSITION OF THE BLOOD

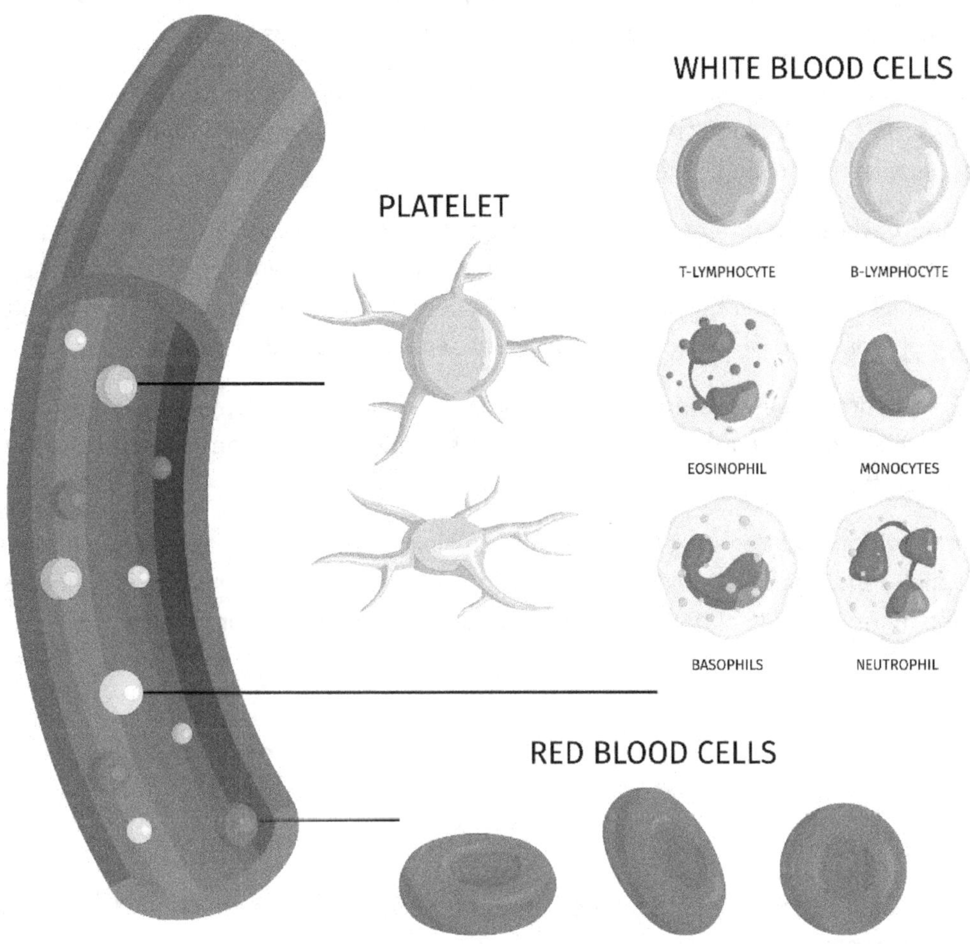

Introduction to hematology and its unique terminology

Hematology is a branch of medicine that focuses on the study of blood, blood-forming organs, and blood diseases. It includes the diagnosis, prognosis, treatment, and prevention of blood diseases that affect the production of blood and its components, such as blood cells, hemoglobin, blood proteins, and the coagulation system.

Here are some key points that you should understand as a beginner in this field:

1. Components of Blood: Blood is composed of several parts: red blood cells (which carry oxygen), white blood cells (which fight infections), platelets (which help blood clot), and plasma (the liquid portion of the blood that carries cells and proteins throughout the body).

2. Common Conditions: Hematologists diagnose and treat many blood disorders. These can include anemias (such as sickle cell anemia and iron deficiency anemia), clotting disorders (such as hemophilia), leukemias and lymphomas (cancers of the blood and lymphatic system), multiple myeloma, and other conditions like thalassemia, myelodysplastic syndromes, and polycythemia vera.

3. Diagnostic Tools: Hematologists use a variety of tools to diagnose blood disorders. These include complete blood counts (CBC), blood smear tests, bone marrow aspirations and biopsies, flow cytometry, genetic testing, coagulation testing, and more.

4. Treatment Approaches: Treatment can vary widely depending on the specific condition and its severity. For example, treatment might involve dietary changes or iron supplements for iron deficiency anemia, clotting factor replacement therapy for hemophilia, chemotherapy or stem cell transplantation for leukemias or lymphomas, and various medications to manage other blood disorders.

5. Hemostasis and Thrombosis: Hemostasis is the process of blood clot formation, and its counterpart, thrombosis, is the abnormal formation of clots. Specialists in this area study and manage diseases related to problems with clotting.

6. Transfusion Medicine and Hematopathology: Transfusion medicine involves the transfusion of blood and blood products, and managing any adverse reactions. Hematopathology is the study of diseases of blood cells, bone marrow, and lymph nodes from a microscopic and molecular perspective.

Blood disorders, diagnostic tests, and treatment modalities

I. Blood Disorders:

1. Anemia: A condition characterized by a decrease in the number of red blood cells or hemoglobin, leading to reduced oxygen-carrying capacity in the blood.

2. Thrombocytopenia: A condition characterized by a low platelet count, which can lead to an increased risk of bleeding.

3. Leukemia: A type of cancer that affects the white blood cells, resulting in an overproduction of abnormal cells in the bone marrow.

4. Hemophilia: A genetic disorder that impairs the body's ability to clot blood, leading to prolonged bleeding and easy bruising.

5. Sickle Cell Disease: An inherited disorder that affects red blood cells, causing them to become misshapen and prone to blockages, leading to pain and organ damage.

6. Thrombophilia: A condition characterized by an increased tendency to develop blood clots.

7. Hemochromatosis: A genetic disorder characterized by excessive absorption and storage of iron in the body, leading to iron overload and organ damage.

8. Polycythemia Vera: A rare blood disorder characterized by the overproduction of red blood cells, white blood cells, and platelets.

9. Idiopathic Thrombocytopenic Purpura (ITP): An autoimmune disorder that leads to a low platelet count and increased risk of bleeding.

10. Aplastic Anemia: A condition characterized by the failure of the bone marrow to produce an adequate number of blood cells.

11. Von Willebrand Disease: A genetic bleeding disorder caused by a deficiency or dysfunction of the von Willebrand factor, an essential protein for normal blood clotting.

12. Myelodysplastic Syndromes: A group of disorders characterized by abnormal production and maturation of blood cells in the bone marrow.

13. Hemolytic Anemia: A condition characterized by the premature destruction of red blood cells, leading to low red blood cell count and symptoms of anemia.

14. Essential Thrombocythemia: A rare blood disorder characterized by the overproduction of platelets, leading to an increased risk of blood clot formation.

15. Coagulation Disorders: Conditions that affect the body's ability to form blood clots or maintain proper clotting function.

16. Hemoglobinopathies: Genetic disorders that affect the structure or production of hemoglobin, leading to abnormal oxygen transport in the blood.

17. Myelofibrosis: A rare bone marrow disorder in which abnormal cells cause fibrosis or scarring, leading to impaired blood cell production.

18. Disseminated Intravascular Coagulation (DIC): A condition characterized by widespread clotting and bleeding, often triggered by an underlying illness or condition.

19. Thalassemia: An inherited blood disorder that affects the production of hemoglobin, leading to anemia and other complications.

20. Paroxysmal Nocturnal Hemoglobinuria (PNH): A rare acquired disorder characterized by the destruction of red blood cells, leading to anemia, blood clots, and other complications.

21. Hematologic Cancers: Cancers that affect the blood cells or bone marrow, including leukemia, lymphoma, and multiple myeloma.

22. Neutropenia: A condition characterized by a low neutrophil count, increasing the risk of infections.

23. Pancytopenia: A condition characterized by low counts of all three blood cell types: red blood cells, white blood cells, and platelets.

24. Hemorrhagic Disorders: Conditions that result in abnormal bleeding or excessive bruising due to defects in blood clotting or blood vessel integrity.

25. Hematologic Autoimmune Disorders: Autoimmune conditions that target blood cells or components, such as autoimmune hemolytic anemia or immune thrombocytopenic purpura.

II. Diagnostic Tests:

1. Complete Blood Count (CBC): A blood test that provides information about the various blood cell types, including red blood cells, white blood cells, and platelets.

2. Blood Smear: A laboratory test in which a blood sample is examined under a microscope to evaluate the size, shape, and characteristics of blood cells.

3. Coagulation Profile: Blood tests that assess the clotting function of the blood, including prothrombin time (PT), activated partial thromboplastin time (aPTT), and international normalized ratio (INR).

4. Bone Marrow Biopsy: A procedure in which a small sample of bone marrow is collected and examined to evaluate blood cell production and detect abnormalities.

5. Genetic Testing: Tests that analyze the genetic material (DNA) to identify specific mutations or abnormalities associated with blood disorders.

6. Hemoglobin Electrophoresis: A test that separates and identifies different types of hemoglobin to diagnose hemoglobinopathies, such as sickle cell disease or thalassemia.

7. Flow Cytometry: A technique used to analyze and identify different types of cells in a blood sample, often used to diagnose and monitor hematologic cancers.

8. Bleeding Time Test: A test that measures the time it takes for bleeding to stop after a small skin puncture, assessing platelet function and overall blood clotting ability.

9. Bone Marrow Aspiration: A procedure in which a small amount of liquid bone marrow is aspirated using a needle for examination and evaluation of blood cell production.

10. Serum Iron Studies: Blood tests that measure the levels of iron, ferritin, transferrin, and other markers to assess iron status and diagnose iron-related disorders.

11. Erythrocyte Sedimentation Rate (ESR): A blood test that measures the rate at which red blood cells settle in a tube, which can be an indicator of inflammation or certain blood disorders.

12. Flow Cytometry Immunophenotyping: A specialized flow cytometry test that helps identify specific cell types and markers on the surface of blood cells, aiding in the diagnosis of hematologic disorders.

13. JAK2 Mutation Analysis: A genetic test that detects mutations in the JAK2 gene, commonly associated with myeloproliferative neoplasms like polycythemia vera and essential thrombocythemia.

14. Serum Protein Electrophoresis: A laboratory test that separates and quantifies the different proteins in the blood, helping to diagnose and monitor conditions like multiple myeloma.

15. Hemoglobin A1C (HbA1c): A blood test that measures the average blood sugar levels over the past two to three months, used for monitoring and diagnosing diabetes mellitus.

16. Ferritin Test: A blood test that measures the level of ferritin, a protein that stores iron, helping to assess iron deficiency or iron overload conditions.

17. Platelet Function Test: Tests that evaluate the ability of platelets to form blood clots and assess platelet function disorders.

18. Coombs Test: A blood test used to detect the presence of antibodies or complement proteins that can cause destruction of red blood cells, helping to diagnose autoimmune hemolytic anemia.

19. Prothrombin Time (PT): A blood test that measures the time it takes for blood to clot, used to assess the function of the clotting factors in the blood.

20. Von Willebrand Factor (vWF) Assay: Tests that measure the quantity and function of von Willebrand factor, aiding in the diagnosis of von Willebrand disease.

21. Hemoglobin Electrophoresis: A test that separates and identifies different types of hemoglobin to diagnose hemoglobinopathies, such as sickle cell disease or thalassemia.

22. Iron Studies: Blood tests that measure the levels of iron, ferritin, transferrin, and other markers to assess iron status and diagnose iron-related disorders.

23. D-Dimer Test: A blood test that measures the level of D-dimer, a substance produced when blood clots break down, helping to diagnose or rule out conditions like deep vein thrombosis or pulmonary embolism.

24. Procalcitonin Test: A blood test that measures the level of procalcitonin, a marker of bacterial infection, aiding in the diagnosis of sepsis or systemic bacterial infections.

25. Complement Levels: Blood tests that measure the levels of complement proteins in the blood, helping to evaluate immune system function and diagnose complement-related disorders.

III. Treatment Modalities:

1. Medications: Various medications may be used to manage blood disorders, including anticoagulants, antiplatelet agents, iron supplements, immunosuppressants, or targeted therapies for specific blood cancers.

2. Blood Transfusion: The administration of donated blood or blood components to replace deficient or abnormal blood cells, improve oxygen-carrying capacity, or address clotting disorders.

3. Bone Marrow Transplantation: A procedure that involves replacing diseased or damaged bone marrow with healthy stem cells to treat certain blood cancers or severe bone marrow disorders.

4. Chemotherapy: The use of powerful medications to destroy cancer cells or suppress abnormal blood cell production.

5. Radiation Therapy: The use of high-energy radiation to target and destroy cancer cells or reduce tumor size in certain blood cancers.

6. Immunotherapy: Treatment approaches that enhance the body's immune response to fight cancer cells, such as monoclonal antibodies or immune checkpoint inhibitors.

7. Surgical Procedures: Surgeries may be performed to treat specific blood disorders, such as splenectomy (removal of the spleen) for certain conditions like hereditary spherocytosis or splenic tumors.

8. Erythropoietin Stimulating Agents (ESAs): Medications that stimulate the production of red blood cells and are used to treat anemia associated with certain conditions like chronic kidney disease.

9. Intravenous Immunoglobulin (IVIG): Infusion of immunoglobulin, a blood product containing antibodies, to boost the immune system or treat certain immune disorders.

10. Plasmapheresis: A procedure in which blood plasma is removed, filtered, and then returned to the body, used to remove harmful antibodies or toxins from the blood in conditions like autoimmune hemolytic anemia or Guillain-Barré syndrome.

11. Hemodialysis: A treatment method that uses a machine to filter and cleanse the blood in individuals with severe kidney dysfunction or kidney failure.

12. Supportive Care: Measures taken to manage symptoms and improve quality of life, including pain management, nutritional support, physical therapy, or psychosocial support.

13. Iron Chelation Therapy: Treatment to remove excess iron from the body in conditions like hereditary hemochromatosis or transfusional iron overload.

14. Targeted Therapy: Treatment approaches that target specific molecular abnormalities or signaling pathways involved in the development or progression of blood cancers.

15. Gene Therapy: Experimental treatment strategies that involve modifying a patient's genes to correct genetic abnormalities or enhance their ability to fight blood disorders.

16. Stem Cell Therapy: The use of stem cells, either from the patient's own body (autologous) or from a donor (allogeneic), to replace damaged or diseased cells and promote blood cell regeneration.

17. Lifestyle Modifications: Recommendations for lifestyle changes, including dietary modifications, regular exercise, smoking cessation, or stress reduction, to manage and prevent blood disorders.

18. Phlebotomy: The therapeutic removal of blood from the body to reduce excess iron levels in conditions like hereditary hemochromatosis or polycythemia vera.

19. Compression Stockings: Elastic stockings or sleeves worn on the legs to improve blood circulation and prevent blood clots in conditions like deep vein thrombosis or venous insufficiency.

20. Splinting or Surgery for Bleeding Disorders: Orthopedic interventions or surgical procedures may be performed to address joint bleeds or correct anatomical abnormalities that contribute to bleeding disorders.

21. Electrolyte Replacement: Intravenous administration of electrolyte solutions to correct imbalances or deficiencies that can arise in certain blood disorders.

22. Phototherapy: The use of specific wavelengths of light to treat conditions like neonatal jaundice or cutaneous T-cell lymphoma.

23. Dietary Modifications: Nutritional adjustments, such as iron-rich diets, vitamin supplementation, or specific dietary restrictions, to support blood health and manage underlying blood disorders.

24. Anti-inflammatory Medications: Medications that reduce inflammation and immune system activity, which can be beneficial in managing certain autoimmune-related blood disorders.

25. Counseling and Support Groups: Psychological counseling, patient education, and support groups can play a vital role in managing the emotional and psychological impact of blood disorders, as well as providing information and support to patients and their families.

Exercises for transcribing hematology reports accurately

Exercise 1: Fill in the blanks

Transcribe the following sentence:

The patient's complete blood count (CBC) showed a low _______ count.

Answer:

The patient's complete blood count (CBC) showed a low platelet count.

Exercise 2: True or False

Indicate whether the following statement is true or false:

Anemia is a condition characterized by a decrease in the number of red blood cells or hemoglobin in the blood.

Answer:

True

Exercise 3: Fill in the blanks

Transcribe the following sentence:

The patient's bone marrow biopsy revealed the presence of _____.

Answer:

The patient's bone marrow biopsy revealed the presence of leukemia.

Exercise 4: Matching

Match the blood disorder with its description:

1. Thrombocytopenia

2. Anemia

3. Leukocytosis

4. Polycythemia vera

A. Abnormal increase in the number of red blood cells

B. Decrease in the number of platelets in the blood

C. Decrease in the number of white blood cells in the blood

D. Decrease in the number of red blood cells or hemoglobin in the blood

Answer:

1. Thrombocytopenia

B. Decrease in the number of platelets in the blood

2. Anemia

D. Decrease in the number of red blood cells or hemoglobin in the blood

3. Leukocytosis

C. Increase in the number of white blood cells in the blood

4. Polycythemia vera

A. Abnormal increase in the number of red blood cells

Exercise 5: Fill in the blanks

Transcribe the following sentence:

The patient's peripheral blood smear showed the presence of _______ cells.

Answer:

The patient's peripheral blood smear showed the presence of sickle cells.

Exercise 6: True or False

Indicate whether the following statement is true or false:

Hemophilia is a genetic disorder that impairs the body's ability to form blood clots.

Answer:

True

Exercise 7: Fill in the blanks

Transcribe the following sentence:

The patient's coagulation profile revealed prolonged _______ time.

Answer:

The patient's coagulation profile revealed prolonged prothrombin time.

Exercise 8: Matching

Match the diagnostic test with its description:

1. Bone marrow aspiration

2. Coombs test

3. Prothrombin time (PT)

4. Flow cytometry

A. Procedure to obtain a sample of bone marrow for examination

B. Blood test to detect the presence of antibodies on red blood cells

C. Blood test to assess blood clotting time

D. Laboratory technique to analyze cell characteristics and identify abnormal cells

Answer:

1. Bone marrow aspiration

A. Procedure to obtain a sample of bone marrow for examination

2. Coombs test

B. Blood test to detect the presence of antibodies on red blood cells

3. Prothrombin time (PT)

C. Blood test to assess blood clotting time

4. Flow cytometry

D. Laboratory technique to analyze cell characteristics and identify abnormal cells

Exercise 9: True or False

Indicate whether the following statement is true or false:

Hematocrit measures the percentage of red blood cells in the total blood volume.

Answer:

True

Exercise 10: Fill in the blanks

Transcribe the following sentence:

The patient's blood film showed the presence of _____.

Answer:

The patient's blood film showed the presence of abnormal cells.

8. ONCOLOGY

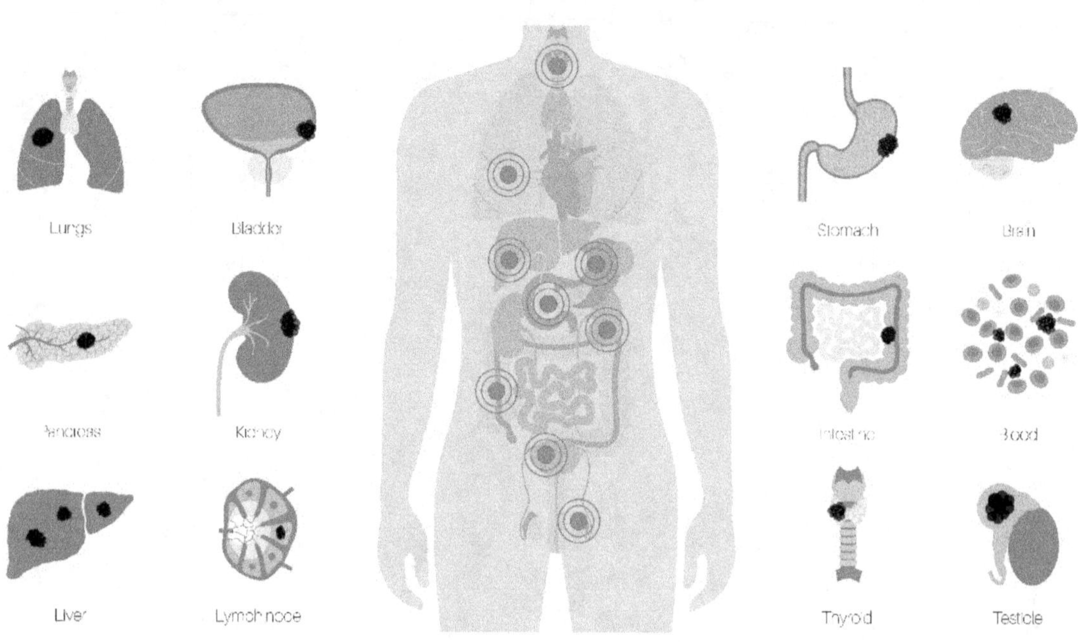

Understanding oncology and its specific terminology

Oncology is a branch of medicine that deals with the prevention, diagnosis, and treatment of cancer. Cancer is a group of diseases characterized by the uncontrolled growth and spread of abnormal cells.

Here are some essential points you need to understand as a beginner in this field:

1. Cancer Development: Cancer occurs when a cell's DNA is damaged, causing the cell to divide and grow uncontrollably, eventually forming a tumor. Not all tumors are cancerous; benign tumors do not spread to other parts of the body and are not life-threatening, while malignant tumors can invade nearby tissues and spread to distant organs, a process called metastasis.

2. Types of Cancer: There are over 200 types of cancer, and they are usually named for the organs or tissues where they form. For example, lung cancer starts in cells of the lung, and brain cancer starts in cells of the brain. Leukemias are cancers that begin in the blood-forming tissue of the bone marrow.

3. Common Treatments: Oncologists use various treatment modalities to manage cancer, including surgery to remove tumors, radiation therapy to kill cancer cells, chemotherapy to stop the growth of cancer cells, targeted therapy to target specific genes or proteins that help cancer cells grow, and immunotherapy to help the body's immune system fight cancer.

4. Diagnostic Tools: Oncologists use a wide range of tools to diagnose cancer, including physical exams, laboratory tests (including blood tests and genetic tests), imaging tests (like X-rays, CT scans, and MRI), and biopsy procedures where a sample of tissue is removed for examination under a microscope.

5. Staging and Grading: Oncologists use staging to describe the extent to which cancer has spread in the body, and grading to describe how abnormal the cancer cells look under a microscope. Both are important factors in determining the most appropriate treatment options and predicting a patient's prognosis.

6. Medical, Surgical, and Radiation Oncology: Medical oncologists treat cancer using chemotherapy, targeted therapies, and immunotherapy. Surgical oncologists remove tumors and nearby tissue during surgery, and they also perform certain types of biopsies. Radiation oncologists treat cancer using radiation therapy.

7. Pediatric Oncology: Pediatric oncologists specialize in diagnosing and treating cancer in children. Types of cancers common in children are often different from those seen in adults.

Cancer types, staging, and treatment approaches

I. Cancer Types:

1. Carcinoma: Cancer that starts in the epithelial cells, which are the cells that line the body's organs and tissues.

2. Sarcoma: Cancer that develops in the connective tissues, such as bones, muscles, or soft tissues.

3. Leukemia: Cancer of the blood or bone marrow, characterized by the overproduction of abnormal white blood cells.

4. Lymphoma: Cancer that affects the lymphatic system, including the lymph nodes, spleen, and bone marrow.

5. Melanoma: A type of skin cancer that originates in the pigment-producing cells called melanocytes.

6. Breast Cancer: Cancer that develops in the breast tissue, commonly affecting women but also occurring in men.

7. Lung Cancer: Cancer that forms in the tissues of the lungs, usually caused by long-term exposure to tobacco smoke.

8. Prostate Cancer: Cancer that develops in the prostate gland, a small organ located below the bladder in men.

9. Colorectal Cancer: Cancer that affects the colon or rectum, often starting as polyps and progressing over time.

10. Ovarian Cancer: Cancer that forms in the ovaries, the female reproductive organs that produce eggs.

11. Pancreatic Cancer: Cancer that arises in the pancreas, an organ responsible for producing enzymes and hormones.

12. Kidney Cancer: Cancer that originates in the kidneys, the organs responsible for filtering waste from the blood.

13. Bladder Cancer: Cancer that occurs in the bladder, the organ that stores urine.

14. Liver Cancer: Cancer that starts in the liver, often associated with underlying liver diseases like cirrhosis or hepatitis.

15. Brain Tumor: A mass or abnormal growth of cells in the brain, which can be cancerous or non-cancerous.

16. Thyroid Cancer: Cancer that develops in the thyroid gland, a butterfly-shaped gland in the neck.

17. Cervical Cancer: Cancer that begins in the cervix, the lower part of the uterus that connects to the vagina.

18. Endometrial Cancer: Cancer that forms in the lining of the uterus, known as the endometrium.

19. Esophageal Cancer: Cancer that occurs in the esophagus, the tube that carries food from the throat to the stomach.

20. Gastric Cancer: Cancer that affects the stomach, often associated with long-term inflammation or Helicobacter pylori infection.

21. Head and Neck Cancer: Cancer that arises in the tissues of the head and neck region, including the mouth, throat, nose, or salivary glands.

22. Bone Cancer: Cancer that starts in the bones, either as primary bone cancer or as a metastatic spread from other cancers.

23. Multiple Myeloma: A cancer of plasma cells, a type of white blood cell, that affects the bone marrow.

24. Soft Tissue Sarcoma: Cancer that develops in the soft tissues of the body, such as muscles, tendons, or fat.

25. Hematologic Malignancies: A group of cancers that affect the blood, bone marrow, and lymphatic system, including leukemia, lymphoma, and myeloma.

II. Staging:

1. Stage 0: Also known as carcinoma in situ, the cancer cells are present only in the layer of cells where they originated and have not invaded nearby tissues.

2. Stage I: The cancer is small and localized, typically limited to the organ where it originated.

3. Stage II: The cancer has grown larger and may have spread to nearby tissues or lymph nodes.

4. Stage III: The cancer has advanced further and has spread to nearby lymph nodes and potentially other tissues or organs.

5. Stage IV: The cancer has metastasized, meaning it has spread to distant organs or distant lymph nodes.

6. Stage X: Cancer cannot be classified into a specific stage due to incomplete information or lack of assessment.

7. Stage M0: Indicates that there is no evidence of distant metastasis.

8. Stage M1: Indicates the presence of distant metastasis.

9. Stage L1: Used to describe cancer that has invaded lymphatic vessels.

10. Stage V: Sometimes used to describe recurrent cancer that has come back after treatment.

11. Stage R0: Indicates that there is no residual tumor after surgery or other treatment.

12. Stage R1: Indicates that microscopic residual tumor cells are present after treatment.

13. Stage R2: Indicates that there is visible residual tumor after treatment.

14. Stage Tis: Used to describe cancer in situ, where abnormal cells are present but have not invaded surrounding tissues.

15. Stage T1: Indicates a small tumor that has not spread beyond the organ of origin.

16. Stage T2: Indicates a larger tumor that may have invaded nearby structures or organs.

17. Stage T3: Indicates a tumor that has further invaded nearby structures or organs.

18. Stage T4: Indicates a large tumor that has invaded nearby structures or organs.

19. Stage N0: Indicates no regional lymph node involvement.

20. Stage N1: Indicates involvement of nearby lymph nodes.

21. Stage N2: Indicates involvement of additional lymph nodes or lymph node regions.

22. Stage N3: Indicates involvement of further lymph nodes or lymph node regions.

23. Stage NX: Indicates that lymph node involvement cannot be assessed or is not known.

24. Stage P0: Indicates no evidence of primary tumor.

25. Stage P1: Indicates evidence of a primary tumor but cannot be classified into a specific stage.

III. Treatment Approaches:

1. Surgery: The removal of cancerous tumors or tissues through surgical procedures.

2. Radiation Therapy: The use of high-energy radiation to kill or shrink cancer cells.

3. Chemotherapy: The administration of drugs that target and destroy cancer cells throughout the body.

4. Targeted Therapy: Treatment that targets specific genetic or molecular changes in cancer cells to disrupt their growth and survival.

5. Immunotherapy: Therapy that stimulates the body's immune system to recognize and destroy cancer cells.

6. Hormone Therapy: Treatment that alters hormone levels or blocks hormone receptors to inhibit the growth of hormone-dependent cancers.

7. Stem Cell Transplantation: The infusion of healthy stem cells to replace damaged or destroyed cells after high-dose chemotherapy or radiation.

8. Precision Medicine: Treatment approaches that involve personalized therapies based on a patient's unique genetic profile.

9. Palliative Care: Supportive care aimed at managing symptoms, providing pain relief, and improving quality of life for patients with advanced cancer.

10. Clinical Trials: Participation in research studies to evaluate new treatments or treatment combinations for cancer.

11. Immunomodulators: Drugs that enhance the immune response against cancer cells by stimulating immune cells or blocking immune checkpoints.

12. Angiogenesis Inhibitors: Medications that prevent the formation of new blood vessels, depriving tumors of necessary nutrients and oxygen.

13. Gene Therapy: Treatment that involves introducing genetic material into cells to repair or replace faulty genes associated with cancer.

14. Photodynamic Therapy: Therapy that uses a photosensitizing agent and light to destroy cancer cells selectively.

15. Cryotherapy: The use of extreme cold temperatures to freeze and destroy cancer cells.

16. Radiofrequency Ablation: A minimally invasive procedure that uses heat generated by radiofrequency energy to destroy cancer cells.

17. Proton Therapy: A type of radiation therapy that uses protons instead of X-rays to deliver targeted radiation to tumors while minimizing damage to surrounding healthy tissues.

18. Watchful Waiting: A strategy that involves closely monitoring the progression of cancer without immediate treatment, particularly for slow-growing or early-stage cancers.

19. Adjuvant Therapy: Additional treatment given after primary treatment, such as surgery or radiation, to eliminate any remaining cancer cells and reduce the risk of recurrence.

20. Neoadjuvant Therapy: Treatment given before the primary treatment, such as chemotherapy or radiation, to shrink tumors and make them more manageable for surgical removal.

21. Supportive Care: Comprehensive care that focuses on managing side effects, pain management, emotional support, and maintaining the overall well-being of cancer patients.

22.   Alternative and Complementary Therapies: Non-traditional treatment approaches, such as acupuncture, herbal remedies, or mind-body techniques, used alongside conventional cancer treatments to improve well-being and alleviate symptoms.

23.   Pain Management: Strategies and medications aimed at alleviating cancer-related pain, including pharmacological interventions, nerve blocks, and palliative care services.

24. Hyperthermia: Treatment that involves exposing the cancerous area to high temperatures to induce cancer cell death.

25. Resection: Surgical removal of cancerous tissue or organs affected by cancer.

Practice activities for transcribing oncology reports effectively

Exercise 1: Fill in the blanks

Transcribe the following sentence:

The patient was diagnosed with _______ cancer.

Answer:

The patient was diagnosed with breast cancer.

Exercise 2: True or False

Indicate whether the following statement is true or false:

Chemotherapy is a common treatment option for cancer that involves the use of drugs to kill cancer cells.

Answer:

True

Exercise 3: Fill in the blanks

Transcribe the following sentence:

The patient underwent a _______ to remove the tumor.

Answer:

The patient underwent a surgery to remove the tumor.

Exercise 4: Matching

Match the type of cancer with its description:

1. Lung cancer

2. Prostate cancer

3. Melanoma

4. Colorectal cancer

A. Cancer that starts in the colon or rectum

B. Cancer that affects the blood and bone marrow

C. Cancer that begins in the lung tissue

D. Cancer that forms in the prostate gland

Answer:

1. Lung cancer

C. Cancer that begins in the lung tissue

2. Prostate cancer

D. Cancer that forms in the prostate gland

3. Melanoma

A. Cancer that starts in the colon or rectum

4. Colorectal cancer

B. Cancer that affects the blood and bone marrow

Exercise 5: Fill in the blanks

Transcribe the following sentence:

The patient's PET-CT scan revealed ______ metastasis.

Answer:

The patient's PET-CT scan revealed liver metastasis.

Exercise 6: True or False

Indicate whether the following statement is true or false:

Radiation therapy uses high-energy rays to kill cancer cells and shrink tumors.

Answer:

True

Exercise 7: Fill in the blanks

Transcribe the following sentence:

The patient's oncologist recommended ______ as the treatment option.

Answer:

The patient's oncologist recommended chemotherapy as the treatment option.

Exercise 8: Matching

Match the treatment modality with its description:

1. Immunotherapy

2. Targeted therapy

3. Hormone therapy

4. Chemotherapy

A. Treatment that uses drugs to slow down the growth of cancer cells

B. Treatment that boosts the body's immune system to fight cancer

C. Treatment that targets specific genetic or molecular changes in cancer cells

D. Treatment that blocks hormones or hormone receptors to stop cancer growth

Answer:

1. Immunotherapy

B. Treatment that boosts the body's immune system to fight cancer

2. Targeted therapy

C. Treatment that targets specific genetic or molecular changes in cancer cells

3. Hormone therapy

D. Treatment that blocks hormones or hormone receptors to stop cancer growth

4. Chemotherapy

A. Treatment that uses drugs to slow down the growth of cancer cells

Exercise 9: True or False

Indicate whether the following statement is true or false:

Metastasis refers to the spread of cancer cells from one part of the body to another.

Answer:

True

Exercise 10: Fill in the blanks

Transcribe the following sentence:

The patient's tumor was classified as ______ stage.

Answer:

The patient's tumor was classified as stage III.

NERVOUS SYSTEM

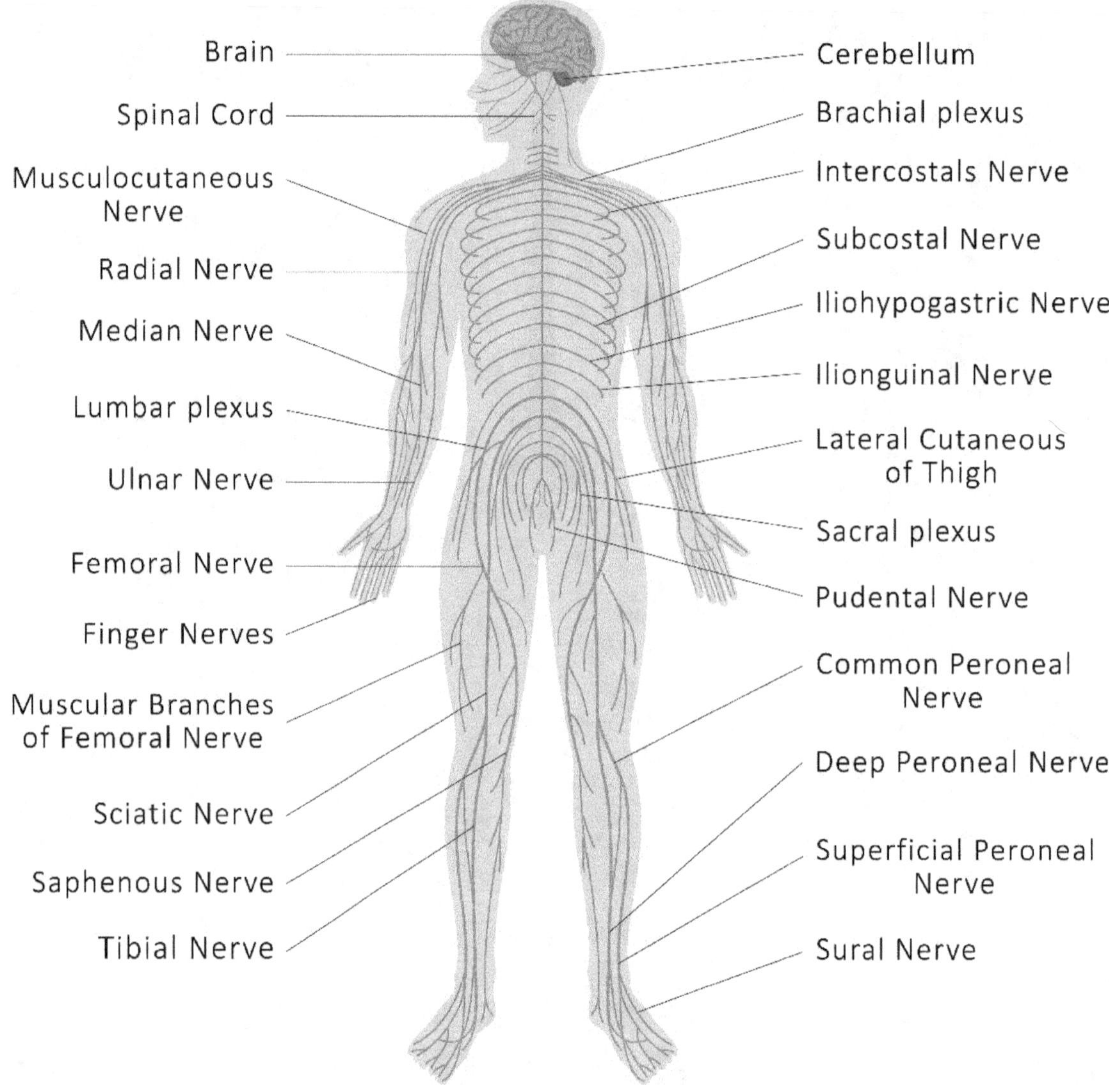

Overview of neurology and its specialized vocabulary

Neurology is a branch of medicine dealing with disorders of the nervous system. The nervous system is a complex, sophisticated system that regulates and coordinates body activities. It has two major divisions: the central nervous system, which includes the brain and spinal cord, and the peripheral nervous system, which includes all other neural elements, such as eyes, ears, skin, and other "sensory receptors".

Here are some key points you should understand as a beginner in this field:

1. Nervous System: The nervous system is responsible for coordinating and controlling many body activities. It allows us to sense the world around us, control our movements, regulate body functions like heart rate and breathing, and allows us to think, learn, and remember.

2. Common Conditions: Neurologists diagnose and treat a wide range of conditions. These include stroke, epilepsy (seizure disorders), headaches and migraines, Alzheimer's disease and other forms of dementia, Parkinson's disease and other movement disorders, multiple sclerosis, and various forms of neuropathy and myopathy.

3. Diagnostic Tools: Neurologists use a variety of tools to diagnose neurological disorders. These include physical and neurological exams, imaging studies (like CT scans, MRIs, and PET scans), electroencephalograms (EEGs) to measure brain electrical activity, electromyograms and nerve conduction studies (EMG/NCS) to assess peripheral nerve and muscle function, and lumbar puncture (spinal tap) to evaluate cerebrospinal fluid.

4. Treatment Approaches: Treatment in neurology can involve lifestyle modifications, physical therapy, medications, and sometimes surgery, which is typically performed by a neurosurgeon. Some neurological disorders, like Parkinson's disease, can be managed with deep brain stimulation (DBS), a surgical procedure to implant a device that sends electrical signals to brain areas responsible for body movement.

5. Neurological Subspecialties: There are many subspecialties within neurology, each focusing on specific types of conditions. These include stroke medicine (vascular neurology), epilepsy, movement disorders, headache medicine, neuromuscular medicine, and neuroimmunology, among others.

6. Neuro-oncology and Neurocritical Care: Neuro-oncology focuses on the management of cancers of the brain and nervous system. Neurocritical care is a field that deals with life-threatening diseases of the nervous system and the management of complications in critically ill neurological and neurosurgical patients.

Neurological conditions, diagnostic tests, and therapeutic interventions

I. Neurological Conditions:

1. Stroke: A neurological condition that occurs when the blood supply to the brain is interrupted, resulting in damage to brain cells.

2. Alzheimer's Disease: A progressive neurodegenerative disorder characterized by memory loss, cognitive decline, and behavioral changes.

3. Parkinson's Disease: A neurodegenerative disorder that affects movement, causing tremors, stiffness, and difficulty with coordination.

4. Multiple Sclerosis: An autoimmune disease that affects the central nervous system, causing damage to the protective covering of nerve fibers.

5. Epilepsy: A neurological disorder characterized by recurrent seizures, which are abnormal electrical disturbances in the brain.

6. Migraine: A neurological condition characterized by severe headache episodes often accompanied by other symptoms such as nausea and sensitivity to light and sound.

7. Amyotrophic Lateral Sclerosis (ALS): A progressive neurodegenerative disease that affects nerve cells responsible for controlling voluntary muscle movements.

8. Neuropathy: Damage or dysfunction of the nerves, resulting in symptoms such as pain, numbness, tingling, or weakness.

9. Huntington's Disease: An inherited neurodegenerative disorder that causes the progressive breakdown of nerve cells in the brain, leading to movement, cognitive, and psychiatric symptoms.

10. Traumatic Brain Injury: Damage to the brain caused by external force or trauma, often resulting in cognitive, physical, and emotional impairments.

11. Cerebral Palsy: A group of permanent movement disorders that appear in early childhood, caused by damage to the developing brain.

12. Guillain-Barré Syndrome: A rare neurological disorder characterized by muscle weakness or paralysis, usually starting in the legs and spreading to the upper body.

13. Tourette Syndrome: A neurodevelopmental disorder characterized by repetitive, involuntary movements and vocalizations known as tics.

14. Restless Legs Syndrome: A condition characterized by an uncontrollable urge to move the legs, often accompanied by uncomfortable sensations.

15. Neuromuscular Disorders: A group of disorders that affect the muscles and the nerves that control them, leading to weakness and muscle wasting.

16. Myasthenia Gravis: A chronic autoimmune disorder that causes muscle weakness and fatigue, often affecting the muscles responsible for eye movements and facial expressions.

17. Cerebellar Ataxia: A condition characterized by problems with coordination, balance, and voluntary movements, usually caused by damage to the cerebellum.

18. Neuralgia: Intense, stabbing pain along the course of a nerve, often caused by irritation or damage to the nerve.

19. Dementia: A syndrome characterized by a decline in memory, thinking, behavior, and the ability to perform everyday activities, often caused by underlying neurological conditions.

20. Epileptic Seizures: Sudden, abnormal electrical activity in the brain, resulting in various types of seizures with different symptoms and characteristics.

21. Bell's Palsy: A condition characterized by sudden weakness or paralysis of the facial muscles, usually affecting one side of the face.

22. Traumatic Spinal Cord Injury: Damage to the spinal cord as a result of trauma, leading to loss of sensation and function below the level of injury.

23. Narcolepsy: A neurological disorder that affects sleep regulation, causing excessive daytime sleepiness and episodes of sudden muscle weakness or loss of muscle control.

24. Encephalitis: Inflammation of the brain, often caused by viral infections, leading to symptoms such as fever, headache, and changes in consciousness.

25. Cerebrovascular Disease: Conditions that affect the blood vessels supplying the brain, including conditions such as aneurysms, arteriovenous malformations, and vascular blockages.

II. Diagnostic Tests:

1. Magnetic Resonance Imaging (MRI): A non-invasive imaging technique that uses magnetic fields and radio waves to generate detailed images of the brain and other parts of the body.

2. Computed Tomography (CT) Scan: A diagnostic imaging technique that uses X-rays to create cross-sectional images of the brain and other body structures.

3. Electroencephalogram (EEG): A test that measures and records the electrical activity of the brain to diagnose and monitor conditions such as epilepsy and sleep disorders.

4. Nerve Conduction Studies (NCS) and Electromyography (EMG): Tests that evaluate the electrical activity and functioning of nerves and muscles to diagnose conditions such as neuropathy and muscular disorders.

5. Lumbar Puncture (Spinal Tap): A procedure in which a needle is inserted into the lower back to collect cerebrospinal fluid for analysis, aiding in the diagnosis of conditions such as meningitis and multiple sclerosis.

6. Neurological Examination: A comprehensive assessment of a patient's nervous system, including evaluating motor function, sensory function, reflexes, and cognitive abilities.

7. Positron Emission Tomography (PET) Scan: A nuclear medicine imaging technique that uses radioactive substances to create images of metabolic activity in the brain and detect abnormalities.

8. Neuropsychological Testing: Assessments that measure cognitive abilities, memory, attention, and other aspects of brain function to aid in the diagnosis and management of neurological conditions.

9. Genetic Testing: Analysis of an individual's DNA to identify genetic variations associated with neurological disorders and provide information about the risk, diagnosis, or treatment of certain conditions.

10. Sleep Studies (Polysomnography): Tests conducted overnight to monitor brain activity, eye movements, muscle activity, heart rhythm, and other physiological parameters to diagnose sleep disorders such as sleep apnea and narcolepsy.

11. Angiography: Imaging of the blood vessels using contrast agents to evaluate the blood supply to the brain and diagnose conditions such as aneurysms and arteriovenous malformations.

12. Neuroimaging Techniques: Various imaging modalities, including functional MRI (fMRI), diffusion tensor imaging (DTI), and magnetoencephalography (MEG), used to study brain structure, function, and connectivity.

13. Biopsy: Surgical removal of a small sample of tissue for examination under a microscope to diagnose conditions such as brain tumors and certain inflammatory disorders.

14. Neurophysiological Testing: Assessments that measure electrical activity in the brain and nerves to evaluate conditions such as epilepsy and nerve disorders.

15. Neurovascular Studies: Imaging techniques such as Doppler ultrasound and transcranial Doppler (TCD) to assess blood flow in the brain and diagnose conditions such as carotid artery disease and stroke risk.

16. Cerebrospinal Fluid Analysis: Examination of the cerebrospinal fluid collected through a lumbar puncture to detect abnormalities related to infections, inflammation, and certain neurological conditions.

17. Evoked Potential Studies: Tests that measure the electrical activity in response to specific stimuli, such as visual or auditory stimuli, to assess the integrity of the sensory pathways in the nervous system.

18. Neurosonography: Ultrasound imaging of the brain and spinal cord in infants to evaluate brain development, detect abnormalities, and monitor conditions such as hydrocephalus.

19. Video Electroencephalography (VEEG): A combination of EEG and video recording to capture and analyze brain activity during seizures and assess epilepsy-related symptoms.

20. Molecular Imaging: Imaging techniques that use specific molecular tracers to visualize and study cellular and molecular processes in the brain associated with neurological disorders.

21. Neurocognitive Testing: Assessments that evaluate cognitive abilities, memory, attention, and executive functions to assess neurological impairments and monitor disease progression.

22. Neurogenetic Testing: Genetic tests designed to detect specific gene mutations or variations associated with inherited neurological disorders.

23. Autonomic Function Testing: Assessments that measure the function of the autonomic nervous system to diagnose conditions such as autonomic neuropathy and dysautonomia.

24. Neurosonology: The use of ultrasound to assess blood flow and vascular abnormalities in the brain and neck, aiding in the diagnosis of conditions such as stroke and carotid artery disease.

25. Neuroendocrine Testing: Tests that assess hormone levels and functioning of the endocrine system to diagnose and manage conditions such as pituitary disorders and hormonal imbalances.

III. Therapeutic Interventions:

1. Medication Management: Prescribing and adjusting medications to manage symptoms, slow disease progression, or treat specific neurological conditions.

2. Physical Therapy: Rehabilitation techniques and exercises to improve movement, balance, strength, and coordination in individuals with neurological conditions.

3. Occupational Therapy: Activities and strategies to improve daily functioning, fine motor skills, and independence in individuals with neurological impairments.

4. Speech and Language Therapy: Techniques to address communication difficulties, speech disorders, and swallowing problems caused by neurological conditions.

5. Cognitive Rehabilitation: Therapeutic approaches to improve cognitive abilities, memory, attention, and problem-solving skills affected by neurological impairments.

6. Neurosurgery: Surgical procedures performed on the brain, spinal cord, or nerves to treat conditions such as brain tumors, epilepsy, and nerve compression syndromes.

7. Deep Brain Stimulation (DBS): A surgical procedure that involves implanting electrodes in specific areas of the brain and delivering electrical impulses to alleviate symptoms of movement disorders such as Parkinson's disease and essential tremor.

8. Interventional Radiology: Minimally invasive procedures using image-guided techniques to treat conditions such as cerebral aneurysms, stroke, and arteriovenous malformations.

9. Neurorehabilitation: Comprehensive rehabilitation programs that combine various therapies and interventions to aid recovery and improve functional outcomes in individuals with neurological conditions.

10. Botulinum Toxin Injections: Injections of botulinum toxin (Botox) to temporarily paralyze specific muscles and reduce spasticity or manage conditions such as dystonia and chronic migraines.

11. Neurostimulation: The use of electrical or magnetic stimulation to modulate neural activity and manage conditions such as chronic pain, migraine, and depression.

12. Palliative Care: Supportive care provided to individuals with advanced or life-limiting neurological conditions to alleviate symptoms, improve quality of life, and provide emotional and psychological support.

13. Rehabilitation Medicine: Specialized medical care focused on restoring function, maximizing independence, and improving quality of life in individuals with neurological disabilities.

14. Pain Management: Multidisciplinary approaches to assess and manage chronic pain associated with neurological conditions, involving medications, physical therapies, psychological interventions, and interventional procedures.

15. Assistive Devices and Adaptive Equipment: The use of mobility aids, communication devices, orthotics, and other assistive technologies to enhance independence and improve quality of life in individuals with neurological impairments.

16. Neuropharmacology: The study and use of medications and drugs that target the nervous system to treat neurological conditions and manage symptoms.

17. Neuro-oncology: The specialized field focused on the diagnosis, treatment, and management of brain and spinal cord tumors.

18. Rehabilitation Robotics: The use of robotic devices and technologies to assist in the rehabilitation process, improve motor function, and enhance recovery outcomes in individuals with neurological conditions.

19. Neurointensive Care: Specialized critical care management for patients with severe neurological conditions, including monitoring and intervention to optimize brain function and prevent secondary complications.

20. Neurobehavioral Therapy: Therapeutic approaches that address behavioral and psychological aspects associated with neurological conditions, such as cognitive-behavioral therapy (CBT) and psychoeducation.

21. Neuroplasticity Training: Techniques and exercises designed to promote the rewiring and adaptation of neural pathways to enhance recovery and functional improvements in individuals with neurological impairments.

22. Gene Therapy: Experimental treatments that involve the introduction of genetic material into cells to correct or modify genetic abnormalities associated with certain neurological disorders.

23. Rehabilitation Counseling: Counseling and support services aimed at helping individuals with neurological conditions and their families cope with emotional and psychological challenges and navigate the rehabilitation process.

24. Sleep Hygiene Education: Education and strategies to promote healthy sleep habits and improve sleep quality in individuals with sleep disorders or neurological conditions affecting sleep.

25. Cognitive-Behavioral Interventions: Psychological interventions aimed at addressing cognitive distortions, promoting adaptive behaviors, and enhancing coping skills in individuals with neurological conditions affecting cognition and emotions.

Exercises for transcribing neurology reports accurately

Exercise 1: Fill in the blanks

Transcribe the following sentence:

The patient presented with _____ weakness in their right arm.

Answer:

The patient presented with muscle weakness in their right arm.

Exercise 2: True or False

Indicate whether the following statement is true or false:

Magnetic resonance imaging (MRI) is a diagnostic test commonly used in neurology to visualize the brain and spinal cord.

Answer:

True

Exercise 3: Fill in the blanks

Transcribe the following sentence:

The patient's EEG showed abnormal _______ activity.

Answer:

The patient's EEG showed abnormal electrical activity.

Exercise 4: Matching

Match the neurological condition with its description:

1. Epilepsy

2. Alzheimer's disease

3. Multiple sclerosis (MS)

4. Parkinson's disease

A. A chronic neurodegenerative disorder that affects movement and coordination

B. A disorder characterized by recurrent seizures

C. A progressive neurological disease that affects memory, thinking, and behavior

D. A condition that causes damage to the protective covering of nerve fibers in the brain and spinal cord

Answer:

1. Epilepsy

B. A disorder characterized by recurrent seizures

2. Alzheimer's disease

C. A progressive neurological disease that affects memory, thinking, and behavior

3. Multiple sclerosis (MS)

D. A condition that causes damage to the protective covering of nerve fibers in the brain and spinal cord

4. Parkinson's disease

A. A chronic neurodegenerative disorder that affects movement and coordination

Exercise 5: Fill in the blanks

Transcribe the following sentence:

The patient exhibited signs of ______ aphasia.

Answer:

The patient exhibited signs of expressive aphasia.

Exercise 6: True or False

Indicate whether the following statement is true or false:

A lumbar puncture is a diagnostic procedure that involves collecting cerebrospinal fluid (CSF) from the spinal canal.

Answer:

True

Exercise 7: Fill in the blanks

Transcribe the following sentence:

The patient's neurological examination revealed _____ reflexes.

Answer:

The patient's neurological examination revealed hyperactive reflexes.

Exercise 8: Matching

Match the diagnostic test with its description:

1. Electromyography (EMG)

2. Electroencephalography (EEG)

3. Nerve conduction study (NCS)

4. Electrocardiogram (ECG)

A. Test that measures brain activity to evaluate epilepsy or other neurological disorders

B. Test that assesses nerve and muscle function to diagnose conditions such as neuropathy or muscle disorders

C. Test that measures the electrical activity of muscles to diagnose neuromuscular disorders

D. Test that evaluates the electrical activity of the heart to detect heart rhythm abnormalities

Answer:

1. Electromyography (EMG)   C. Test that measures the electrical activity of muscles to diagnose neuromuscular disorders

2. Electroencephalography (EEG) A. Test that measures brain activity to evaluate epilepsy or other neurological disorders

3. Nerve conduction study (NCS) B. Test that assesses nerve and muscle function to diagnose conditions such as neuropathy or muscle disorders

4. Electrocardiogram (ECG)   D. Test that evaluates the electrical activity of the heart to detect heart rhythm abnormalities

Exercise 9: True or False

Indicate whether the following statement is true or false:

A cerebrovascular accident (CVA) is commonly known as a stroke.

Answer:

True

Exercise 10: Fill in the blanks

Transcribe the following sentence:

The patient's MRI scan showed _____ lesions in the white matter.

Answer:

The patient's MRI scan showed multiple lesions in the white matter.

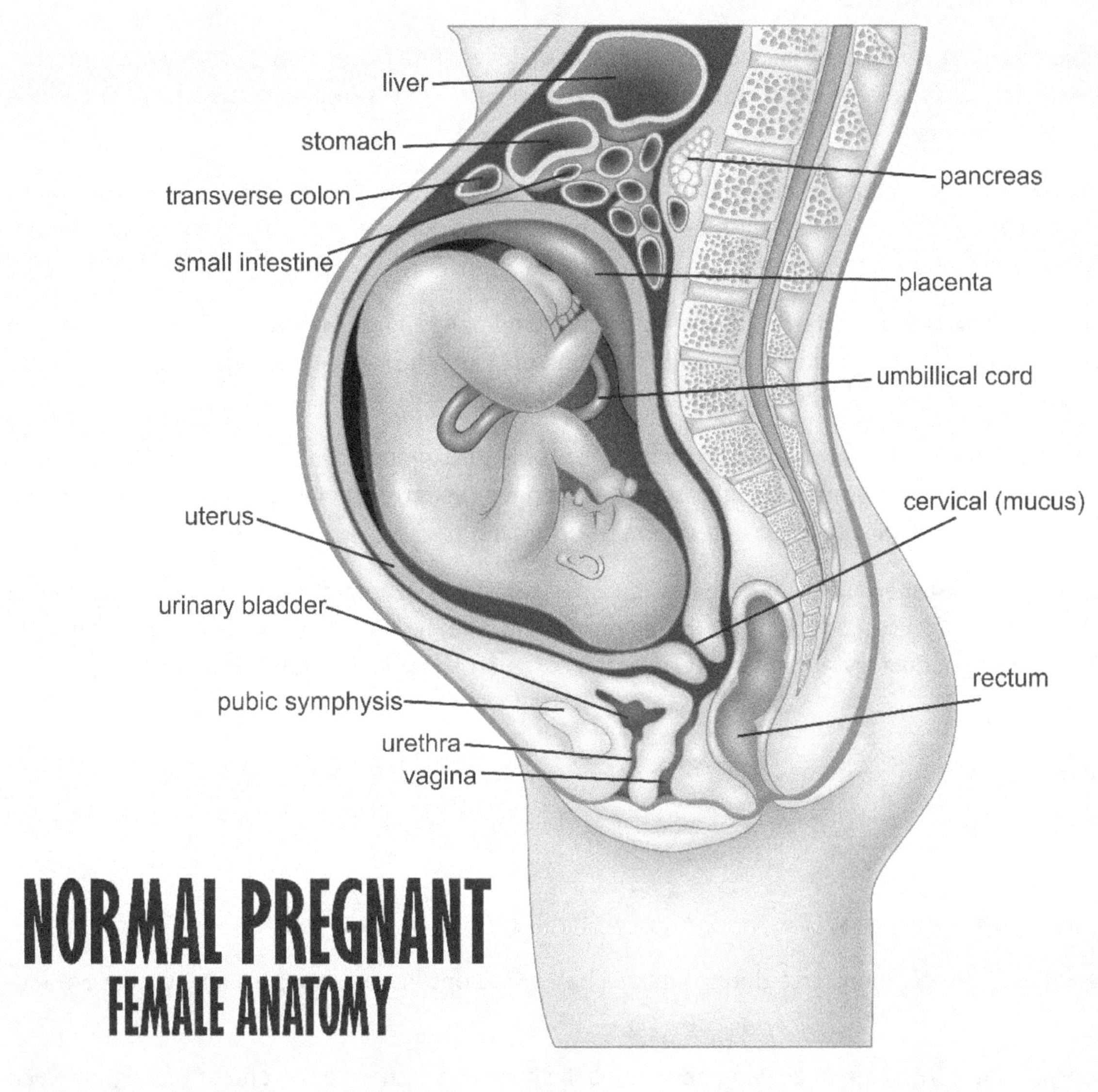

Introduction to obstetrics and its unique terminology

Obstetrics is a branch of medicine that focuses on the care of women during pregnancy, childbirth, and the recovery period following delivery, known as the postpartum period. This specialty encompasses all aspects of reproductive health from conception to the postnatal period.

Here are some essential points to understand as a beginner in this field:

1. Pregnancy Care: Obstetricians provide medical and surgical care to women during pregnancy and childbirth. They monitor both the mother and the fetus, provide prenatal care, and manage any complications that may arise.

2. Childbirth: Obstetricians are involved in all aspects of delivering a baby. They can carry out both vaginal deliveries and Cesarean sections (C-sections), where the baby is delivered through a surgical incision in the mother's abdomen.

3. Postpartum Care: After the baby is born, obstetricians continue to care for the mother. They manage any surgical wounds from childbirth, monitor for postpartum depression, and provide advice on infant care, breastfeeding, and contraception.

4. Common Conditions: Obstetricians manage many conditions and complications related to pregnancy, including ectopic pregnancy, preeclampsia (high blood pressure during pregnancy), gestational diabetes, preterm labor, and various complications during labor and delivery.

5. Diagnostic Tools: Obstetricians use a variety of tools to diagnose conditions related to pregnancy. These include blood and urine tests, ultrasound to monitor the fetus's development, and amniocentesis or chorionic villus sampling (CVS) to detect genetic disorders.

6. Obstetrical Subspecialties: There are subspecialties within obstetrics, including maternal-fetal medicine, which focuses on high-risk pregnancies and the health of the mother and fetus, and reproductive endocrinology and infertility, which focuses on the management of complex reproductive problems.

Pregnancy-related terms, prenatal care, and delivery procedures

I. Pregnancy-Related Terms:

1. Gestation: The period of time during which a baby develops in the womb, usually lasting around 40 weeks.

2. Embryo: The early stage of development of a baby from conception to the end of the eighth week of pregnancy.

3. Fetus: The developing baby from the ninth week of pregnancy until birth.

4. Placenta: An organ that develops in the uterus during pregnancy and provides oxygen and nutrients to the fetus.

5. Amniotic Fluid: The fluid surrounding the fetus within the amniotic sac, which helps protect and cushion the baby.

6. Braxton Hicks Contractions: Irregular contractions of the uterus that can occur during pregnancy, often referred to as "false labor."

7. Preterm Labor: The onset of labor before 37 weeks of pregnancy.

8. Ectopic Pregnancy: A pregnancy that occurs outside of the uterus, typically in the fallopian tube.

9. Placenta Previa: A condition in which the placenta partially or completely covers the cervix, leading to potential complications during delivery.

10. Preeclampsia: A pregnancy-related condition characterized by high blood pressure and damage to organs, typically occurring after 20 weeks of gestation.

11. Gestational Diabetes: Diabetes that develops during pregnancy and usually resolves after delivery.

12. Miscarriage: The spontaneous loss of a pregnancy before 20 weeks gestation.

13. Stillbirth: The loss of a baby after 20 weeks gestation, before delivery.

14. Multiple Gestation: A pregnancy with two or more fetuses, such as twins or triplets.

15. Fetal Movement: The sensation of the baby's movements within the womb, which typically increases as pregnancy progresses.

16. Maternal Weight Gain: The recommended weight gain for a pregnant woman based on pre-pregnancy body mass index (BMI).

17. Cervical Dilation: The opening of the cervix during labor to allow the baby to pass through the birth canal.

18. Episiotomy: A surgical incision made in the perineum (area between the vagina and anus) during childbirth to facilitate delivery.

19. Postpartum Depression: A mood disorder that can occur after childbirth, characterized by feelings of sadness, anxiety, and exhaustion.

20. Neonate: A newborn baby, typically within the first 28 days of life.

21. Umbilical Cord: A flexible cord-like structure that connects the fetus to the placenta, supplying nutrients and oxygen.

22. Colostrum: The first milk produced by the breasts during late pregnancy and the early days after childbirth, rich in antibodies and nutrients.

23. Lochia: Vaginal discharge that occurs after childbirth, consisting of blood, mucus, and tissue.

24. Engorgement: Swelling and enlargement of the breasts as milk production increases after childbirth.

25. Lactation: The process of producing and secreting milk from the breasts after childbirth.

II. Prenatal Care:

1. Ultrasound: A diagnostic imaging technique that uses high-frequency sound waves to create images of the developing fetus.

2. Blood Tests: Various blood tests performed during pregnancy to assess the health of the mother and baby, including blood typing, genetic screening, and glucose tolerance tests.

3. Urine Analysis: Testing urine samples for signs of infection, protein, glucose, or other abnormalities during prenatal visits.

4. Fetal Monitoring: Monitoring the baby's heart rate and movement during prenatal visits to ensure proper growth and well-being.

5. Blood Pressure Monitoring: Regular measurement of the mother's blood pressure to detect and manage conditions such as preeclampsia.

6. Fundal Height Measurement: Measuring the distance from the pubic bone to the top of the uterus to monitor fetal growth and development.

7. Group B Streptococcus (GBS) Screening: Testing for the presence of GBS bacteria in the mother's vagina and rectum, which can cause infections in newborns.

8. Genetic Counseling: Counseling and testing to assess the risk of genetic disorders or birth defects in the baby.

9. Nutritional Guidance: Providing information and guidance on maintaining a healthy diet during pregnancy to support the growth and development of the baby.

10. Rh Factor Testing: Testing to determine if a pregnant woman's blood is Rh-negative or Rh-positive, which can impact the health of the baby.

11. Antenatal Classes: Educational classes that prepare expectant parents for childbirth, breastfeeding, and newborn care.

12. Maternal Weight Monitoring: Monitoring the mother's weight gain during pregnancy to ensure it is within a healthy range.

13. Gestational Diabetes Screening: Testing for gestational diabetes, a form of diabetes that develops during pregnancy and can affect the health of the baby.

14. Iron Supplementation: Prescribing iron supplements to prevent or treat iron deficiency anemia in pregnant women.

15. Folic Acid Supplementation: Recommending folic acid supplements to reduce the risk of neural tube defects in the developing baby.

16. Infection Screening: Testing for sexually transmitted infections and other infections that can affect pregnancy and the health of the baby.

17. Vaccinations: Administering vaccines, such as the flu vaccine and Tdap vaccine, to protect the mother and baby from certain diseases.

18. Rh Immunoglobulin (RhIg) Administration: Administering RhIg to Rh-negative mothers to prevent Rh sensitization, a condition that can harm future pregnancies.

19. Group Support: Providing opportunities for expectant mothers to connect with other women going through similar experiences and share information and support.

20. Mental Health Screening: Assessing and addressing mental health concerns during pregnancy, including depression and anxiety.

21. Dental Care: Encouraging regular dental check-ups and oral hygiene to maintain oral health, which is linked to overall pregnancy health.

22. Preterm Labor Assessment: Monitoring and assessing the risk of preterm labor to take necessary interventions and precautions.

23. Maternal Immunizations: Administering vaccines, such as the COVID-19 vaccine or varicella vaccine, to protect the mother and baby from infectious diseases.

24. Genetic Testing: Conducting genetic tests, such as non-invasive prenatal testing (NIPT), to detect chromosomal abnormalities or genetic disorders in the developing baby.

25. Cord Blood Banking: Providing information and options for preserving the baby's umbilical cord blood for potential future medical use.

III. Delivery Procedures:

1. Vaginal Delivery: The natural process of childbirth through the birth canal, typically assisted by contractions and pushing.

2. Cesarean Section (C-Section): A surgical procedure in which the baby is delivered through an incision in the mother's abdomen and uterus.

3. Epidural Anesthesia: Pain relief medication administered through a catheter placed in the epidural space of the spine during labor.

4. Forceps-Assisted Delivery: Using a medical instrument called forceps to gently guide and assist the baby's delivery during vaginal birth.

5. Vacuum-Assisted Delivery: Using a vacuum device attached to the baby's head to facilitate delivery during vaginal birth.

6. Induction of Labor: The artificial initiation of labor using medications or other methods to stimulate uterine contractions.

7. Water Birth: Delivering the baby in a pool or tub of warm water, providing pain relief and a soothing environment.

8. Episiotomy Repair: Surgical repair of an episiotomy or perineal tear that may occur during childbirth.

9. Umbilical Cord Clamping: The timing and method of clamping and cutting the umbilical cord after the baby is born.

10. Placenta Delivery: The delivery of the placenta and fetal membranes after the birth of the baby.

11. Neonatal Resuscitation: Emergency medical procedures performed on a newborn if there are signs of distress or difficulty breathing.

12. Skin-to-Skin Contact: Placing the baby directly on the mother's chest immediately after birth to promote bonding and breastfeeding.

13. Delayed Cord Clamping: Allowing the umbilical cord to remain unclamped for a period of time after birth to enhance blood flow to the baby.

14. Perineal Massage: Gentle massage of the perineal area during pregnancy to prepare the tissues for childbirth and reduce the risk of tearing.

15. Cord Blood Banking: Collecting and storing umbilical cord blood for potential future medical use.

16. Tocodynamometer Monitoring: Monitoring uterine contractions using a tocodynamometer device during labor.

17. External Cephalic Version (ECV): A procedure to manually turn a breech baby into a head-down position before delivery.

18. Amniotomy: Artificial rupture of the amniotic sac to induce or augment labor.

19. Controlled Cord Traction: Controlled pulling on the umbilical cord to assist in the delivery of the placenta.

20. Perineal Cooling: Applying cold packs or cooling measures to the perineal area after childbirth to reduce swelling and discomfort.

21. Lithotomy Position: Positioning the mother on her back with legs raised and feet in stirrups for childbirth.

22. Placental Examination: Examination of the placenta after delivery to assess its health and identify any abnormalities.

23. Fetal Scalp Electrode Placement: Placing an electrode on the baby's scalp to monitor the fetal heart rate more accurately during labor.

24. Fetal Blood Sampling: Collecting a small sample of blood from the baby's scalp for testing during labor.

25. Cesarean Scar Revision: Surgical correction of a previous cesarean section scar for subsequent pregnancies or cosmetic purposes.

Practice activities for transcribing obstetrics reports effectively

Exercise 1: Fill in the blanks

Transcribe the following sentence:

The patient is currently _______ weeks pregnant.

Answer:

The patient is currently 24 weeks pregnant.

Exercise 2: True or False

Indicate whether the following statement is true or false:

Amniocentesis is a diagnostic procedure performed during pregnancy to collect and analyze amniotic fluid.

Answer:

True

Exercise 3: Fill in the blanks

Transcribe the following sentence:

The fetal heart rate was recorded as _______ beats per minute.

Answer:

The fetal heart rate was recorded as 140 beats per minute.

Exercise 4: Matching

Match the prenatal test with its description:

1. Ultrasound

2. Amniocentesis

3. Chorionic villus sampling

4. First-trimester screening

A. A blood test performed in early pregnancy to assess the risk of certain chromosomal abnormalities

B. A diagnostic imaging technique that uses sound waves to create images of the developing fetus

C. A procedure that involves sampling the chorionic villi (placental tissue) to diagnose genetic conditions

D. A test that measures specific hormones and proteins in the mother's blood to assess the risk of certain birth defects

Answer:

1. Ultrasound

B. A diagnostic imaging technique that uses sound waves to create images of the developing fetus

2. Amniocentesis

C. A procedure that involves sampling the chorionic villi (placental tissue) to diagnose genetic conditions

3. Chorionic villus sampling

D. A test that measures specific hormones and proteins in the mother's blood to assess the risk of certain birth defects

4. First-trimester screening

A. A blood test performed in early pregnancy to assess the risk of certain chromosomal abnormalities

Exercise 5: Fill in the blanks

Transcribe the following sentence:

The patient experienced ______ contractions during labor.

Answer:

The patient experienced regular contractions during labor.

Exercise 6: True or False

Indicate whether the following statement is true or false:

Gestational diabetes is a form of diabetes that occurs during pregnancy and usually resolves after childbirth.

Answer:

True

Exercise 7: Fill in the blanks

Transcribe the following sentence:

The patient's prenatal bloodwork showed normal levels of _____.

Answer:

The patient's prenatal bloodwork showed normal levels of hemoglobin and hematocrit.

Exercise 8: Matching

Match the delivery procedure with its description:

1. Vaginal delivery

2. Cesarean section (C-section)

3. Vacuum extraction

4. Forceps delivery

A. Delivery of the baby through a surgical incision in the mother's abdomen and uterus

B. Delivery of the baby through the birth canal without the use of surgical intervention

C. Assisted vaginal delivery using a vacuum device to help guide the baby's head out of the birth canal

D. Assisted vaginal delivery using forceps (medical instruments) to help guide the baby's head out of the birth canal

Answer:

1. Vaginal delivery

B. Delivery of the baby through the birth canal without the use of surgical intervention

2. Cesarean section (C-section)

A. Delivery of the baby through a surgical incision in the mother's abdomen and uterus

3. Vacuum extraction

C. Assisted vaginal delivery using a vacuum device to help guide the baby's head out of the birth canal

4. Forceps delivery

D. Assisted vaginal delivery using forceps (medical instruments) to help guide the baby's head out of the birth canal

Exercise 9: True or False

Indicate whether the following statement is true or false:

The Apgar score is a quick assessment of a newborn's overall well-being and is performed at one minute and five minutes after birth.

Answer:

True

Exercise 10: Fill in the blanks

Transcribe the following sentence:

The newborn's birth weight was _______ grams.

Answer:

The newborn's birth weight was 3,250 grams.

Human reproductive system

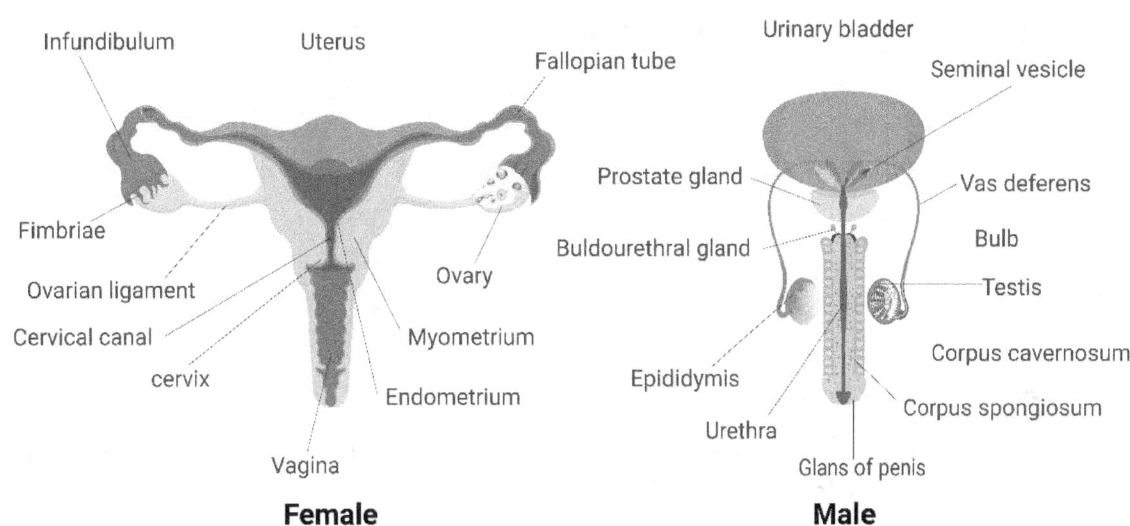

Understanding gynecology and its specific terminology

Gynecology is a branch of medicine that focuses on the health of the female reproductive system, which includes the uterus, ovaries, fallopian tubes, cervix, vagina, and breasts. It's often practiced alongside obstetrics, a field focused on pregnancy and childbirth.

Here are some key points to understand as a beginner in this field:

1. Women's Health: Gynecologists provide medical and surgical care with a focus on diseases and disorders that impact female reproductive organs. They also provide routine health services such as pap smears, mammograms, and family planning advice.

2. Common Conditions: Gynecologists diagnose and treat a wide range of conditions related to female reproductive health. These can include menstrual and hormonal disorders, pelvic inflammatory disease, endometriosis, uterine fibroids, sexually transmitted infections, infertility, and gynecological cancers such as ovarian and cervical cancer.

3. Diagnostic Tools: Gynecologists use various diagnostic tools, including pelvic examinations, ultrasounds, and lab tests. Biopsies of tissue may also be taken for examination. For certain diseases like cervical or ovarian cancer, specialized tests such as Pap smears or transvaginal ultrasounds are used.

4. Treatment Approaches: Treatment can involve lifestyle modifications, medication, or surgery. For example, hormonal disorders can often be managed with medication, while conditions like uterine fibroids or cancers may require surgical intervention. Gynecologists are trained in surgical procedures including laparoscopic surgery, hysteroscopy, and larger surgeries like hysterectomy (removal of the uterus).

5. Subspecialties: There are several subspecialties within gynecology, including reproductive endocrinology and infertility (dealing with issues of fertility and hormonal function), gynecologic oncology (focusing on gynecological cancers), and urogynecology (concentrating on pelvic floor disorders and associated urinary problems).

6. Reproductive Health: Gynecologists play an important role in reproductive health, providing advice on contraception, sexual health, preconception care, and fertility.

Reproductive system disorders, diagnostic tests, and surgical interventions

I. Reproductive System Disorders:

1. Polycystic Ovary Syndrome (PCOS): A hormonal disorder in women characterized by the presence of cysts on the ovaries, irregular periods, and fertility issues.

2. Endometriosis: A condition in which the tissue lining the uterus grows outside of it, leading to pelvic pain and infertility.

3. Uterine Fibroids: Noncancerous growths that develop in the uterus, often causing heavy menstrual bleeding and pelvic pressure.

4. Ovarian Cysts: Fluid-filled sacs that form on or within the ovaries, which can sometimes cause pain or fertility problems.

5. Pelvic Inflammatory Disease (PID): An infection of the female reproductive organs, usually caused by sexually transmitted bacteria, resulting in pelvic pain and potential infertility.

6. Polycystic Breast Disease: A condition characterized by the presence of multiple cysts in the breast tissue, which may cause breast pain or discomfort.

7. Premenstrual Syndrome (PMS): A group of physical and emotional symptoms that occur in the days leading up to menstruation, such as bloating, mood swings, and breast tenderness.

8. Amenorrhea: The absence of menstruation, which can be caused by various factors such as hormonal imbalances, pregnancy, or certain medical conditions.

9. Menorrhagia: Excessive or prolonged menstrual bleeding, often resulting in heavy flow and longer periods.

10. Dysmenorrhea: Painful menstrual periods, typically accompanied by cramping and lower abdominal pain.

11. Vulvodynia: Chronic pain or discomfort in the vulva, the external female genitalia, without an identifiable cause.

12. Vaginal Infections: Infections of the vagina, such as yeast infections or bacterial vaginosis, leading to symptoms like itching, discharge, and odor.

13. Cervical Dysplasia: Abnormal changes in the cells of the cervix, often detected through Pap smears and associated with the human papillomavirus (HPV).

14. Pelvic Organ Prolapse: The descent or dropping of pelvic organs, such as the uterus or bladder, into the vaginal canal due to weakened pelvic floor muscles.

15. Infertility: The inability to conceive or carry a pregnancy to term, often caused by various factors such as hormonal imbalances, blocked fallopian tubes, or sperm-related issues.

16. Ectopic Pregnancy: A pregnancy that occurs outside of the uterus, usually in the fallopian tube, which can be life-threatening and requires immediate medical attention.

17. Ovarian Cancer: Cancer that originates in the ovaries, with symptoms that may include abdominal bloating, pelvic pain, and changes in bowel habits.

18. Cervical Cancer: Cancer that develops in the cervix, often caused by certain strains of HPV, and may be detected through Pap smears or HPV testing.

19. Uterine Cancer: Cancer that forms in the uterus, usually in the endometrium (inner lining), and may cause abnormal vaginal bleeding or pelvic pain.

20. Vaginal Atrophy: Thinning, drying, and inflammation of the vaginal walls, typically occurring during menopause due to decreased estrogen levels.

21. Ovarian Hyperstimulation Syndrome (OHSS): A condition that can occur as a side effect of fertility treatments, causing enlarged ovaries and fluid accumulation in the abdomen.

22. Premature Ovarian Failure (POF): A condition in which the ovaries stop functioning normally before the age of 40, leading to infertility and hormonal imbalances.

23. Pelvic Congestion Syndrome: Chronic pelvic pain caused by varicose veins in the pelvis, resulting in discomfort and a feeling of heaviness.

24. Vulvar Cancer: Cancer that develops in the external genital area, including the labia, clitoris, and vaginal opening.

25. Uterine Prolapse: The downward displacement of the uterus into the vaginal canal, often occurring due to weakened pelvic floor muscles and connective tissues.

II. Diagnostic Tests:

1. Pelvic Ultrasound: Imaging technique that uses sound waves to create pictures of the pelvic organs, helping to diagnose conditions such as fibroids, ovarian cysts, and endometriosis.

2. Pap Smear: A screening test that involves collecting cells from the cervix to detect early signs of cervical cancer or other abnormalities.

3. Hysteroscopy: A procedure in which a thin, lighted tube is inserted into the uterus to examine the uterine lining and diagnose conditions like fibroids or polyps.

4. Hormone Level Testing: Blood tests to measure hormone levels, such as estrogen and progesterone, which can help evaluate fertility issues or hormonal imbalances.

5. Colposcopy: Examination of the cervix, vagina, and vulva using a special magnifying instrument to detect and evaluate abnormal cells or lesions.

6. Transvaginal Ultrasound: A type of pelvic ultrasound that uses a probe inserted into the vagina to obtain detailed images of the reproductive organs, useful in evaluating conditions such as ovarian cysts or uterine abnormalities.

7. Saline Infusion Sonohysterography (SIS): A procedure that involves injecting saline solution into the uterus during an ultrasound to enhance visualization of the uterine cavity and detect abnormalities.

8. Genetic Testing: Testing performed to assess the risk of inherited genetic conditions that may impact fertility or reproductive health.

9. Endometrial Biopsy: A procedure in which a small sample of the uterine lining is collected and examined to evaluate abnormal bleeding, diagnose endometrial cancer, or assess the menstrual cycle.

10. Hormone Panel: A comprehensive blood test that measures multiple hormone levels, providing insights into hormonal imbalances or conditions affecting fertility and reproductive health.

11. Sonohysterogram: Similar to SIS, this procedure involves injecting sterile fluid into the uterus during ultrasound to visualize the uterine cavity and identify abnormalities.

12. STD Testing: Testing for sexually transmitted infections that can affect the reproductive system, such as chlamydia, gonorrhea, or syphilis.

13. Anti-Müllerian Hormone (AMH) Test: A blood test that helps assess ovarian reserve and provides insights into a woman's fertility potential.

14. Ovarian Reserve Testing: Various tests, including AMH, follicle-stimulating hormone (FSH), and estradiol levels, to evaluate the quantity and quality of a woman's eggs.

15. Thyroid Function Tests: Blood tests to assess thyroid hormone levels, as imbalances can affect fertility and menstrual regularity.

16. Laparoscopy: A minimally invasive surgical procedure that uses a small camera inserted through a small incision in the abdomen to visualize and diagnose conditions such as endometriosis, pelvic adhesions, or ovarian cysts.

17. Mammogram: A specialized X-ray of the breasts used for screening and diagnosing breast conditions, including breast cancer.

18. Genetic Carrier Screening: Testing performed to determine if individuals carry genetic mutations that could be passed on to their children and potentially impact reproductive health.

19. Chromosomal Analysis: Testing performed to assess chromosomal abnormalities that may affect fertility or cause reproductive system disorders, such as Turner syndrome or Klinefelter syndrome.

20. Transrectal Ultrasound: An ultrasound examination that uses a probe inserted into the rectum to visualize the prostate gland and assess for conditions such as prostate cancer or benign prostatic hyperplasia.

21. Urodynamic Testing: Diagnostic tests performed to evaluate urinary system function and identify issues such as urinary incontinence or bladder dysfunction that may contribute to reproductive health concerns.

22. Cervical Biopsy: A procedure that involves removing a small sample of cervical tissue for examination, often performed to assess abnormal Pap smear results or detect cervical cancer.

23. Semen Analysis: Testing performed to evaluate male fertility by analyzing the quantity, quality, and movement of sperm in a semen sample.

24. Hysterosalpingography: A radiologic procedure that uses contrast dye injected into the uterus and fallopian tubes to evaluate the structure and patency of the reproductive organs.

25. Molecular Genetic Testing: Advanced genetic testing techniques that analyze DNA or RNA for specific gene mutations or abnormalities related to reproductive system disorders.

III. Surgical Interventions:

1. Hysterectomy: Surgical removal of the uterus, either partially or entirely, which may be performed to treat conditions such as fibroids, endometriosis, or cancer.

2. Myomectomy: Surgical removal of uterine fibroids while preserving the uterus, often performed for women who wish to retain their fertility.

3. Oophorectomy: Surgical removal of one or both ovaries, typically performed to treat ovarian cysts, endometriosis, or ovarian cancer.

4. Tubal Ligation: A surgical procedure in which the fallopian tubes are sealed or cut to prevent pregnancy permanently.

5. Assisted Reproductive Technologies (ART): Procedures such as in vitro fertilization (IVF), intracytoplasmic sperm injection (ICSI), or gamete intrafallopian transfer (GIFT) that help individuals or couples overcome infertility by facilitating fertilization and implantation of embryos.

6. Laparoscopy: A minimally invasive surgical procedure in which a small incision is made in the abdomen to examine or treat conditions affecting the reproductive organs, such as endometriosis or tubal blockages.

7. Uterine Artery Embolization (UAE): A nonsurgical procedure that involves blocking the blood supply to uterine fibroids, causing them to shrink and alleviate symptoms.

8. Endometrial Ablation: A procedure to remove or destroy the uterine lining, often performed to manage heavy menstrual bleeding or certain uterine conditions.

9. Hysterosalpingography (HSG): A diagnostic procedure in which a contrast dye is injected into the uterus and fallopian tubes to evaluate their structure and detect any blockages.

10. Cervical Cerclage: A surgical procedure in which a stitch is placed around the cervix to prevent premature birth in women at risk of cervical insufficiency.

11. Salpingectomy: Surgical removal of one or both fallopian tubes, often performed to treat conditions such as ectopic pregnancy, tubal blockages, or reduce the risk of ovarian cancer.

12. Vulvectomy: Surgical removal of part or all of the external female genitalia (vulva), typically performed to treat vulvar cancer or precancerous conditions.

13. Pelvic Organ Prolapse Surgery: Surgical procedures to repair and restore pelvic organs, such as the uterus, bladder, or rectum, which may have descended or prolapsed due to weakened pelvic floor muscles.

14. Cervical Conization: A surgical procedure in which a cone-shaped piece of tissue is removed from the cervix, often performed to treat precancerous or cancerous conditions.

15. Uterine Suspension: A surgical procedure to reposition and support the uterus, often performed to alleviate symptoms of uterine prolapse.

16. Vesicovaginal Fistula Repair: Surgical correction of an abnormal connection between the bladder and the vagina, which can result from childbirth complications or other causes.

17. Rectovaginal Fistula Repair: Surgical correction of an abnormal connection between the rectum and vagina, often caused by trauma, surgery, or inflammatory bowel disease.

18. Vaginoplasty: Surgical reconstruction or tightening of the vagina, typically performed for functional or cosmetic purposes.

19. Labiaplasty: Surgical alteration of the labia minora or labia majora for aesthetic or functional reasons.

20. Clitoroplasty: Surgical reconstruction or reshaping of the clitoris, sometimes performed as part of gender-affirming surgeries or to treat certain conditions.

21. Fertility Preservation Procedures: Surgical interventions to preserve fertility in individuals undergoing treatments that may impact reproductive function, such as cancer treatments.

22. Transvaginal Mesh Procedures: Surgical implantation of a synthetic mesh to provide support for weakened or damaged vaginal tissues, often used to treat pelvic organ prolapse or stress urinary incontinence.

23. Fallopian Tube Recanalization: A procedure to open blocked or damaged fallopian tubes, allowing for improved fertility and natural conception.

24. Clitoral Hood Reduction: Surgical reduction of excess tissue covering the clitoral hood, typically performed to improve sexual sensation or aesthetics.

25. Vaginal Rejuvenation: A collective term for various surgical or non-surgical procedures aimed at improving the appearance, function, or sensation of the vaginal area.

Exercises for transcribing gynecology reports accurately

Exercise 1: Fill in the blanks

Transcribe the following sentence:

The patient presented with complaints of _______ and _______.

Answer:

The patient presented with complaints of pelvic pain and abnormal uterine bleeding.

Exercise 2: True or False

Indicate whether the following statement is true or false:

Endometriosis is a condition in which the tissue that lines the uterus grows outside of it.

Answer:

True

Exercise 3: Fill in the blanks

Transcribe the following sentence:

The patient underwent a _______ to remove an ovarian cyst.

Answer:

The patient underwent a laparoscopic surgery to remove an ovarian cyst.

Exercise 4: Matching

Match the gynecological procedure with its description:

1. Hysteroscopy

2. Colposcopy

3. Loop electrosurgical excision procedure (LEEP)

4. Myomectomy

A. A procedure to visualize and examine the inside of the uterus using a thin, lighted tube

B. A diagnostic procedure to examine the cervix, vagina, and vulva for abnormalities

C. A surgical procedure to remove abnormal or precancerous tissue from the cervix

D. Surgical removal of uterine fibroids while preserving the uterus

Answer:

1. Hysteroscopy

A. A procedure to visualize and examine the inside of the uterus using a thin, lighted tube

2. Colposcopy

B. A diagnostic procedure to examine the cervix, vagina, and vulva for abnormalities

3. Loop electrosurgical excision procedure (LEEP)

C. A surgical procedure to remove abnormal or precancerous tissue from the cervix

4. Myomectomy

D. Surgical removal of uterine fibroids while preserving the uterus

Exercise 5: Fill in the blanks

Transcribe the following sentence:

The patient's pap smear results were ______.

Answer:

The patient's pap smear results were normal.

Exercise 6: True or False

Indicate whether the following statement is true or false:

Polycystic ovary syndrome (PCOS) is a hormonal disorder characterized by the presence of multiple cysts on the ovaries.

Answer:

True

Exercise 7: Fill in the blanks

Transcribe the following sentence:

The patient's mammogram showed no evidence of ______.

Answer:

The patient's mammogram showed no evidence of breast abnormalities or malignancy.

Exercise 8: Matching

Match the contraceptive method with its description:

1. Oral contraceptives

2. Condoms

3. Intrauterine device (IUD)

4. Hormonal implants

A. A small, T-shaped device inserted into the uterus to prevent pregnancy

B. Barrier method of contraception that prevents sperm from reaching the egg

C. Hormonal pills taken daily to prevent pregnancy

D. Small, flexible rods implanted under the skin that release hormones to prevent pregnancy

Answer:

1. Oral contraceptives

C. Hormonal pills taken daily to prevent pregnancy

2. Condoms

B. Barrier method of contraception that prevents sperm from reaching the egg

3. Intrauterine device (IUD)

A. A small, T-shaped device inserted into the uterus to prevent pregnancy

4. Hormonal implants

D. Small, flexible rods implanted under the skin that release hormones to prevent pregnancy

Exercise 9: True or False

Indicate whether the following statement is true or false:

Endometrial ablation is a procedure to remove or destroy the lining of the uterus and is performed to manage heavy menstrual bleeding.

Answer:

True

Exercise 10: Fill in the blanks

Transcribe the following sentence:

The patient underwent a bilateral _____ for sterilization.

Answer:

The patient underwent a bilateral tubal ligation for sterilization.

12. ORTHOPEDICS

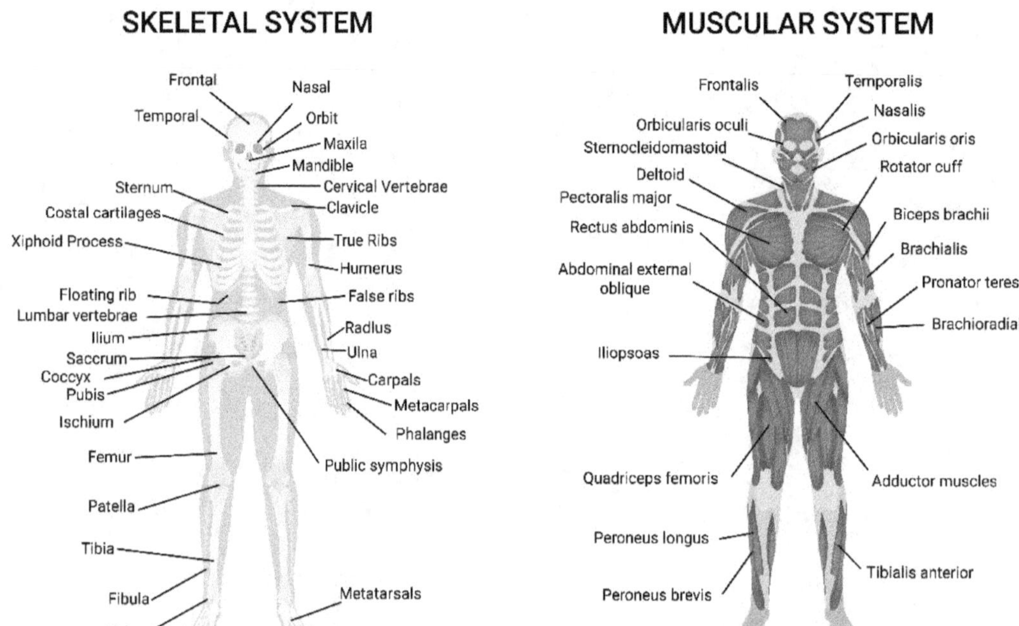

Overview of orthopedics and its specialized vocabulary

Orthopedics, also spelled orthopaedics, is a branch of medicine that deals with the prevention, diagnosis, and treatment of conditions related to the musculoskeletal system. This includes disorders of the bones, joints, ligaments, tendons, muscles, and nerves, which allow you to move, work, and be active.

Here are some key points to understand as a beginner in this field:

1. Musculoskeletal System: This system gives humans the ability to move using muscular and skeletal systems. It provides form, support, stability, and movement to the body.

2. Common Conditions: Orthopedic physicians treat a multitude of conditions that range from congenital (present at birth) and developmental (occurring in childhood) conditions, to injuries and diseases that can develop at any age. These can include fractures and dislocations, back pain, arthritis, strains, sprains, osteoporosis, spinal deformities, and musculoskeletal tumors.

3. Diagnostic Tools: Orthopedic physicians use a variety of methods to help diagnose conditions, including physical exams, medical histories, and imaging tests such as X-rays, CT scans, and MRI scans. In some cases, they may use arthroscopy to visualize, diagnose, and treat problems inside a joint.

4. Treatment Approaches: Orthopedic physicians utilize both surgical and non-surgical means to treat musculoskeletal conditions. Non-surgical treatments can include medication, physical therapy, and lifestyle changes. Surgical treatments can range from minimally invasive procedures, often using arthroscopy, to major joint repair or replacement surgeries, such as hip or knee replacements.

5. Orthopedic Subspecialties: There are several subspecialties within orthopedics, including sports medicine (focusing on musculoskeletal conditions related to sports injuries), pediatric orthopedics (focusing on musculoskeletal issues in children), and orthopedic oncology (focusing on the diagnosis and treatment of tumors of the musculoskeletal system).

6. Sports Medicine and Rehabilitation: Apart from managing acute injuries, orthopedic physicians often work in rehabilitation, helping patients regain mobility and strength after injury or surgery. They also advise on injury prevention and promote overall health and fitness.

Musculoskeletal conditions, orthopedic procedures, and rehabilitation

I. Musculoskeletal Conditions:

1. Osteoarthritis: A degenerative joint disease characterized by the breakdown of cartilage, resulting in joint pain, stiffness, and reduced mobility.

2. Rheumatoid Arthritis: An autoimmune disease that causes chronic inflammation in the joints, leading to joint pain, swelling, and deformity.

3. Fracture: A break or crack in a bone, often caused by trauma or osteoporosis.

4. Sprain: Injury to a ligament, the fibrous tissue connecting bones at a joint, resulting in pain, swelling, and instability.

5. Strain: Injury to a muscle or tendon, often caused by overstretching or overuse, leading to pain, swelling, and limited movement.

6. Herniated Disc: A condition where the soft tissue cushion between spinal vertebrae protrudes, causing back or neck pain and potentially affecting nerve function.

7. Scoliosis: Abnormal curvature of the spine, often diagnosed during adolescence, which may cause back pain and postural issues.

8. Tendinitis: Inflammation of a tendon, usually caused by repetitive motion or overuse, resulting in pain, swelling, and difficulty moving the affected joint.

9. Bursitis: Inflammation of a bursa, a fluid-filled sac that cushions and reduces friction between tendons, muscles, and bones, leading to pain and swelling.

10. Carpal Tunnel Syndrome: Compression of the median nerve in the wrist, causing hand numbness, tingling, and weakness.

11. Tennis Elbow (Lateral Epicondylitis): Pain and inflammation on the outer side of the elbow, commonly caused by repetitive wrist and arm movements.

12. Frozen Shoulder (Adhesive Capsulitis): Stiffness and pain in the shoulder joint, often resulting from inflammation and thickening of the shoulder capsule.

13. Rotator Cuff Tear: Damage or tear to the tendons of the rotator cuff in the shoulder, causing pain, weakness, and limited shoulder movement.

14. Plantar Fasciitis: Inflammation of the plantar fascia, a thick band of tissue on the bottom of the foot, leading to heel pain and difficulty walking.

15. Achilles Tendonitis: Inflammation of the Achilles tendon, the large tendon connecting the calf muscles to the heel bone, causing pain and stiffness.

16. Osteoporosis: A condition characterized by low bone density and increased risk of fractures, particularly in postmenopausal women and older adults.

17. Gout: A form of arthritis caused by the buildup of uric acid crystals in the joints, resulting in sudden and severe joint pain, often in the big toe.

18. Fibromyalgia: A chronic pain disorder characterized by widespread musculoskeletal pain, fatigue, and tenderness.

19. Osteomyelitis: Infection of the bone, typically caused by bacteria, leading to bone pain, swelling, and fever.

20. Paget's Disease of Bone: A condition characterized by abnormal bone remodeling, leading to enlarged and weakened bones, often causing pain and fractures.

21. Ankylosing Spondylitis: An inflammatory disease primarily affecting the spine, causing chronic back pain and stiffness.

22. Bunion (Hallux Valgus): A bony bump that forms at the base of the big toe, often causing pain and difficulty wearing certain shoes.

23. Kyphosis: Excessive forward curvature of the upper spine, resulting in a rounded or hunched back.

24. Lordosis: Excessive inward curvature of the lower spine, leading to a pronounced arch in the lower back.

25. Osteomalacia: Softening of the bones due to vitamin D deficiency or problems with calcium absorption, resulting in bone pain and increased risk of fractures.

II. Orthopedic Procedures:

1. Total Knee Replacement: Surgical procedure to replace a damaged or arthritic knee joint with an artificial implant to restore joint function and alleviate pain.

2. Total Hip Replacement: Surgical procedure to replace a damaged or arthritic hip joint with an artificial implant to improve hip mobility and reduce pain.

3. Arthroscopy: Minimally invasive procedure that uses a small camera and surgical instruments inserted through tiny incisions to diagnose and treat various joint conditions, such as torn cartilage or ligaments.

4. Spinal Fusion: Surgical procedure to permanently join two or more vertebrae in the spine to provide stability and reduce pain caused by spinal conditions, such as degenerative disc disease or spinal fractures.

5. ACL Reconstruction: Surgical procedure to repair or replace a torn anterior cruciate ligament (ACL) in the knee, often using grafts from the patient's own tissues or donor tissues.

6. Rotator Cuff Repair: Surgical procedure to repair a torn rotator cuff tendon in the shoulder, often performed arthroscopically or through an open incision.

7. Carpal Tunnel Release: Surgical procedure to relieve pressure on the median nerve in the wrist by cutting the transverse carpal ligament, reducing symptoms of carpal tunnel syndrome.

8. Meniscus Repair: Surgical procedure to repair or remove damaged or torn meniscus cartilage in the knee, promoting joint stability and reducing pain.

9. Lumbar Discectomy: Surgical procedure to remove a herniated or damaged disc in the lower back to alleviate pressure on spinal nerves and reduce pain.

10. Joint Arthroplasty: Surgical procedure to replace a damaged joint, such as the knee, hip, or shoulder, with an artificial prosthesis to improve joint function and reduce pain.

11. Fracture Fixation: Surgical procedure to align and stabilize broken bones using various methods, such as plates, screws, rods, or external fixation devices.

12. Laminectomy: Surgical procedure to remove a portion of the vertebral bone called the lamina to relieve pressure on the spinal cord or nerves, often performed to treat spinal stenosis or herniated discs.

13. Achilles Tendon Repair: Surgical procedure to repair a ruptured or torn Achilles tendon, often requiring suturing or reattachment of the tendon ends.

14. Joint Arthroscopy: Minimally invasive procedure using a small camera and specialized instruments to visualize and treat joint conditions, such as removing loose bodies or repairing damaged tissues.

15. Debridement: Surgical procedure to remove damaged or infected tissue from a wound or joint, promoting healing and preventing further complications.

16. Osteotomy: Surgical procedure to cut and reposition a bone to correct deformities or improve alignment, often performed in cases of joint malalignment or bone fractures.

17. Open Reduction and Internal Fixation (ORIF): Surgical procedure to realign and stabilize fractured bones using open incisions and internal fixation devices, such as plates, screws, or pins.

18. Arthroplasty: Surgical procedure to restore or reconstruct a joint by reshaping or replacing the joint surfaces with prosthetic components.

19. Joint Revision Surgery: Surgical procedure to replace or repair a previously implanted artificial joint that has become worn, loose, or infected.

20. Synovectomy: Surgical procedure to remove the inflamed synovial lining of a joint, often performed in cases of rheumatoid arthritis or synovial joint disorders.

21. Joint Replacement Revision: Surgical procedure to replace a previously implanted artificial joint that has failed or worn out, requiring removal and replacement with a new prosthesis.

22. Hip Resurfacing: Surgical procedure that involves removing the damaged surface of the hip joint and capping it with a metal prosthesis, preserving more of the patient's natural bone compared to a total hip replacement.

23. Arthroplasty for Osteoarthritis: Surgical procedure to replace or resurface the damaged joint surfaces affected by osteoarthritis, reducing pain and improving joint function.

24. Elbow Arthroscopy: Minimally invasive procedure using a small camera and specialized instruments to diagnose and treat various elbow conditions, such as tennis elbow or loose bodies in the joint.

25. Limb Lengthening: Surgical procedure to increase the length of a bone in cases of congenital limb length discrepancies, skeletal deformities, or traumatic injuries, involving the gradual distraction of bone segments with external fixation devices.

III. Rehabilitation:

1. Physical Therapy: Rehabilitation program designed to improve physical function, mobility, strength, and flexibility through exercises, stretches, and manual therapy techniques.

2. Occupational Therapy: Rehabilitation therapy focused on helping individuals regain independence and functional skills necessary for daily activities, such as self-care, work, and leisure.

3. Speech Therapy: Rehabilitation therapy aimed at improving communication, language, speech, and swallowing abilities in individuals with speech or language disorders.

4. Aquatic Therapy: Rehabilitation therapy performed in a pool or water environment to reduce weight-bearing stress, improve mobility, and enhance physical function.

5. Balance and Vestibular Rehabilitation: Rehabilitation program targeting balance, coordination, and inner ear or vestibular disorders to improve stability and reduce dizziness or vertigo symptoms.

6. Pulmonary Rehabilitation: Rehabilitation program for individuals with respiratory conditions, focusing on improving lung function, breathing techniques, and overall endurance.

7. Cardiac Rehabilitation: Rehabilitation program for individuals recovering from heart-related conditions or procedures, aiming to improve cardiovascular health, strength, and endurance.

8. Neurorehabilitation: Rehabilitation program for individuals with neurological conditions, such as stroke, traumatic brain injury, or spinal cord injury, to restore or improve motor and cognitive function.

9. Orthotic and Prosthetic Rehabilitation: Rehabilitation program involving the use of orthotic or prosthetic devices to support or replace lost or impaired limb function, improving mobility and quality of life.

10. Sports Rehabilitation: Rehabilitation program tailored to athletes or individuals recovering from sports-related injuries, focusing on specific sport-specific movements, strength, and conditioning.

11. Geriatric Rehabilitation: Rehabilitation program for older adults to address age-related impairments, functional decline, and promote independence in daily activities.

12. Pediatric Rehabilitation: Rehabilitation program for children with developmental delays, congenital conditions, or injuries, aiming to enhance their physical, cognitive, and social abilities.

13. Cognitive Rehabilitation: Rehabilitation program targeting cognitive impairments or deficits following neurological conditions or brain injuries, helping individuals regain cognitive function and daily living skills.

14. Vocational Rehabilitation: Rehabilitation program assisting individuals with disabilities or injuries in transitioning back to work or finding suitable employment through vocational training and support services.

15. Pain Management Rehabilitation: Rehabilitation program focused on helping individuals manage chronic pain through various techniques, such as physical therapy, cognitive-behavioral therapy, and relaxation techniques.

16. Hand Therapy: Rehabilitation program specifically designed for hand and upper extremity conditions, involving exercises, splinting, and functional activities to improve hand function and dexterity.

17. Gait Training: Rehabilitation program targeting walking and gait abnormalities, utilizing specialized exercises and assistive devices to improve walking patterns and stability.

18. Assistive Technology Training: Rehabilitation program teaching individuals how to effectively use assistive devices, such as wheelchairs, walkers, or communication aids, to enhance independence and functionality.

19. Vocational Rehabilitation: Rehabilitation program assisting individuals with disabilities or injuries in transitioning back to work or finding suitable employment through vocational training and support services.

20. Group Therapy: Rehabilitation program conducted in a group setting, providing support, motivation, and camaraderie among individuals going through similar challenges.

21. Pain Management Techniques: Rehabilitation program incorporating various techniques to manage and alleviate pain, such as hot/cold therapy, transcutaneous electrical nerve stimulation (TENS), and relaxation exercises.

22. Assistive Device Training: Rehabilitation program focusing on teaching individuals how to effectively use assistive devices, such as canes, crutches, or mobility scooters, to enhance mobility and independence.

23. Aquatic Therapy: Rehabilitation program conducted in a pool or water environment to reduce weight-bearing stress, improve range of motion, and promote relaxation and overall well-being.

24. Constraint-Induced Movement Therapy: Rehabilitation technique used to improve motor function in individuals with limb weakness or paralysis, involving the restriction of movement in unaffected limbs to encourage the use and recovery of affected limbs.

25. Home Modification and Adaptive Equipment: Rehabilitation program providing guidance and recommendations for modifying the home environment and incorporating adaptive equipment to enhance safety and accessibility for individuals with disabilities or mobility limitations.

Practice activities for transcribing orthopedics reports effectively

Exercise 1: Fill in the blanks

Transcribe the following sentence:

The patient complained of _____ in the right knee.

Answer:

The patient complained of pain in the right knee.

Exercise 2: True or False

Indicate whether the following statement is true or false:

Arthroscopy is a surgical procedure used to visualize, diagnose, and treat joint problems.

Answer:

True

Exercise 3: Fill in the blanks

Transcribe the following sentence:

The patient underwent an _____ to repair a fractured bone.

Answer:

The patient underwent an open reduction internal fixation (ORIF) to repair a fractured bone.

Exercise 4: Matching

Match the orthopedic procedure with its description:

1. Total hip replacement

2. Arthroplasty

3. Spinal fusion

4. Knee arthroscopy

A. Surgical removal of damaged cartilage and bone in the knee joint and replacement with an artificial joint

B. Surgical procedure to replace a damaged or diseased hip joint with an artificial joint

C. Surgical procedure to join two or more vertebrae to stabilize the spine and reduce pain

D. Minimally invasive procedure to visualize and treat knee joint conditions using an arthroscope

Answer:

1. Total hip replacement

B. Surgical procedure to replace a damaged or diseased hip joint with an artificial joint

2. Arthroplasty

B. Surgical procedure to replace a damaged or diseased hip joint with an artificial joint

3. Spinal fusion

C. Surgical procedure to join two or more vertebrae to stabilize the spine and reduce pain

4. Knee arthroscopy

D. Minimally invasive procedure to visualize and treat knee joint conditions using an arthroscope

Exercise 5: Fill in the blanks

Transcribe the following sentence:

The patient's X-ray revealed a _____ fracture in the left arm.

Answer:

The patient's X-ray revealed a comminuted fracture in the left arm.

Exercise 6: True or False

Indicate whether the following statement is true or false:

Carpal tunnel syndrome is a condition that causes numbness, tingling, and weakness in the hand and arm due to compression of the median nerve.

Answer:

True

Exercise 7: Fill in the blanks

Transcribe the following sentence:

The patient was advised to use a _____ to support the injured ankle.

Answer:

The patient was advised to use a ankle brace to support the injured ankle.

Exercise 8: Matching

Match the orthopedic device with its description:

1. Cervical collar

2. Knee brace

3. Walking boot

4. Spinal brace

A. Brace worn to immobilize and support the spine after spinal surgery or injury

B. Device used to stabilize and immobilize the cervical spine in cases of neck injury or fracture

C. Device worn to provide support and stability to the knee joint during activities

D. Boot-like device used to protect and immobilize the foot and ankle after injury or surgery

Answer:

1. Cervical collar

B. Device used to stabilize and immobilize the cervical spine in cases of neck injury or fracture

2. Knee brace

C. Device worn to provide support and stability to the knee joint during activities

3. Walking boot

D. Boot-like device used to protect and immobilize the foot and ankle after injury or surgery

4. Spinal brace

A. Brace worn to immobilize and support the spine after spinal surgery or injury

Exercise 9: True or False

Indicate whether the following statement is true or false:

Rotator cuff tears are common injuries affecting the shoulder joint and can cause pain, weakness, and limited range of motion.

Answer:

True

Exercise 10: Fill in the blanks

Transcribe the following sentence:

The patient was referred to a physical therapist for ______ exercises to improve shoulder strength and flexibility.

Answer:

The patient was referred to a physical therapist for therapeutic exercises to improve shoulder strength and flexibility.

13. OTORHINOLARYNGOLOGY (ENT)

Anatomy of human ear

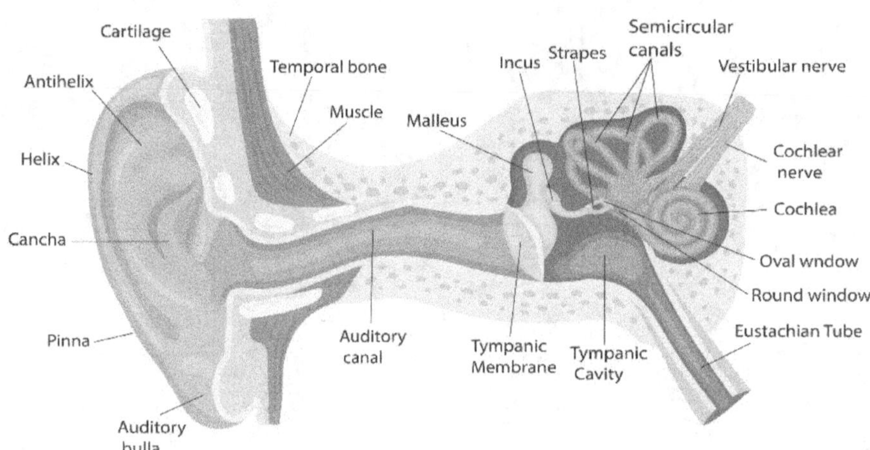

NOSE ANATOMY

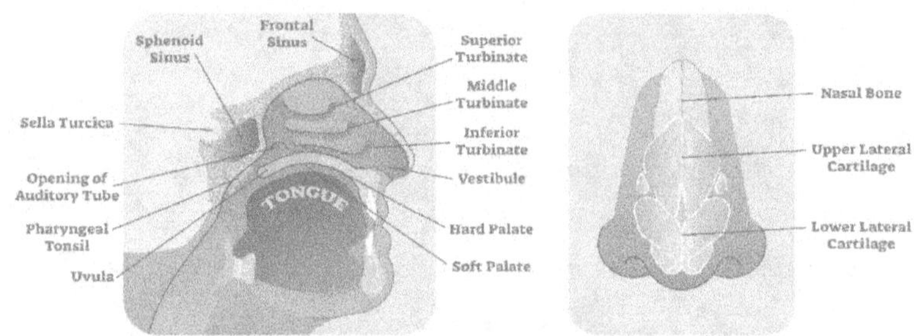

ANATOMY OF ORAL CAVITY

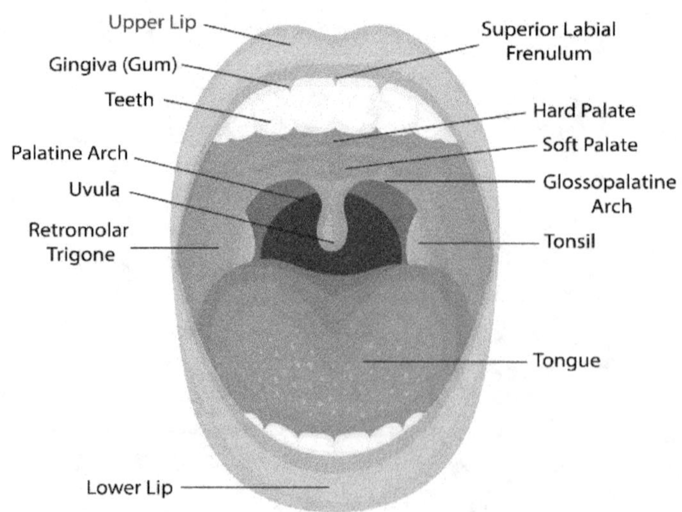

Otorhinolaryngology, often referred to as Ear, Nose, and Throat (ENT) medicine, is a medical specialty that focuses on the diagnosis and treatment of conditions affecting the ears, nose, throat, head, and neck.

Here are some key points to understand as a beginner in this field:

1. Ears, Nose, and Throat: The specialty got its common name from its focus on the three main anatomical areas it covers - the ears, nose, and throat. However, otolaryngologists also address conditions affecting the neck and head, including trauma, tumors, and deformities.

2. Common Conditions: Otolaryngologists diagnose and treat a wide range of conditions. These can include hearing loss, ear infections, balance disorders, tinnitus (ringing in the ears), congenital disorders of the outer and inner ear, sinusitis, allergies, disorders of the voice, swallowing disorders, and conditions affecting the larynx (voice box) and esophagus. They also manage diseases of the nasal cavity, paranasal sinuses, and conditions affecting the head and neck, including cancer.

3. Diagnostic Tools: Otolaryngologists use a variety of diagnostic tools, including physical exams, audiology tests, balance tests, endoscopes (a tool that allows the visualization of the structures inside the nose, throat, and ears), imaging studies like CT scans and MRIs, and biopsies for diagnosing cancer.

4. Treatment Approaches: Treatment in otolaryngology can involve medication, lifestyle modifications, and both minor and major surgery. This can range from simple procedures such as ear tube placement or tonsillectomy, to complex head and neck surgery and reconstruction.

5. Subspecialties: There are several subspecialties within otolaryngology, including pediatric otolaryngology (children's ear, nose, and throat disorders), otology/neurotology (ears, balance, and tinnitus), allergy, facial plastic and reconstructive surgery, head and neck (treatment of cancerous and noncancerous tumors), laryngology (throat, voice, and swallowing), and rhinology (nose and sinuses).

6. Head and Neck Surgery: Otolaryngologists are trained to perform both cosmetic and reconstructive surgery in the head and neck region, manage problems with the upper aero-digestive tract, and treat cancers of the head and neck, including the thyroid and parathyroid.

Ear, nose, and throat conditions, diagnostic procedures, and surgeries

I. Ear, Nose, and Throat Conditions:

1. Otitis Media: Inflammation of the middle ear, often caused by bacterial or viral infections. It can result in ear pain, hearing loss, and fluid accumulation behind the eardrum.

2. Sinusitis: Inflammation of the sinuses, commonly caused by viral, bacterial, or fungal infections. Symptoms include facial pain, congestion, and nasal discharge.

3. Tonsillitis: Inflammation of the tonsils, usually due to bacterial or viral infections. It can lead to sore throat, difficulty swallowing, and swollen tonsils.

4. Pharyngitis: Inflammation of the throat, often caused by viral or bacterial infections. It presents as a sore throat, difficulty swallowing, and swollen lymph nodes.

5. Allergic Rhinitis: An allergic reaction to airborne allergens, causing nasal congestion, sneezing, and itching. It can be seasonal (hay fever) or perennial (year-round).

6. Deviated Septum: A structural abnormality in the nasal septum, which can cause nasal congestion, frequent sinus infections, and difficulty breathing.

7. Sleep Apnea: A sleep disorder characterized by pauses in breathing during sleep. It can result in excessive daytime sleepiness, loud snoring, and interrupted sleep.

8. Laryngitis: Inflammation of the larynx or voice box, often due to viral infections or overuse of the voice. It leads to hoarseness, loss of voice, and throat discomfort.

9. Tinnitus: The perception of ringing or buzzing sounds in the ears, which can be caused by various factors, including exposure to loud noise or certain medical conditions.

10. Vertigo: A sensation of spinning or dizziness, usually associated with inner ear disorders such as benign paroxysmal positional vertigo (BPPV) or Meniere's disease.

11. Nasal Polyps: Soft, noncancerous growths on the lining of the nose or sinuses. They can cause nasal congestion, runny nose, and a decreased sense of smell.

12. Epistaxis: Commonly known as a nosebleed, it occurs when blood vessels in the nose rupture, resulting in bleeding from the nostrils.

13. Laryngeal Cancer: Cancer that develops in the tissues of the larynx. Symptoms may include hoarseness, persistent cough, and difficulty swallowing.

14. Chronic Rhinosinusitis: Ongoing inflammation of the nasal passages and sinuses, lasting for at least 12 weeks. It causes nasal congestion, facial pain, and postnasal drip.

15. Glue Ear: A condition in which thick fluid accumulates in the middle ear, causing hearing loss, particularly in children.

16. Adenoiditis: Inflammation of the adenoids, located in the back of the throat. It can lead to breathing difficulties, snoring, and recurrent ear infections.

17. Otitis Externa: Inflammation of the ear canal, often called swimmer's ear. It causes ear pain, itching, and discharge.

18. Thyroid Nodules: Abnormal growths or lumps in the thyroid gland. Most nodules are benign, but they may require further evaluation and treatment.

19. Hoarseness: A change in voice quality, often characterized by a raspy, strained, or weak voice. It can result from vocal cord polyps, laryngitis, or vocal cord paralysis.

20. Salivary Gland Stones: Hard deposits that form in the salivary glands, causing pain and swelling, particularly when eating or drinking.

21. Meniere's Disease: A disorder of the inner ear characterized by episodes of vertigo, hearing loss, tinnitus, and a feeling of fullness in the ear.

22. Adenoid Hypertrophy: Enlargement of the adenoids, commonly seen in children. It can cause nasal congestion, snoring, and recurrent ear infections.

23. Nasal Fracture: A break or crack in the bones of the nose, often resulting from trauma or injury. It causes pain, swelling, and difficulty breathing through the nose.

24. Nasal Vestibulitis: Inflammation of the nasal vestibule, typically caused by bacterial infection. It presents as redness, tenderness, and crusting of the nasal lining.

25. Nasal Septal Perforation: A hole or opening in the nasal septum, usually resulting from injury, previous surgeries, or certain medical conditions. It can cause nasal obstruction, nosebleeds, and whistle-like breathing.

II. Diagnostic Procedures:

1. Otoscopy: Examination of the ear using an otoscope to visualize the ear canal, eardrum, and middle ear structures.

2. Audiometry: Assessment of hearing ability using various tests, such as pure-tone audiometry and speech audiometry.

3. Rhinoscopy: Visualization of the nasal cavity and nasal passages using a nasal endoscope or speculum.

4. Nasal Smear: Collection of nasal secretions for laboratory analysis to identify allergens or infection-causing agents.

5. Tympanometry: Measurement of middle ear pressure and eardrum movement to assess middle ear function.

6. Laryngoscopy: Examination of the larynx and vocal cords using a laryngoscope to detect abnormalities or assess vocal cord function.

7. Flexible Laryngoscopy: Visualization of the larynx and vocal cords using a flexible endoscope passed through the nose or mouth.

8. Videostroboscopy: A specialized form of laryngoscopy that uses strobe light to visualize vocal cord movement and assess vocal cord function.

9. Fiberoptic Bronchoscopy: Insertion of a thin, flexible tube with a camera (bronchoscope) through the nose or mouth to examine the airways and lungs.

10. Sinus CT Scan: Imaging of the paranasal sinuses using computed tomography (CT) to evaluate sinus conditions, such as sinusitis or nasal polyps.

11. Fine Needle Aspiration (FNA): The extraction of cells or fluid from a suspicious lump or swollen lymph node using a thin needle for further evaluation.

12. Allergy Testing: Various tests, including skin prick tests or blood tests (specific IgE), to identify allergens causing allergic reactions.

13. Barium Swallow: X-ray examination of the esophagus and upper digestive tract after swallowing barium contrast material to detect abnormalities or swallowing difficulties.

14. pH Monitoring: Measurement of acid levels in the esophagus using a pH probe to diagnose gastroesophageal reflux disease (GERD).

15. Esophagoscopy: Visual examination of the esophagus using an endoscope to evaluate swallowing difficulties, strictures, or abnormal growths.

16. Sleep Study (Polysomnography): Evaluation of sleep patterns, breathing, and oxygen levels during sleep to diagnose sleep disorders such as sleep apnea.

17. Videonystagmography (VNG): Assessment of eye movements and balance function using infrared goggles to diagnose vestibular disorders or evaluate dizziness.

18. Biopsy: Removal of a small tissue sample for microscopic examination to determine if abnormal growths or lesions are cancerous or noncancerous.

19. Nasal Endoscopy: Insertion of a thin, flexible tube with a camera (endoscope) into the nose to visualize the nasal cavity and detect abnormalities.

20. Tilt Table Test: Evaluation of the cardiovascular response to changes in body position to diagnose conditions like orthostatic hypotension or syncope.

21. Skin Prick Test: Allergy testing method involving the application of small amounts of allergens to the skin surface to identify specific allergies.

22. Patch Test: A test performed to identify contact allergies by applying patches containing potential allergens to the skin.

23. Computed Tomography Angiography (CTA): A specialized CT scan that visualizes the blood vessels to evaluate conditions like vascular malformations or tumors.

24. Magnetic Resonance Imaging (MRI): Imaging technique that uses magnetic fields and radio waves to generate detailed images of the structures within the head and neck.

25. Video Fluoroscopy Swallow Study: Real-time X-ray examination of swallowing function and the passage of food or liquid through the throat to detect swallowing disorders.

III. Surgeries:

1. Tonsillectomy: Surgical removal of the tonsils to treat recurrent tonsillitis or sleep-disordered breathing.

2. Adenoidectomy: Surgical removal of the adenoids, located at the back of the nose, to address chronic infection or obstruction.

3. Septoplasty: Correction of a deviated septum to improve nasal airflow and alleviate breathing difficulties.

4. Sinus Surgery: Various surgical procedures, such as functional endoscopic sinus surgery (FESS), to remove nasal polyps, treat chronic sinusitis, or address sinus blockages.

5. Myringotomy: Incision made in the eardrum to drain fluid from the middle ear and insert ventilation tubes for recurrent ear infections.

6. Mastoidectomy: Surgical removal of infected mastoid air cells, usually performed to treat chronic ear infections or cholesteatoma.

7. Tympanoplasty: Reconstruction of the eardrum or middle ear bones (ossicles) to restore hearing and treat eardrum perforations.

8. Cochlear Implant Surgery: Surgical implantation of a device to restore hearing in individuals with severe hearing loss or deafness.

9. Laryngectomy: Surgical removal of the larynx (voice box) to treat laryngeal cancer, usually followed by a tracheostomy to create a stoma for breathing.

10. Thyroidectomy: Surgical removal of all or part of the thyroid gland to treat thyroid disorders, including thyroid nodules or thyroid cancer.

11. Parathyroidectomy: Surgical removal of one or more parathyroid glands to address hyperparathyroidism or parathyroid tumors.

12. Neck Dissection: Surgical removal of lymph nodes and surrounding tissues in the neck to treat head and neck cancers.

13. Uvulopalatopharyngoplasty (UPPP): Surgical procedure to remove excess tissue in the throat, such as the uvula and parts of the soft palate, to alleviate snoring and sleep apnea.

14. Vocal Cord Surgery: Various surgical procedures, such as vocal cord polyp removal or vocal cord injection, to address voice disorders or vocal cord lesions.

15. Salivary Gland Surgery: Surgical interventions to remove salivary gland tumors, manage salivary duct stones, or address salivary gland infections.

16. Maxillofacial Surgery: Surgical procedures involving the jaw, face, or oral cavity, such as corrective jaw surgery, facial reconstruction, or dental implant placement.

17. Turbinate Reduction Surgery: Surgical reduction or removal of the nasal turbinates to alleviate nasal congestion and improve airflow.

18. Tonsillotomy: Partial removal of the tonsils to treat obstructive sleep apnea in select cases.

19. Rhinoplasty: Cosmetic or functional surgery to reshape or reconstruct the nose, addressing structural abnormalities or improving nasal aesthetics.

20. Laryngeal Framework Surgery: Surgical procedures to correct vocal cord paralysis or improve vocal cord function and voice quality.

21. Stapedectomy: Surgical replacement of the stapes bone in the middle ear to improve hearing in cases of otosclerosis.

22. Nasal Valve Repair: Surgical interventions to address nasal valve collapse, improving nasal breathing and airflow.

23. Parotidectomy: Surgical removal of the parotid gland, usually performed to treat parotid tumors or manage chronic infections.

24. Endoscopic Skull Base Surgery: Minimally invasive surgical procedures to address skull base tumors or lesions, often utilizing endoscopes.

25. Tracheal Reconstruction: Surgical procedures to repair or reconstruct the trachea (windpipe), usually done to address tracheal stenosis or tracheal damage.

Exercises for transcribing otolaryngology reports accurately

Exercise 1: Fill in the blanks

Transcribe the following sentence:

The patient complained of _______ in the left ear.

Answer:

The patient complained of pain in the left ear.

Exercise 2: True or False

Indicate whether the following statement is true or false:

Tonsillectomy is a surgical procedure to remove the tonsils.

Answer:

True

Exercise 3: Fill in the blanks

Transcribe the following sentence:

The patient was diagnosed with ______, an inflammation of the middle ear.

Answer:

The patient was diagnosed with otitis media, an inflammation of the middle ear.

Exercise 4: Matching

Match the otolaryngology procedure with its description:

1. Rhinoplasty

2. Tympanoplasty

3. Adenoidectomy

4. Septoplasty

A. Surgical procedure to correct a deviated nasal septum and improve nasal airflow

B. Surgical procedure to reshape or reconstruct the nose for cosmetic or functional purposes

C. Surgical removal of the adenoids, often performed to relieve chronic nasal congestion or recurrent ear infections

D. Surgical procedure to repair a perforated eardrum and restore hearing

Answer:

1. Rhinoplasty

B. Surgical procedure to reshape or reconstruct the nose for cosmetic or functional purposes

2. Tympanoplasty

D. Surgical procedure to repair a perforated eardrum and restore hearing

3. Adenoidectomy

C. Surgical removal of the adenoids, often performed to relieve chronic nasal congestion or recurrent ear infections

4. Septoplasty

A. Surgical procedure to correct a deviated nasal septum and improve nasal airflow

Exercise 5: Fill in the blanks

Transcribe the following sentence:

The patient underwent a _______ to remove nasal polyps.

Answer:

The patient underwent a polypectomy to remove nasal polyps.

Exercise 6: True or False

Indicate whether the following statement is true or false:

Laryngitis is an inflammation of the vocal cords that can cause hoarseness or loss of voice.

Answer:

True

Exercise 7: Fill in the blanks

Transcribe the following sentence:

The patient was advised to use _______ drops to relieve ear pain.

Answer:

The patient was advised to use ear drops to relieve ear pain.

Exercise 8: Matching

Match the otolaryngology condition with its description:

1. Sinusitis

2. Epistaxis

3. Tonsillitis

4. Vertigo

A. Inflammation of the sinuses, often causing facial pain, nasal congestion, and sinus pressure

B. Medical term for a nosebleed

C. Inflammation of the tonsils, resulting in a sore throat, difficulty swallowing, and swollen tonsils

D. A sensation of spinning or dizziness, often associated with inner ear problems

Answer:

1. Sinusitis

A. Inflammation of the sinuses, often causing facial pain, nasal congestion, and sinus pressure

2. Epistaxis

B. Medical term for a nosebleed

3. Tonsillitis

C. Inflammation of the tonsils, resulting in a sore throat, difficulty swallowing, and swollen tonsils

4. Vertigo

D. A sensation of spinning or dizziness, often associated with inner ear problems

Exercise 9: True or False

Indicate whether the following statement is true or false:

Otoplasty is a surgical procedure to correct prominent or misshapen ears.

Answer:

True

Exercise 10: Fill in the blanks

Transcribe the following sentence:

The patient was referred to a ______ for speech therapy to address voice disorders.

Answer:

The patient was referred to a speech-language pathologist for speech therapy to address voice disorders.

HUMAN RESPIRATORY SYSTEM

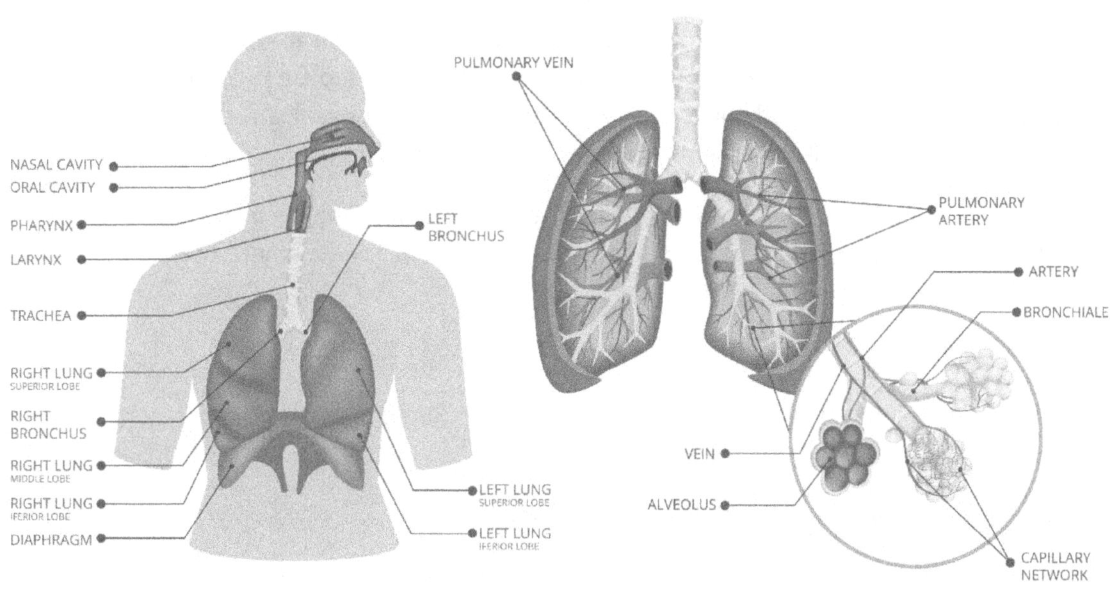

Understanding pulmonology and its specific terminology

Pulmonology, also known as pneumology or respiratory medicine, is a medical specialty that deals with diseases involving the respiratory tract. This specialty is generally classified as a subspecialty of internal medicine.

Here are some key points to understand as a beginner in this field:

1. Respiratory System: The respiratory system consists of the organs and tissues that allow us to breathe, including the nasal passages, pharynx, larynx, trachea, bronchi, and lungs. Its primary function is to supply the blood with oxygen so it can be delivered to all parts of the body.

2. Common Conditions: Pulmonologists diagnose and treat a wide range of conditions that affect the respiratory system. These include chronic obstructive pulmonary disease (COPD), asthma, pneumonia, tuberculosis, lung cancers, pulmonary fibrosis, and acute and chronic respiratory failure, among others.

3. Diagnostic Tools: Pulmonologists use various diagnostic tools, including pulmonary function tests (PFTs) to assess how well your lungs work, imaging studies such as chest X-rays and CT scans to visualize the lungs, and bronchoscopy to examine the airways. They may also use laboratory tests to identify infections or other diseases affecting the lungs.

4. Treatment Approaches: Treatment in pulmonology can involve lifestyle modifications (like smoking cessation), medications (like inhalers for asthma or antibiotics for infections), and occasionally, surgery. For instance, severe conditions such as lung cancer or end-stage lung disease may require surgical interventions, including lung transplantation.

5. Pulmonary Subspecialties: There are several subspecialties within pulmonology, including interventional pulmonology (using endoscopic techniques to diagnose and treat conditions), pulmonary rehabilitation (improving function and quality of life in those with lung disease), and critical care (managing patients in the intensive care unit, often with severe respiratory problems).

6. Sleep Medicine: Many pulmonologists also specialize in sleep medicine, as many sleep disorders are linked to respiratory function. This can include conditions like sleep apnea, where breathing repeatedly stops and starts during sleep.

Respiratory system disorders, pulmonary function tests, and interventions

I. Respiratory System Disorders:

1. Asthma: A chronic respiratory condition characterized by inflammation and narrowing of the airways, leading to recurring episodes of wheezing, shortness of breath, and coughing. It is often triggered by allergies, exercise, or exposure to irritants.

2. Chronic Obstructive Pulmonary Disease (COPD): A progressive lung disease that causes airflow limitation, including conditions such as chronic bronchitis and emphysema. It is commonly caused by smoking or exposure to harmful substances.

3. Pneumonia: Infection in one or both lungs, usually caused by bacteria, viruses, or fungi, leading to inflammation and fluid buildup in the air sacs. It can cause symptoms such as cough, fever, chest pain, and difficulty breathing.

4. Tuberculosis (TB): An infectious disease caused by Mycobacterium tuberculosis bacteria, primarily affecting the lungs and causing symptoms such as cough, chest pain, and fatigue. It can be transmitted through the air.

5. Pulmonary Fibrosis: A condition characterized by the scarring and thickening of lung tissue, leading to reduced lung function and shortness of breath. It can be caused by various factors, including exposure to environmental toxins or certain medications.

6. Lung Cancer: Malignant growths in the lungs that can arise from various factors, including smoking, exposure to toxins, or genetic predisposition. It can cause symptoms such as persistent cough, chest pain, and unexplained weight loss.

7. Pulmonary Embolism: A blockage in the pulmonary arteries, usually caused by a blood clot that travels from elsewhere in the body, leading to reduced blood flow to the lungs. It can result in sudden onset of chest pain, difficulty breathing, and even life-threatening complications.

8. Sleep Apnea: A sleep disorder characterized by pauses in breathing or shallow breathing during sleep, often accompanied by loud snoring and daytime sleepiness. It can lead to fatigue, poor sleep quality, and increased risk of cardiovascular problems.

9. Cystic Fibrosis: A genetic disorder that affects the production of mucus, leading to the buildup of thick, sticky mucus in the lungs and other organs. It can cause recurrent lung infections, cough, and difficulty breathing.

10. Interstitial Lung Disease: A group of lung disorders characterized by progressive scarring of the lung tissue, impairing lung function and gas exchange. It can cause symptoms such as cough, shortness of breath, and fatigue.

11. Bronchiectasis: A condition characterized by abnormal widening and scarring of the bronchial tubes, leading to chronic cough, mucus production, and recurrent respiratory infections.

12. Pleural Effusion: The accumulation of fluid in the pleural space, the thin space between the lungs and the chest wall, causing difficulty in breathing. It can result from various causes, including infections, heart failure, or cancer.

13. Pulmonary Hypertension: High blood pressure in the arteries of the lungs, resulting in increased resistance and strain on the heart. It can lead to symptoms such as shortness of breath, fatigue, and chest pain.

14. Allergic Rhinitis: Inflammation of the nasal passages caused by an allergic response to substances such as pollen, dust mites, or animal dander. It can cause symptoms like sneezing, itching, nasal congestion, and runny nose.

15. Pneumothorax: The presence of air or gas in the pleural cavity, causing the lung to collapse partially or completely. It can result from trauma, underlying lung diseases, or spontaneous rupture of air-filled sacs in the lungs.

16. Chronic Rhinosinusitis: Inflammation of the nasal passages and sinuses that lasts for an extended period, often characterized by nasal congestion, facial pain or pressure, and postnasal drip.

17. Pulmonary Edema: The buildup of fluid in the air sacs of the lungs, leading to difficulty breathing, coughing, and wheezing. It can be caused by heart problems, infections, or exposure to certain toxins.

18. Obstructive Sleep Apnea: A form of sleep apnea characterized by repeated episodes of partial or complete blockage of the upper airway during sleep, resulting in disrupted breathing and frequent awakening.

19. Occupational Lung Diseases: Lung conditions caused by exposure to specific substances in the workplace, such as asbestos, silica dust, or chemicals, leading to respiratory symptoms and lung damage.

20. Pleurisy: Inflammation of the pleura, the thin membrane that lines the chest cavity and covers the lungs, causing sharp chest pain that worsens with deep breathing or coughing.

21. Pulmonary Fibrosis: A progressive lung disease characterized by the formation of scar tissue in the lungs, leading to stiffness and reduced lung capacity.

22. Pulmonary Nodules: Small, round growths or lesions in the lungs, often incidentally detected on imaging studies. They can be benign or indicative of underlying conditions such as lung cancer.

23. Rhinosinusitis: Inflammation of the nasal passages and sinuses, causing symptoms such as nasal congestion, facial pain or pressure, and thick nasal discharge.

24. Pleuritic Chest Pain: Sharp, stabbing chest pain that worsens with breathing, often associated with inflammation of the pleura or other underlying conditions.

25. Upper Respiratory Tract Infections: Infections affecting the nose, throat, sinuses, or larynx, commonly caused by viruses and resulting in symptoms such as nasal congestion, sore throat, and cough.

II. Pulmonary Function Tests:

1. Spirometry: A common pulmonary function test that measures how much air you can breathe in and out and how quickly you can exhale.

2. Peak Expiratory Flow (PEF) Test: A simple test that measures how fast you can exhale forcefully, often used to monitor and manage asthma.

3. Lung Volume Measurements: Tests that measure the total lung capacity, residual volume, and other lung volumes to assess lung function and diagnose conditions such as restrictive lung disease.

4. Diffusion Capacity Test: A test that measures how well oxygen moves from the lungs into the bloodstream, helping to evaluate lung health and detect conditions such as pulmonary fibrosis.

5. Arterial Blood Gas (ABG) Test: A blood test that measures oxygen and carbon dioxide levels in the blood, providing information about respiratory function and acid-base balance.

6. Exercise Stress Test: A test that evaluates lung function during physical exertion, usually performed on a treadmill or stationary bike.

7. Methacholine Challenge Test: A test used to diagnose and assess the severity of asthma by measuring how sensitive the airways are to a specific medication (methacholine) that can cause airway constriction.

8. Fractional Exhaled Nitric Oxide (FeNO) Test: A non-invasive test that measures the level of nitric oxide in breath, which can indicate airway inflammation and help manage conditions like asthma.

9. Bronchial Provocation Test: A test that assesses airway hyperresponsiveness by exposing the patient to specific triggers (such as allergens or chemicals) to provoke bronchospasm.

10. Lung Clearance Index (LCI): A test used primarily in children to assess small airway function and detect early signs of lung disease.

11. Maximal Inspiratory and Expiratory Pressures: Tests that measure the strength of the respiratory muscles, helping to evaluate respiratory muscle function and diagnose conditions such as neuromuscular disorders.

12. Pulse Oximetry: A non-invasive test that measures oxygen saturation levels in the blood, often performed using a small device attached to a finger or earlobe.

13. Bronchoscopy: A procedure in which a flexible tube with a light and camera is inserted into the airways to visually examine the lungs and collect samples for further analysis.

14. Fractional Carbon Monoxide Diffusing Capacity (DLCO): A test that measures the ability of the lungs to transfer carbon monoxide from inhaled air to the bloodstream, providing information about gas exchange in the lungs.

15. Sleep Studies: Tests conducted during sleep to evaluate respiratory function, assess sleep disorders such as sleep apnea, and monitor oxygen levels.

16. Forced Oscillation Technique (FOT): A non-invasive test that measures the resistance and reactance of the respiratory system, providing information about airway function and respiratory mechanics.

17. Exercise Oximetry: A test that monitors oxygen saturation levels during exercise to assess how well the lungs and cardiovascular system deliver oxygen to the body.

18. Capnography: A test that measures the level of carbon dioxide in exhaled breath, helping to monitor respiratory status and assess ventilation.

19. Respiratory Muscle Strength Testing: Tests such as maximal inspiratory pressure (MIP) and maximal expiratory pressure (MEP) that assess the strength and function of the respiratory muscles.

20. High-Altitude Simulation Test: A test that mimics the effects of high altitude on the body to evaluate respiratory adaptation and identify individuals at risk of altitude-related complications.

21. Provocative Testing: Tests that involve exposure to specific substances or stimuli to assess respiratory allergies, irritant sensitivity, or exercise-induced bronchoconstriction.

22. Fractional Exhaled Hydrogen Peroxide (FeH2O2) Test: A test used to assess airway inflammation by measuring the level of hydrogen peroxide in exhaled breath condensate.

23. Maximal Voluntary Ventilation (MVV) Test: A test that measures the maximum amount of air a person can breathe in and out within a specific time frame, providing information about overall lung function.

24. Impulse Oscillometry (IOS): A non-invasive test that measures lung resistance and reactance using small pressure waves, helping to evaluate airway function and detect respiratory abnormalities.

25. Exercise-induced Bronchospasm (EIB) Test: A test that assesses airway responsiveness during exercise to diagnose exercise-induced bronchospasm, a common symptom in individuals with asthma or exercise-induced asthma.

III. Interventions:

1. Bronchodilators: Medications that relax the muscles surrounding the airways, helping to open up the air passages and improve airflow in conditions such as asthma and chronic obstructive pulmonary disease (COPD).

2. Inhaled Corticosteroids: Medications that reduce inflammation in the airways, helping to manage chronic respiratory conditions such as asthma and COPD.

3. Oxygen Therapy: Administration of supplemental oxygen to individuals with low blood oxygen levels, providing support for respiratory function and improving oxygenation.

4. Respiratory Physiotherapy: Techniques and exercises aimed at improving lung function, clearing mucus from the airways, and enhancing breathing efficiency.

5. Mechanical Ventilation: The use of a machine to support or replace spontaneous breathing in individuals with severe respiratory failure or during surgical procedures.

6. Chest Physiotherapy: Manual techniques, such as chest percussion and vibration, to help loosen and remove mucus from the lungs in conditions like cystic fibrosis and bronchiectasis.

7. Pulmonary Rehabilitation: A comprehensive program that combines exercise training, education, and support to improve lung function, reduce symptoms, and enhance quality of life in individuals with chronic respiratory conditions.

8. Smoking Cessation: Assistance and support to help individuals quit smoking, as smoking cessation is crucial for preventing and managing respiratory disorders.

9. Antibiotic Therapy: Medications prescribed to treat respiratory infections caused by bacteria, helping to eliminate the infection and alleviate symptoms.

10. Lung Transplantation: Surgical replacement of a diseased lung with a healthy lung from a donor, typically reserved for individuals with end-stage lung disease who have not responded to other treatments.

11. Pulmonary Artery Catheterization: Insertion of a catheter into the pulmonary artery to monitor heart and lung function, especially in critically ill patients.

12. Respiratory Support: Various methods to provide respiratory support, including non-invasive ventilation (e.g., continuous positive airway pressure, bilevel positive airway pressure) or invasive mechanical ventilation in critical care settings.

13. Immunotherapy: Treatment options, such as allergen immunotherapy or monoclonal antibody therapy, to address specific respiratory conditions like allergic rhinitis or severe asthma.

14. Airway Clearance Devices: Devices designed to assist with clearing mucus from the airways, improving lung function and preventing respiratory complications.

15. Lifestyle Modifications: Encouraging individuals to adopt healthy lifestyle habits, such as regular exercise, weight management, and avoiding respiratory irritants, to optimize respiratory health and prevent exacerbations.

16. Thoracentesis: A procedure to remove fluid or air from the pleural space around the lungs, relieving symptoms and improving lung function.

17. Bronchoscopy: A procedure that uses a thin, flexible tube with a light and camera to visualize the airways and collect samples for diagnosis or treat specific respiratory conditions.

18. Lung Volume Reduction Surgery: Surgical removal of damaged or diseased portions of the lung to improve lung function and relieve symptoms in individuals with severe emphysema.

19. Pulmonary Rehabilitation: A comprehensive program that combines exercise training, education, and support to improve lung function, reduce symptoms, and enhance quality of life in individuals with chronic respiratory conditions.

20. Tracheostomy: Surgical creation of an opening in the neck into the windpipe to assist with breathing, often performed in cases of severe airway obstruction or long-term ventilator support.

21. Pulmonary Rehabilitation: A comprehensive program that combines exercise training, education, and support to improve lung function, reduce symptoms, and enhance quality of life in individuals with chronic respiratory conditions.

22. Non-invasive Positive Pressure Ventilation (NIPPV): The use of a mask or nasal device to deliver pressurized air to the lungs, supporting breathing and improving oxygenation in conditions such as obstructive sleep apnea or respiratory failure.

23. Chest Tube Insertion: Placement of a tube into the chest to drain fluid, air, or blood from the pleural space, helping to re-expand the lung and relieve symptoms.

24. Lung Resection: Surgical removal of a portion of the lung affected by a tumor, infection, or other respiratory conditions.

25. Respiratory Medications: Various medications, such as bronchodilators, corticosteroids, antibiotics, and mucolytics, prescribed to manage respiratory symptoms, reduce inflammation, treat infections, and improve lung function.

Practice activities for transcribing pulmonology reports effectively

Exercise 1: Fill in the blanks

Transcribe the following sentence:

The patient presented with ______ and shortness of breath.

Answer:

The patient presented with cough and shortness of breath.

Exercise 2: True or False

Indicate whether the following statement is true or false:

Spirometry is a diagnostic test used to measure lung function.

Answer:

True

Exercise 3: Fill in the blanks

Transcribe the following sentence:

The chest X-ray revealed _______ in the right lung.

Answer:

The chest X-ray revealed consolidation in the right lung.

Exercise 4: Matching

Match the pulmonology procedure with its description:

1. Bronchoscopy

2. Pulmonary function test

3. Thoracentesis

4. Sleep study

A. Diagnostic test to evaluate the airways and collect samples for further examination

B. Noninvasive test to measure the volume and flow of air during breathing

C. Procedure to remove excess fluid or air from the pleural space surrounding the lungs

D. Procedure to examine the airways using a flexible tube with a light and camera

Answer:

1. Bronchoscopy

D. Procedure to examine the airways using a flexible tube with a light and camera

2. Pulmonary function test

B. Noninvasive test to measure the volume and flow of air during breathing

3. Thoracentesis

C. Procedure to remove excess fluid or air from the pleural space surrounding the lungs

4. Sleep study

A. Diagnostic test to evaluate the airways and collect samples for further examination

Exercise 5: Fill in the blanks

Transcribe the following sentence:

The patient was prescribed _______ to manage their asthma symptoms.

Answer:

The patient was prescribed inhalers to manage their asthma symptoms.

Exercise 6: True or False

Indicate whether the following statement is true or false:

Pneumonia is an infection that causes inflammation in the air sacs of the lungs.

Answer:

True

Exercise 7: Fill in the blanks

Transcribe the following sentence:

The patient's oxygen saturation level was ______%.

Answer:

The patient's oxygen saturation level was 95%.

Exercise 8: Matching

Match the pulmonology condition with its description:

1. Chronic obstructive pulmonary disease (COPD)

2. Asthma

3. Pneumothorax

4. Pulmonary embolism

A. A chronic lung condition characterized by difficulty breathing and reduced lung function

B. Inflammatory lung disease causing narrowing of the airways and difficulty breathing

C. Collapse of the lung due to the accumulation of air in the pleural space

D. Blockage of a pulmonary artery by a blood clot, leading to reduced blood flow to the lungs

Answer:

1. Chronic obstructive pulmonary disease (COPD)

A. A chronic lung condition characterized by difficulty breathing and reduced lung function

2. Asthma

B. Inflammatory lung disease causing narrowing of the airways and difficulty breathing

3. Pneumothorax

C. Collapse of the lung due to the accumulation of air in the pleural space

4. Pulmonary embolism

D. Blockage of a pulmonary artery by a blood clot, leading to reduced blood flow to the lungs

Exercise 9: True or False

Indicate whether the following statement is true or false:

Lung cancer is the most common cause of cancer-related deaths worldwide.

Answer:

True

Exercise 10: Fill in the blanks

Transcribe the following sentence:

The patient's _______ revealed a high eosinophil count.

Answer:

The patient's blood test revealed a high eosinophil count.

Common Laboratory Values

CBC			
Test	Normal value	Function	Significance
Hemoglobin	12-18 g/100 mL	Measures oxygen carrying capacity of blood	Low: hemorrhage, anemia High: polycythemia
Hematocrit	35%-50%	Measures relative volume of cells and plasma in blood	Low: hemorrhage, anemia High: polycythemia, dehydration
Red blood cell	4-6 million/mm³	Measures oxygen-carrying capacity of blood	Low: hemorrhage, anemia High: polycythemia, heart disease, pulmonary disease
White blood cell Infant 4-7 y 8-18 y	 8,000-15,000/mm³ 6,000-15,000/mm³ 4,500-13,500/mm³	Measures host defense against inflammatory agents	Low: aplastic anemia, drug toxicity, specific infections High: inflammation, trauma, toxicity, leukemia

Diffential Count		
Test	Normal value	Significance
Neutrophils	54%-62%	Increase in bacterial infections, hemorrhage, diabetic acidosis
Lymphocytes	25%-30%	Viral and bacterial infections, acute and chronic lymphocytic leukemia, antigen reaction
Eosinophils	1%-3%	Increase in parasitic and allergic conditions, blood dyscrasias, pernicious anemia
Basophils	1%	Increase in types of blood dyscrasias
Monocytes	0%-9%	Hodgkin's disease, lipid storage disease, recovery from severe infections, monocytic leukemia

Absolute Neutrophil Count (ANC)		
Calculation	Normal value	Significance
$\dfrac{(\%\ \text{Polymorphonuclear Leukocytes} + \%\ \text{Bands}) \times \text{Total White Cell Count}}{100}$	>1500	<1000 Patient at increased risk for infection; defer elective dental care

Bleeding Screen			
Test	Normal value	Function	Significance
Prothrombin time	1-18 sec	Measures extrinsic	Prolonged in liver disease, impaired Vitamin K production, surgical trauma with blood loss
Partial thromboplastin time	By laboratory control	Measures intrinsic clotting of blood, congenital clotting disorders	Prolonged in hemophilia A, B, and C and Von Willebrand's disease
Platelets	140,000-340,000/mL	Measures clotting potential	Increased in polycythemia, leukemia, severe hemorrhage; decreased in thrombocytopenia purpura
Bleeding time	1-6 min	Measures quality of platelets	Prolonged in thrombocytopenia
International Normalized Ratio (INR)	Without anticoagulant therapy: 1; Anticoagulant therapy target range: 2-3	Measures extrinsic clotting function	Increased with anticoagulant therapy

Urinalysis			
Test	Normal value	Function	Significance
Volume	1,000-2,000 mL/day		Increase in diabetes mellitus, chronic nephritis
Specific gravity	1.015-1.025	Measures the degree of tubular reabsorption and dehydration	Increase in diabetes mellitus; decrease in acute nephritis, diabetes insipidus, aldosteronism
pH	6-8	Reflects acidosis and alkalosis	Acidic: diabetes, acidosis, prolonged fever Alkaline: urinary tract infection, alkalosis
Casts	1-2 per high power field		Renal tubule degeneration occurring in cardiac failure, pregnancy, and hemogobinuric-nephrosis

Electrolytes			
Test	Normal value	Function	Significance
Sodium (Na)	135-147 mEq		Increase in Crushing's syndrome
Potassium (K)	3.5-5 mEq		Increase in tissue breakdown
Bicarbonate (HCO_3)	24-30 mEq	Reflects acid-base balance	
Chloride (Cl)	100-106 mEq		Increase in renal disease and hypertension

Radiology is a medical specialty that uses imaging to diagnose and treat diseases seen within the body. It involves various types of modalities, including X-ray, computed tomography (CT), magnetic resonance imaging (MRI), ultrasound, and nuclear medicine.

Here are some key points to understand as a beginner in this field:

1. Medical Imaging: Radiologists use a range of imaging technologies to see inside the body, identify medical conditions, and guide treatment. The choice of technology depends on the symptoms and the part of the body being examined.

2. Common Conditions: Radiologists assist in diagnosing a vast array of conditions, from broken bones and cancer to vascular diseases and neurological conditions. They also play a crucial role in monitoring the progression of diseases and the effect of treatments.

3. Diagnostic and Interventional Radiology: Radiology has two main areas of focus - diagnostic and interventional. Diagnostic radiology helps to identify diseases through medical imaging, while interventional radiology involves minimally invasive, targeted treatments using imaging for guidance. This can include procedures like angioplasty (opening blocked blood vessels), biopsies, and delivering targeted radiation therapy for tumors.

4. Radiation Safety: Radiologists are experts in managing the risks associated with radiation exposure from imaging studies. They ensure that any potential risk is outweighed by the benefits of diagnosing and treating medical conditions.

5. Subspecialties: There are several subspecialties within radiology, including breast imaging, cardiovascular radiology, emergency radiology, musculoskeletal radiology, neuroradiology, pediatric radiology, and others. Each focuses on specific types of conditions or areas of the body.

6. Teleradiology: With the advancements in technology, teleradiology has become increasingly common. This involves transmitting radiological images from one location to another for interpretation by appropriately trained and qualified personnel. It allows for faster interpretation of studies, even in remote areas, and outside of regular working hours.

I. Imaging Modalities:

1. X-ray: A commonly used imaging modality that uses ionizing radiation to produce images of bones, lungs, and other internal structures.

2. Computed Tomography (CT): A specialized X-ray technique that generates detailed cross-sectional images of the body.

3. Magnetic Resonance Imaging (MRI): A non-invasive imaging technique that uses magnetic fields and radio waves to produce detailed images of soft tissues, organs, and blood vessels.

4. Ultrasound: A diagnostic imaging technique that uses high-frequency sound waves to create images of internal organs, blood vessels, and other structures.

5. Positron Emission Tomography (PET): A nuclear medicine imaging technique that uses radioactive tracers to visualize metabolic activity in the body.

6. Single-Photon Emission Computed Tomography (SPECT): Another nuclear medicine imaging technique that uses radioactive tracers to create three-dimensional images of organ function.

7. Fluoroscopy: Real-time X-ray imaging that captures moving images of internal structures, often used for procedures such as angiography or barium studies.

8. Mammography: X-ray imaging specifically used for screening and diagnosing breast conditions, including breast cancer.

9. Nuclear Medicine Scans: Various imaging techniques that use small amounts of radioactive materials to visualize organ function and detect abnormalities.

10. Angiography: Imaging of blood vessels using contrast material and X-rays to evaluate their structure and identify blockages or abnormalities.

11. Endoscopy: A procedure that uses a thin, flexible tube with a light and camera to visualize the inside of the body, such as the digestive tract or airways.

12. Magnetic Resonance Cholangiopancreatography (MRCP): A specialized MRI technique used to visualize the bile ducts and pancreatic ducts.

13. Arthrography: Imaging of joints using contrast material to evaluate joint abnormalities, such as tears or inflammation.

14. Bone Densitometry: A specialized X-ray technique used to measure bone density and assess the risk of osteoporosis or bone fractures.

15. Dual-Energy X-ray Absorptiometry (DXA): A low-dose X-ray technique used to measure bone mineral density and assess the risk of osteoporosis.

16. Intravenous Pyelogram (IVP): X-ray imaging of the urinary system after injecting a contrast material to evaluate the kidneys, ureters, and bladder.

17. Myelography: X-ray imaging of the spinal cord and nerve roots after injecting a contrast material into the spinal canal.

18. Interventional Radiology: A subspecialty of radiology that uses imaging guidance to perform minimally invasive procedures, such as angioplasty or embolization.

19. Cone Beam Computed Tomography (CBCT): A specialized CT technique that provides three-dimensional imaging of specific regions, often used in dentistry or maxillofacial imaging.

20. Optical Coherence Tomography (OCT): A high-resolution imaging technique that uses light waves to visualize and evaluate the retina and other structures in the eye.

21. Cystoscopy: Endoscopic examination of the urinary bladder and urethra to detect abnormalities or perform procedures.

22. Bronchoscopy: Endoscopic examination of the airways to visualize the lungs and collect tissue samples for further analysis.

23. Hysterosalpingography: X-ray imaging of the uterus and fallopian tubes after injecting a contrast material to evaluate their structure and detect any blockages.

24. Cholangiography: Imaging of the bile ducts using contrast material to assess the structure and detect any abnormalities or blockages.

25. Radionuclide Scintigraphy: A nuclear medicine imaging technique that uses radioactive tracers to visualize organ function and detect diseases, such as thyroid scans or bone scans.

II. Radiographic Findings:

1. Fracture: A break or crack in a bone, which can be visualized as a discontinuity in the bone structure on the radiograph.

2. Dislocation: The displacement of a joint or bone from its normal position, often evident as an abnormal relationship between adjacent bones on the radiograph.

3. Degenerative changes: Age-related changes in the joints or spine, such as osteoarthritis, which can be seen as joint space narrowing, bone spurs, or changes in bone density.

4. Infiltrate: The presence of abnormal density or opacities in the lungs, suggestive of conditions like pneumonia or pulmonary edema.

5. Nodule: A small, round opacity or mass in the lungs, which may be benign or indicative of a tumor or infection.

6. Atelectasis: Partial or complete collapse of a lung or a portion of a lung, characterized by a loss of air space and increased opacity on the radiograph.

7. Effusion: The accumulation of fluid in a body cavity, such as the pleural cavity (pleural effusion) or joint space (joint effusion), visible as an area of increased density.

8. Mass: An abnormal growth or tumor, which appears as a localized area of increased density or opacity on the radiograph.

9. Pneumothorax: The presence of air in the pleural space, resulting in a collapsed lung and visible as a dark area with absent lung markings on the radiograph.

10. Consolidation: The replacement of normal air-filled lung tissue with fluid, pus, or other substances, causing increased opacity or opacities on the radiograph.

11. Calcification: The deposition of calcium within tissues, such as blood vessels or organs, leading to increased radiographic density.

12. Foreign body: The presence of a foreign object, such as a swallowed coin or an embedded splinter, visible as an abnormal density on the radiograph.

13. Bowel obstruction: The blockage of the intestines, often caused by a mass, adhesions, or hernias, leading to dilated bowel loops seen on the radiograph.

14. Pneumonia: Inflammation and infection of the lung tissue, characterized by opacities, consolidation, or patchy infiltrates on the radiograph.

15. Pleural thickening: The thickening of the pleural lining of the lungs, often due to scarring from conditions like asbestos exposure or tuberculosis, seen as increased density or irregularities on the radiograph.

16. Hiatal hernia: The protrusion of a portion of the stomach through the diaphragm into the chest, visible as an abnormality in the upper abdomen on the radiograph.

17. Osteophytes: Bony outgrowths or spurs commonly associated with degenerative joint diseases, such as osteoarthritis, seen as bony projections on the radiograph.

18. Cavity or cyst: A fluid-filled or air-filled space within a tissue or organ, such as a lung cyst or an abscess, seen as a well-defined rounded area on the radiograph.

19. Scoliosis: Abnormal sideways curvature of the spine, visible as a lateral deviation on the radiograph.

20. Hemorrhage: The presence of blood in tissues or cavities, visualized as areas of increased density or opacities on the radiograph.

21. Emphysema: A condition characterized by the destruction of lung tissue and air sacs, resulting in increased lung size and reduced lung markings on the radiograph.

22. Enlarged lymph nodes: Abnormal enlargement of lymph nodes, often suggestive of infection or malignancy, seen as round or oval opacities on the radiograph.

23. Soft tissue swelling: Swelling or edema in the soft tissues, such as around a joint or in an infected area, visible as an area of increased density on the radiograph.

24. Atherosclerosis: The buildup of plaque in the arteries, causing narrowing or blockage, which may be visualized as calcifications or irregularities in the vessel walls on the radiograph.

25. Osteoporosis: A condition characterized by reduced bone density and increased risk of fractures, seen as loss of bone mass and increased radiolucency on the radiograph.

III. Radiology Reports:

1. Radiolucent: Refers to structures or areas that allow X-rays to pass through easily, appearing dark or black on the radiograph. Examples include air-filled spaces, such as lungs or the bowel.

2. Radiodense: Refers to structures or areas that absorb X-rays and appear white or light on the radiograph. Examples include bones and calcifications.

3. Mass: Refers to an abnormal growth or lesion observed on the radiograph. It may indicate a tumor or other abnormal tissue.

4. Lesion: Refers to any abnormal area or tissue change detected on the radiograph, which may require further investigation for proper diagnosis.

5. Enhancement: Refers to an increase in the contrast or visibility of certain structures or areas after the administration of contrast agents, often indicating vascularity or pathology.

6. Fluid collection: Refers to the presence of fluid in a specific area or cavity, such as an abscess or seroma.

7. Hemorrhage: Refers to the presence of blood outside the normal blood vessels, often seen as an area of increased density or opacity on the radiograph.

8. Nodule: Refers to a small, rounded opacity observed on the radiograph, which may indicate a mass, infection, or granuloma.

9. Consolidation: Refers to the replacement of air-filled lung tissue with fluid, pus, or other substances, resulting in increased radiographic density.

10. Effusion: Refers to the accumulation of fluid in a body cavity, such as the pleural cavity or joint space, visible as an area of increased density on the radiograph.

11. Dilatation: Refers to the enlargement or widening of a tubular structure, such as blood vessels, ducts, or hollow organs.

12. Fracture: Refers to a break or crack in a bone, often indicated by a disruption in the normal bone contour or alignment on the radiograph.

13. Dislocation: Refers to the displacement of a joint or bone from its normal position, often characterized by an abnormal relationship between adjacent bones.

14. Subluxation: Refers to a partial dislocation of a joint, where the articulating surfaces are partially displaced but still in contact with each other.

15. Malalignment: Refers to an abnormal positioning or alignment of bones or joints, often indicating a joint instability or injury.

16. Calcification: Refers to the deposition of calcium in tissues, resulting in increased radiodensity or opacities on the radiograph.

17. Atrophy: Refers to the wasting or shrinkage of tissues or organs, often seen as a decrease in size or volume on the radiograph.

18. Erosion: Refers to the loss or wearing away of bone or tissue surfaces, often seen as irregular areas of bone loss on the radiograph.

19. Osteophyte: Refers to a bony outgrowth or spur, commonly seen in degenerative joint diseases, such as osteoarthritis.

20. Pneumothorax: Refers to the presence of air in the pleural cavity, resulting in a collapsed lung and visible as a dark area with absent lung markings on the radiograph.

21. Atelectasis: Refers to the partial or complete collapse of a lung or a portion of a lung, resulting in increased radiographic density in the affected area.

22. Foreign body: Refers to the presence of an object that is not normally found within the body, visible as an abnormal density or opacity on the radiograph.

23. Impression: Refers to the radiologist's summary or conclusion regarding the findings observed on the radiograph, providing a diagnostic opinion or recommended further actions.

24. Comparison with prior studies: Refers to a comparison of the current radiographic findings with previous studies to assess for changes or progression of a condition.

25. Clinical correlation recommended: Indicates that further clinical evaluation or correlation with the patient's symptoms and medical history is necessary to reach a definitive diagnosis.

These terms are commonly used in radiology reports to describe and communicate findings observed on radiographic images, providing valuable information for patient management and treatment decisions.

Exercises for transcribing radiology reports accurately

Exercise 1: Fill in the blanks

Transcribe the following sentence:

The chest X-ray showed _______ in the left lower lobe.

Answer:

The chest X-ray showed consolidation in the left lower lobe.

Exercise 2: True or False

Indicate whether the following statement is true or false:

An MRI uses magnetic fields and radio waves to produce detailed images of the body.

Answer:

True

Exercise 3: Fill in the blanks

Transcribe the following sentence:

The CT scan revealed a _______ in the liver.

Answer:

The CT scan revealed a mass in the liver.

Exercise 4: Matching

Match the radiology procedure with its description:

1. X-ray

2. MRI

3. CT scan

4. Nuclear medicine scan

A. Imaging technique that uses a radioactive tracer to visualize the structure and function of organs and tissues

B. Imaging technique that uses a powerful magnetic field and radio waves to create detailed images of the body

C. Imaging technique that uses X-rays to create cross-sectional images of the body

D. Imaging technique that uses high-frequency sound waves to create images of the body's internal structures

Answer:

1. X-ray

C. Imaging technique that uses X-rays to create cross-sectional images of the body

2. MRI

B. Imaging technique that uses a powerful magnetic field and radio waves to create detailed images of the body

3. CT scan

C. Imaging technique that uses X-rays to create cross-sectional images of the body

4. Nuclear medicine scan

A. Imaging technique that uses a radioactive tracer to visualize the structure and function of organs and tissues

Exercise 5: Fill in the blanks

Transcribe the following sentence:

The ultrasound examination showed _______ in the right kidney.

Answer:

The ultrasound examination showed a renal cyst in the right kidney.

Exercise 6: True or False

Indicate whether the following statement is true or false:

A mammogram is a type of imaging test used to screen for breast cancer.

Answer:

True

Exercise 7: Fill in the blanks

Transcribe the following sentence:

The MRI report indicated a _______ in the lumbar spine.

Answer:

The MRI report indicated a herniated disc in the lumbar spine.

Exercise 8: Matching

Match the radiology finding with its description:

1. Fracture

2. Nodule

3. Mass

4. Aneurysm

A. Break or crack in a bone

B. Small abnormal growth or lump

C. Abnormal enlargement or swelling

D. Ballooning or bulging of a blood vessel

Answer:

1. Fracture

A. Break or crack in a bone

2. Nodule

B. Small abnormal growth or lump

3. Mass

C. Abnormal enlargement or swelling

4. Aneurysm

D. Ballooning or bulging of a blood vessel

Exercise 9: True or False

Indicate whether the following statement is true or false:

A bone scan is a nuclear medicine imaging test used to diagnose and monitor bone conditions.

Answer:

True

Exercise 10: Fill in the blanks

Transcribe the following sentence:

The radiograph revealed _________ in the left hip joint.

Answer:

The radiograph revealed degenerative changes in the left hip joint.

ANATOMY OF THE URINARY SYSTEM

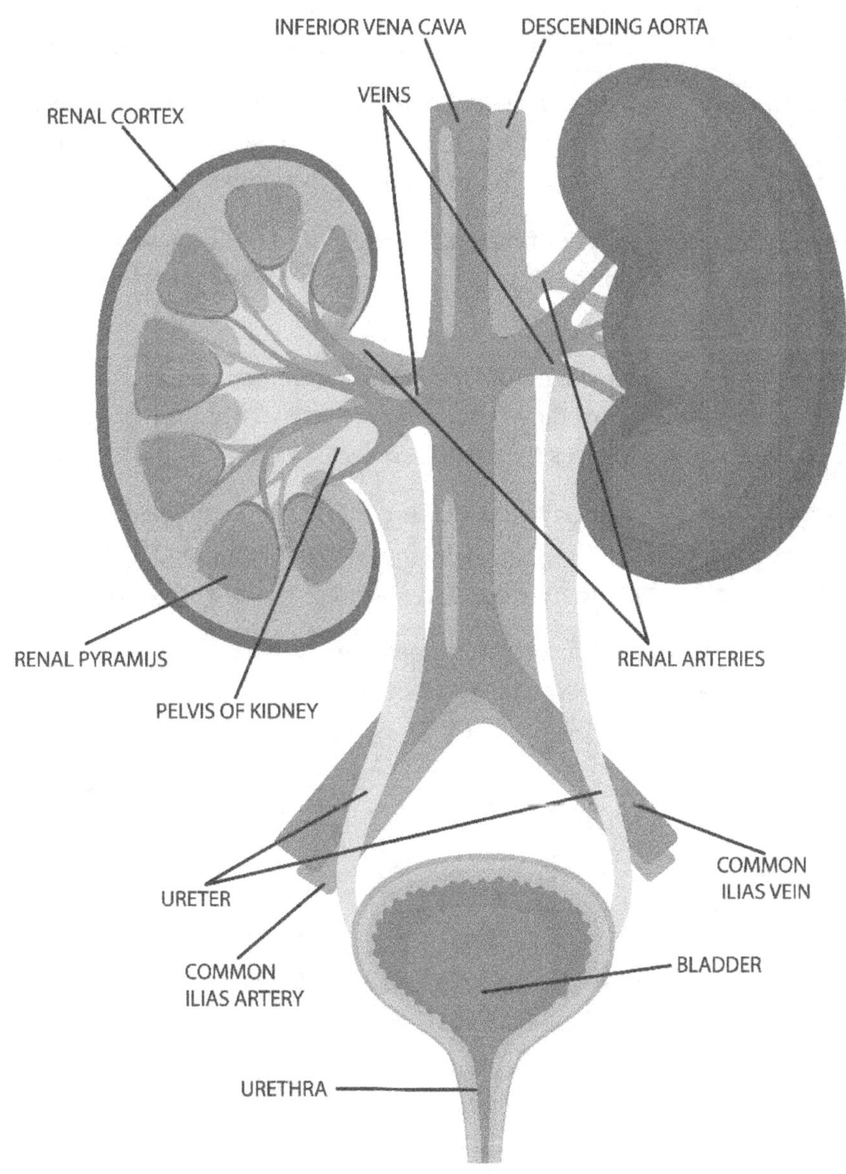

Introduction to urology and its unique terminology

Urology is a branch of medicine that focuses on the health of the urinary tract in both males and females, as well as the male reproductive system. The urinary tract includes kidneys, bladder, ureters, and urethra. In males, the reproductive system involves the prostate, testes, and associated ducts.

Here are some key points to understand as a beginner in this field:

1. Urinary and Male Reproductive System: Urologists diagnose and treat diseases of the urinary tract in both men and women, along with male reproductive disorders. They have expertise in managing diseases involving kidney function, urinary tract infections, urinary incontinence, and prostatic conditions.

2. Common Conditions: Urologists handle a range of conditions, including kidney stones, urinary tract infections (UTIs), bladder control problems, and prostate disorders. They also treat conditions related to male fertility and sexual function, such as erectile dysfunction and male infertility.

3. Diagnostic Tools: Urologists use a variety of diagnostic tools to identify these conditions, including urine tests, imaging studies like ultrasounds or CT scans, cystoscopies to look inside the urinary tract, and biopsies to test tissue for disease.

4. Treatment Approaches: Treatment can range from medication to surgery, depending on the condition. Urologists perform a variety of surgical procedures, from minimally invasive procedures using scopes to enter the urinary tract, to larger open surgeries for conditions such as kidney or bladder cancer.

5. Subspecialties: There are several subspecialties within urology, including pediatric urology (children's urology), urologic oncology (urologic cancers), renal (kidney) transplantation, male infertility, calculi (urinary tract stones), female urology, and neurourology (nerve disorders affecting urinary organs).

6. Men's Health: Urologists play a significant role in men's health, addressing conditions like benign prostatic hyperplasia (BPH), prostate cancer, erectile dysfunction, and issues of male fertility.

Urinary system disorders, diagnostic procedures, and surgical interventions

I. Urinary System Disorders:

1. Urinary Tract Infection (UTI): An infection in any part of the urinary system, commonly caused by bacteria entering the urethra.

2. Kidney Stones: Hard mineral and salt deposits that form in the kidneys and can cause severe pain when passing through the urinary tract.

3. Urinary Incontinence: Involuntary leakage of urine, often due to weakened bladder muscles or urinary sphincter dysfunction.

4. Urinary Retention: Inability to completely empty the bladder, leading to discomfort and frequent urination.

5. Urinary Tract Obstruction: Blockage in the urinary tract, which can be caused by various factors such as kidney stones, tumors, or enlarged prostate.

6. Bladder Infection (Cystitis): Inflammation of the bladder usually caused by a bacterial infection, resulting in frequent and painful urination.

7. Interstitial Cystitis: A chronic condition characterized by bladder pain, pressure, and discomfort, often accompanied by urinary frequency and urgency.

8. Overactive Bladder: A condition characterized by an uncontrollable urge to urinate and frequent urination, sometimes with urinary incontinence.

9. Benign Prostatic Hyperplasia (BPH): Non-cancerous enlargement of the prostate gland, commonly causing urinary symptoms such as frequent urination and weak urine flow.

10. Prostatitis: Inflammation of the prostate gland, typically caused by bacterial infection and characterized by urinary symptoms and pelvic pain.

11. Bladder Cancer: Cancer that develops in the cells of the bladder lining, often leading to symptoms such as blood in the urine and frequent urination.

12. Kidney Cancer: Cancer that originates in the kidneys and can cause symptoms such as blood in the urine, pain, and weight loss.

13. Urinary Tract Fistula: An abnormal connection between the urinary tract and nearby organs, leading to urinary leakage or recurrent infections.

14. Urinary Diversion: Surgical procedure that reroutes urine flow when normal urinary function is compromised, such as after bladder removal surgery.

15. Vesicoureteral Reflux (VUR): A condition in which urine flows backward from the bladder into the ureters, increasing the risk of kidney infections.

16. Hydronephrosis: Swelling of the kidneys due to the backup of urine caused by an obstruction or abnormality in the urinary tract.

17. Nephrolithiasis: The formation of kidney stones, which can cause intense pain and discomfort when passing through the urinary system.

18. Renal Failure: Impaired kidney function that results in the accumulation of waste products and fluids in the body, requiring dialysis or kidney transplantation.

19. Polycystic Kidney Disease: A genetic disorder characterized by the growth of numerous cysts in the kidneys, leading to kidney enlargement and potential renal impairment.

20. Glomerulonephritis: Inflammation of the glomeruli, the tiny blood vessels in the kidneys, often caused by immune system abnormalities or infections.

21. Renal Hypertension: High blood pressure caused by kidney disease or dysfunction, which can lead to further damage to the kidneys and other organs.

22. Renal Calculi: Another term for kidney stones, hard deposits that form in the kidneys and can cause pain and blockages in the urinary system.

23. Urethritis: Inflammation of the urethra, often caused by infections such as sexually transmitted infections or irritation.

24. Renal Cysts: Fluid-filled sacs that develop in the kidneys, often harmless, but can lead to complications if they grow large or cause obstruction.

25. Renal Cell Carcinoma: The most common type of kidney cancer that originates in the cells of the renal tubules and can spread to other organs.

II. Diagnostic Procedures:

1. Urinalysis: Examination of urine for the presence of abnormalities, such as infection, blood, or protein.

2. Urine Culture: Culturing urine to identify the specific bacteria causing a urinary tract infection (UTI) and determine the most effective antibiotic treatment.

3. Imaging Modalities:

  - Ultrasonography: Use of high-frequency sound waves to create images of the urinary system, providing information about the kidneys, bladder, and other structures.

  - CT Scan: Cross-sectional imaging that uses X-rays to create detailed images of the urinary system, helping to detect tumors, stones, or other abnormalities.

  - MRI: Magnetic resonance imaging that uses powerful magnets and radio waves to generate detailed images of the urinary system, providing valuable information about the kidneys and surrounding tissues.

  - Intravenous Pyelogram (IVP): X-ray examination of the kidneys, ureters, and bladder after injecting a contrast dye, allowing visualization of the urinary tract.

  - Cystoscopy: Insertion of a thin, flexible tube with a camera into the urethra and bladder to visually examine the urinary tract for abnormalities.

  - Retrograde Pyelogram: X-ray imaging of the urinary tract after injecting a contrast dye through a catheter inserted into the ureters.

  - Nuclear Medicine Scans: Various imaging techniques that use radioactive materials to evaluate kidney function and blood flow.

4. Renal Biopsy: A procedure in which a small piece of kidney tissue is obtained for microscopic examination, helping to diagnose and determine the extent of kidney diseases.

5. Urodynamic Testing: Assessment of bladder and urethral function to evaluate conditions such as urinary incontinence, measuring factors like bladder pressure and urine flow rate.

6. Cystometry: Evaluation of bladder function by measuring bladder pressure and capacity during filling and voiding.

7. Uroflowmetry: Measurement of urine flow rate and pattern during voiding to assess bladder emptying.

8. Cystourethroscopy: Visual examination of the bladder and urethra using a thin, flexible tube with a camera to identify abnormalities or obstructions.

9. Ureteroscopy: Examination of the ureter using a thin, flexible tube with a camera to detect and remove stones, tumors, or other obstructions.

10. Video Urodynamics: Combination of urodynamic testing with fluoroscopy or video recording to assess bladder and urethral function in real-time.

11. Kidney Function Tests:

  - Blood Urea Nitrogen (BUN) and Creatinine: Blood tests to evaluate kidney function and determine the filtration rate and waste product levels in the blood.

  - Glomerular Filtration Rate (GFR): A calculation based on blood creatinine levels and other factors that assesses the kidney's ability to filter waste products.

  - Renal Clearance Tests: Tests that measure the rate at which the kidneys eliminate a specific substance from the blood, providing insight into kidney function.

12. Urography: Imaging technique that uses X-rays or CT scans with a contrast dye to visualize the urinary system and identify any abnormalities.

13. Bladder Diary: A record of fluid intake, urinary frequency, and voiding volumes over a designated period to evaluate bladder function and urinary patterns.

14. Urethral Pressure Profiles: Measurement of pressure changes along the length of the urethra to assess urethral function and diagnose conditions like urinary incontinence.

15. Urinary Cytology: Microscopic examination of urine to detect abnormal cells that may indicate the presence of urinary system cancers.

16. Electromyography (EMG): Testing that assesses the electrical activity and function of the muscles involved in bladder control.

17. Cystogram: X-ray examination of the bladder, usually after filling it with a contrast dye, to detect structural abnormalities or bladder reflux.

18. Voiding Cystourethrogram (VCUG): X-ray imaging of the bladder and urethra during voiding, often used to assess urinary reflux or anatomical abnormalities.

19. Magnetic Resonance Urography (MRU): A specialized MRI scan that focuses on visualizing the urinary system, including the kidneys, ureters, and bladder.

20. Percutaneous Nephrostomy: Placement of a catheter through the skin into the kidney to drain urine in cases of blockage or obstruction.

21. Kidney Scan (Renal Scan): Nuclear medicine imaging that assesses kidney function, blood flow, and drainage by injecting a radioactive substance.

22. Urethral Retroresistance Pressure Profile (URPP): Measurement of the pressure required to keep the urethra closed, used to diagnose stress urinary incontinence.

23. Biometry: Ultrasound-based measurements of various parameters, such as kidney size, bladder volume, or ureteral diameter, to assess urinary system health.

24. Bladder Ultrasound: Use of ultrasound to visualize the bladder, measure its volume, and identify abnormalities such as tumors or stones.

25. Voiding Pressure Study: Measurement of pressure changes in the bladder during voiding to evaluate bladder function and diagnose conditions like urinary obstruction or neurogenic bladder.

III. Surgical Interventions:

1. Transurethral Resection of the Prostate (TURP): Surgical removal of excess prostate tissue to alleviate urinary symptoms caused by an enlarged prostate.

2. Nephrectomy: Surgical removal of a kidney, either partially or completely, usually performed to treat conditions such as kidney cancer, severe kidney damage, or kidney donation.

3. Pyeloplasty: Surgical reconstruction of the renal pelvis and ureter to correct a blockage or narrowing, typically caused by a congenital condition or scarring.

4. Cystectomy: Surgical removal of all or part of the bladder, often performed to treat bladder cancer or other bladder conditions.

5. Urinary Diversion: Surgical creation of an alternate pathway for urine to bypass a dysfunctional or surgically removed bladder, usually involving the construction of a stoma or an internal pouch.

6. Ureteral Reimplantation: Surgical procedure to reposition and reattach the ureters to the bladder, often performed to correct vesicoureteral reflux or ureteral obstruction.

7. Urethroplasty: Surgical reconstruction of the urethra to treat strictures or abnormalities that obstruct the normal flow of urine.

8. Sacral Nerve Stimulation: Implantation of a device that delivers electrical stimulation to the sacral nerves, helping to control urinary incontinence or overactive bladder.

9. Bladder Neck Suspension: Surgical procedure to provide support and stability to the bladder neck and urethra, commonly performed to treat stress urinary incontinence.

10. Augmentation Cystoplasty: Surgical procedure to increase the size and capacity of the bladder by using a segment of the intestine, performed when the bladder cannot adequately store urine.

11. Percutaneous Nephrolithotomy (PCNL): Minimally invasive procedure to remove large kidney stones by making a small incision in the back and accessing the kidney directly.

12. Ureteroscopy with Laser Lithotripsy: Minimally invasive procedure using a thin tube with a camera to visualize and remove stones in the ureter or kidney, often using laser energy to break up the stones.

13. Extracorporeal Shockwave Lithotripsy (ESWL): Non-invasive procedure that uses shockwaves to break up kidney stones, allowing them to pass more easily through the urinary tract.

14. Renal Artery Angioplasty and Stenting: Procedure to open narrowed or blocked renal arteries, usually performed to treat renal artery stenosis or hypertension.

15. Renal Autotransplantation: Surgical procedure in which a kidney is removed, repaired, and then reimplanted into a different location in the body, often to treat complex renal artery or ureteral disorders.

16. Hemodialysis Access Surgery: Placement of a vascular access device, such as an arteriovenous fistula or graft, to facilitate hemodialysis treatment for individuals with end-stage renal disease.

17. Peritoneal Dialysis Catheter Placement: Surgical implantation of a catheter into the abdomen to allow for peritoneal dialysis, a method of removing waste and excess fluid from the body.

18. Urethral Sling Surgery: Placement of a synthetic sling around the urethra to provide support and improve bladder control in cases of stress urinary incontinence.

19. Artificial Urinary Sphincter Implantation: Surgical placement of a device that helps control the flow of urine by mimicking the function of the natural urinary sphincter, typically used to treat severe urinary incontinence.

20. Renal Cryoablation: Minimally invasive procedure that uses extreme cold temperatures to destroy cancerous kidney tumors, often an alternative to surgical removal.

21. Renal Transplantation: Surgical procedure to replace a failed or non-functioning kidney with a healthy kidney from a living or deceased donor.

22. Ureteral Stent Placement: Insertion of a small tube (stent) into the ureter to relieve obstructions or strictures and promote the flow of urine.

23. Antegrade Ureteral Stenting: Placement of a stent directly into the kidney through a percutaneous approach to bypass ureteral obstructions.

24. Bladder Augmentation with Continent Urinary Diversion: Surgical procedure that combines bladder augmentation with the creation of a continent reservoir to manage bladder dysfunction and provide continence.

25. Robot-Assisted Urologic Surgery: Minimally invasive surgical procedures performed with the assistance of robotic systems, allowing for enhanced precision and dexterity in complex urologic surgeries.

Practice activities for transcribing urology reports effectively

Exercise 1: Fill in the blanks

Transcribe the following sentence:

The patient presented with _______ and difficulty urinating.

Answer:

The patient presented with hematuria and difficulty urinating.

Exercise 2: True or False

Indicate whether the following statement is true or false:

A urinary tract infection (UTI) is commonly caused by a viral infection.

Answer:

False

Exercise 3: Fill in the blanks

Transcribe the following sentence:

The uroflowmetry test showed a _______ flow rate.

Answer:

The uroflowmetry test showed a decreased flow rate.

Exercise 4: Matching

Match the urology procedure with its description:

1. Cystoscopy

2. Urinalysis

3. Ultrasonography

4. Urodynamic testing

A. Imaging technique that uses sound waves to create images of the urinary tract

B. Visual examination of the bladder and urethra using a thin, flexible tube with a camera

C. Laboratory test that analyzes the urine for the presence of abnormalities or infections

D. Assessment of the bladder and urethral function during urine storage and voiding

Answer:

1. Cystoscopy

B. Visual examination of the bladder and urethra using a thin, flexible tube with a camera

2. Urinalysis

C. Laboratory test that analyzes the urine for the presence of abnormalities or infections

3. Ultrasonography

A. Imaging technique that uses sound waves to create images of the urinary tract

4. Urodynamic testing

D. Assessment of the bladder and urethral function during urine storage and voiding

Exercise 5: Fill in the blanks

Transcribe the following sentence:

The renal ultrasound showed _______ in the right kidney.

Answer:

The renal ultrasound showed a renal cyst in the right kidney.

Exercise 6: True or False

Indicate whether the following statement is true or false:

A ureteroscopy is a procedure used to examine and treat conditions affecting the urethra.

Answer:

False

Exercise 7: Fill in the blanks

Transcribe the following sentence:

The urologist recommended a _______ for the patient's kidney stones.

Answer:

The urologist recommended a lithotripsy for the patient's kidney stones.

Exercise 8: Matching

Match the urology finding with its description:

1. Hematuria

2. Urinary incontinence

3. Urethral stricture

4. Urinary retention

A. Presence of bacteria in the urine, indicating a urinary tract infection

B. Involuntary leakage of urine

C. Narrowing of the urethra, leading to difficulty urinating

D. Inability to empty the bladder completely

Answer:

1. Hematuria

A. Presence of blood in the urine

2. Urinary incontinence

B. Involuntary leakage of urine

3. Urethral stricture

C. Narrowing of the urethra, leading to difficulty urinating

4. Urinary retention

D. Inability to empty the bladder completely

Exercise 9: True or False

Indicate whether the following statement is true or false:

A prostate-specific antigen (PSA) test is commonly used to screen for prostate cancer.

Answer:

True

Exercise 10: Fill in the blanks

Transcribe the following sentence:

The urodynamics study revealed ________ bladder function.

Answer:

The urodynamics study revealed impaired bladder function.

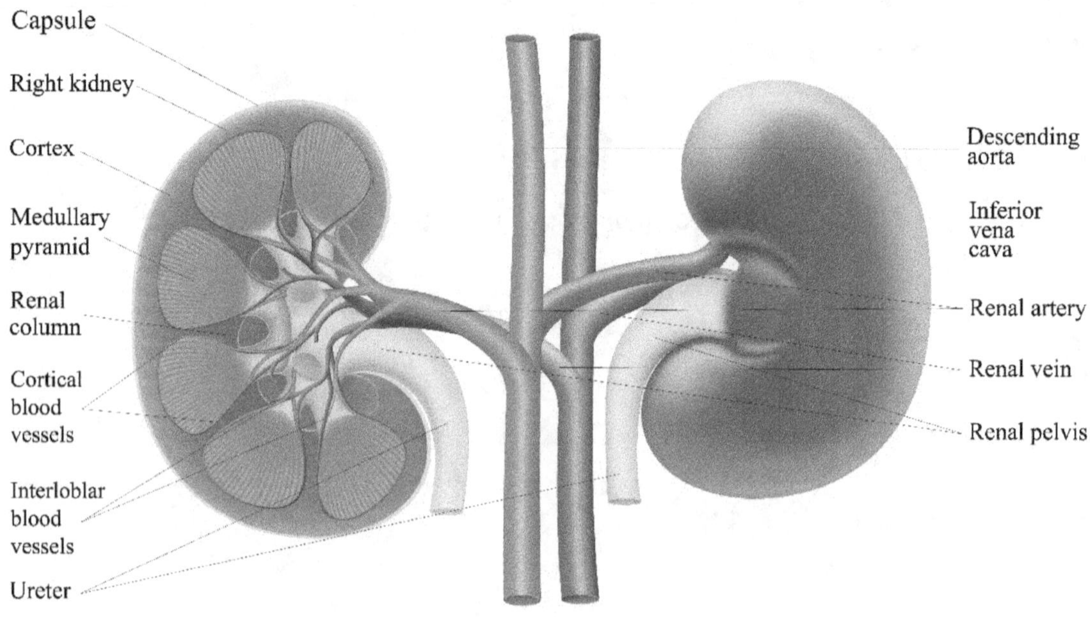

Understanding nephrology and its specialized vocabulary

Nephrology is a medical specialty that focuses on the diagnosis and treatment of diseases affecting the kidneys. The kidneys perform several crucial functions, including filtering waste products from the blood, regulating blood pressure, maintaining electrolyte balance, and stimulating red blood cell production.

Here are some key points to understand as a beginner in this field:

1. Kidneys and their Function: Nephrologists are doctors who specialize in managing diseases that affect the function of the kidneys. They have a deep understanding of how kidney disease or dysfunction can affect other parts of the body.

2. Common Conditions: Nephrologists diagnose and treat a variety of kidney diseases, from kidney stones to chronic kidney disease (CKD) and end-stage renal disease (ESRD). They manage conditions such as glomerulonephritis and polycystic kidney disease and oversee the care of patients requiring renal replacement therapy, including dialysis and kidney transplant patients.

3. Diagnostic Tools: Nephrologists use several diagnostic tools to identify kidney diseases, including blood tests to measure kidney function, urine tests to identify abnormalities, kidney biopsy to evaluate disease severity, and imaging tests like ultrasounds or CT scans to visualize the kidneys.

4. Treatment Approaches: Treatment in nephrology can involve lifestyle changes, medications, and procedures like kidney dialysis, which artificially filters waste from the blood when the kidneys are not functioning adequately. If kidney function is severely diminished, a kidney transplant may be required, and the nephrologist will oversee the patient's care before and after the transplant.

5. Subspecialties: Nephrology also includes several subspecialties, such as pediatric nephrology (kidney diseases in children), renal pathology (microscopic study of kidney disease), and interventional nephrology (procedures involving the kidneys, like kidney biopsies and treatments for kidney stones).

6. Hypertension: Since the kidneys play a vital role in regulating blood pressure, nephrologists often manage patients with hypertension, especially when it's secondary to kidney disease.

Kidney-related conditions, dialysis, and transplantation

I. Kidney-Related Conditions:

1. Chronic Kidney Disease (CKD): A progressive condition in which the kidneys gradually lose their ability to function properly, leading to the accumulation of waste and fluid in the body.

2. Acute Kidney Injury (AKI): Sudden and temporary loss of kidney function, often caused by factors such as dehydration, infection, or medication side effects.

3. Kidney Stones: Hard deposits formed in the kidneys due to the crystallization of minerals and salts, causing severe pain and potential blockage of the urinary tract.

4. Polycystic Kidney Disease (PKD): A genetic disorder characterized by the growth of numerous cysts in the kidneys, leading to kidney enlargement and eventual loss of function.

5. Glomerulonephritis: Inflammation of the glomeruli, the tiny filtering units in the kidneys, which can be caused by infections, autoimmune diseases, or other factors.

6. Nephrotic Syndrome: A condition characterized by increased protein levels in the urine, low levels of protein in the blood, swelling, and elevated cholesterol levels, indicating damage to the kidney's filtering units.

7. Renal Failure: The complete loss of kidney function, requiring renal replacement therapy such as dialysis or kidney transplantation.

8. Urinary Tract Infections (UTIs): Infections that can occur in any part of the urinary system, including the kidneys, bladder, ureters, or urethra, often caused by bacteria.

9. Renal Hypertension: High blood pressure that is specifically caused by kidney-related factors, such as narrowing of the renal arteries or hormonal imbalances.

10. Renal Cysts: Fluid-filled sacs that can develop in the kidneys, usually noncancerous, but may cause discomfort or affect kidney function if they grow large or become infected.

11. Hydronephrosis: Swelling or enlargement of the kidney due to a backup of urine, often caused by blockages in the urinary tract.

12. Renal Cell Carcinoma: The most common type of kidney cancer, originating in the cells of the kidney tubules.

13. Diabetic Nephropathy: Kidney damage caused by long-term uncontrolled diabetes, resulting in impaired kidney function and the excretion of excessive amounts of protein in the urine.

14. Lupus Nephritis: Kidney inflammation caused by systemic lupus erythematosus (SLE), an autoimmune disease affecting various organs and tissues.

15. Alport Syndrome: A genetic disorder characterized by kidney disease, hearing loss, and eye abnormalities, caused by mutations in genes encoding for collagen proteins in the kidney and other tissues.

16. Renal Artery Stenosis: Narrowing of the renal arteries that supply blood to the kidneys, often leading to high blood pressure and reduced kidney function.

17. Hemolytic Uremic Syndrome (HUS): A condition characterized by the destruction of red blood cells, low platelet count, and kidney failure, often caused by certain bacterial infections or medications.

18. Renal Tubular Acidosis (RTA): A group of disorders in which the kidneys are unable to maintain the proper acid-base balance in the blood, leading to imbalances in electrolytes and acidity levels.

19. Autosomal Recessive Polycystic Kidney Disease (ARPKD): A rare genetic disorder characterized by the formation of cysts in the kidneys and other organs, often leading to kidney failure in childhood.

20. Nephrogenic Diabetes Insipidus: A condition in which the kidneys are unable to properly concentrate urine, resulting in excessive thirst and urination.

21. Goodpasture Syndrome: An autoimmune disorder characterized by the presence of autoantibodies that attack the kidneys and lungs, leading to kidney damage and respiratory problems.

22. Fanconi Syndrome: A rare disorder in which the kidneys are unable to properly reabsorb essential substances, such as glucose, amino acids, and electrolytes, leading to their excretion in the urine.

23. Bartter Syndrome: A group of genetic disorders that affect the kidneys' ability to reabsorb salt and maintain electrolyte balance, leading to electrolyte imbalances and fluid loss.

24. Medullary Sponge Kidney: A congenital disorder characterized by the presence of cysts in the inner parts of the kidneys' collecting ducts, which can lead to the formation of kidney stones and recurrent urinary tract infections.

25. Interstitial Nephritis: Inflammation of the kidney's interstitial tissue, often caused by medications, infections, or autoimmune diseases, leading to impaired kidney function.

II. Dialysis:

1. Hemodialysis: A method of dialysis that involves using a machine called a dialyzer to remove waste products and excess fluids from the blood outside the body.

2. Peritoneal Dialysis: A method of dialysis that involves using the peritoneal membrane in the abdominal cavity as a natural filter to remove waste and excess fluid from the body.

3. End-Stage Renal Disease (ESRD): The final stage of kidney disease, where the kidneys have lost their ability to function adequately, often requiring dialysis or kidney transplantation.

4. Arteriovenous (AV) Fistula: A surgically created connection between an artery and a vein, typically in the forearm, to provide access for hemodialysis.

5. Dialysis Catheter: A soft, flexible tube inserted into a large vein, often in the neck or chest, to provide access for hemodialysis or peritoneal dialysis.

6. Dialysate: A solution containing electrolytes and other substances used in dialysis to help remove waste products and balance fluid and electrolyte levels.

7. Ultrafiltration: The process during hemodialysis where excess fluid is removed from the blood by applying pressure across the semipermeable membrane of the dialyzer.

8. Dialysis Machine: A medical device used to control and monitor the dialysis process, including blood flow rate, dialysate composition, and ultrafiltration.

9. Kt/V: A parameter used to measure the effectiveness of dialysis in removing waste products from the blood. It represents the dialyzer clearance (K) multiplied by the treatment time (t) divided by the volume of distribution (V).

10. Continuous Ambulatory Peritoneal Dialysis (CAPD): A type of peritoneal dialysis that is manually performed by the patient, requiring multiple exchanges of dialysate throughout the day.

11. Automated Peritoneal Dialysis (APD): A type of peritoneal dialysis that uses a machine called a cycler to perform the exchanges of dialysate automatically while the patient sleeps.

12. Dialysis Access Complications: Complications that can arise from dialysis access, such as infection, clotting, stenosis, or aneurysm formation, which may require interventions or surgical repair.

13. Hemodialysis Technician: A healthcare professional trained to operate and maintain hemodialysis machines, monitor patients during dialysis, and ensure the safety and effectiveness of the procedure.

14. Dialysis Nurse: A registered nurse specializing in the care of patients undergoing dialysis, including assessing patient's condition, monitoring vital signs, administering medications, and providing patient education.

15. Dialysis Adequacy: Refers to the degree to which dialysis effectively removes waste products and excess fluid from the body, ensuring the patient's overall well-being and optimal health.

16. Residual Renal Function: The remaining ability of the kidneys to filter waste products and maintain fluid balance in patients undergoing dialysis.

17. Dialysis Dose: The amount of dialysis delivered to a patient, measured by parameters such as Kt/V or urea reduction ratio (URR), to assess the adequacy of dialysis treatment.

18. Dialysis-Related Amyloidosis: A condition characterized by the accumulation of abnormal protein deposits, called amyloid fibrils, in the joints and tissues of patients on long-term dialysis.

19. Electrolyte Imbalance: Imbalances in electrolyte levels, such as sodium, potassium, calcium, and phosphate, can occur during dialysis and may require adjustment through dialysate composition or medication administration.

20. Dialysis-Related Hypotension: A drop in blood pressure that can occur during or after dialysis due to fluid removal and changes in blood volume, requiring interventions to stabilize blood pressure.

21. Dialysis-Associated Infections: Infections that can occur in patients on dialysis, such as catheter-related bloodstream infections or peritonitis in peritoneal dialysis, which require prompt diagnosis and appropriate antibiotic treatment.

22. Dialysis Diet: A specialized diet that helps maintain proper nutrition and manage fluid and electrolyte balance for individuals on dialysis, typically low in sodium, potassium, and phosphorus.

23. Dialysis Fistula Care: Proper care and monitoring of an arteriovenous fistula, including regular assessment for signs of infection, maintaining good hygiene, and avoiding activities that may damage the access site.

24. Dialysis Complications: Various complications can arise during dialysis, including hypotension, muscle cramps, access-related issues, infections, electrolyte imbalances, and cardiovascular events.

25. Dialysis Patient Education: The provision of education and support to patients undergoing dialysis, including information on diet and fluid restrictions, medication management, vascular access care, and self-monitoring to promote self-care and optimal treatment outcomes.

III. Transplantation:

1. Organ Transplantation: The surgical procedure of replacing a failed or damaged organ with a healthy organ from a donor.

2. Kidney Transplantation: The most common type of organ transplantation, where a healthy kidney is transplanted into a recipient with end-stage renal disease.

3. Liver Transplantation: A surgical procedure to replace a diseased liver with a healthy liver from a deceased or living donor.

4. Heart Transplantation: The surgical replacement of a failing or diseased heart with a healthy heart from a deceased donor.

5. Lung Transplantation: The transplantation of one or both lungs from a deceased donor into a recipient with severe lung disease.

6. Pancreas Transplantation: The transplantation of a healthy pancreas from a deceased donor into a recipient with diabetes mellitus.

7. Intestinal Transplantation: The transplantation of the small intestine or a combined small intestine and liver from a deceased donor into a recipient with intestinal failure.

8. Tissue Transplantation: The transplantation of various tissues, such as corneas, skin, bone, tendons, and heart valves, to restore function or enhance healing.

9. Living Donor Transplantation: A type of organ transplantation where a living individual donates an organ or a part of an organ, such as a kidney or liver lobe, to a recipient.

10. Deceased Donor Transplantation: Organ transplantation that involves the use of organs from deceased individuals who have chosen to be organ donors.

11. Human leukocyte antigen (HLA): A group of proteins that play a crucial role in the body's immune response and compatibility between donor and recipient in organ transplantation.

12. Organ Procurement: The process of retrieving organs from deceased donors for transplantation, ensuring proper preservation and transportation to the recipient's transplant center.

13. Immunosuppression: The use of medications to suppress the immune system and prevent organ rejection after transplantation.

14. Rejection: The immune system's response to a transplanted organ, which may occur when the immune system recognizes the transplanted organ as foreign and attempts to attack it.

15. Graft-versus-Host Disease (GVHD): A complication that can occur in certain types of transplantation, where immune cells from the donor attack the recipient's tissues.

16. Induction Therapy: The use of potent immunosuppressive medications at the time of transplantation to prevent early organ rejection.

17. Maintenance Therapy: The long-term use of immunosuppressive medications to prevent organ rejection and ensure the survival of the transplanted organ.

18. Acute Rejection: Rejection of a transplanted organ that occurs within the first few months after transplantation, usually requiring prompt treatment and adjustment of immunosuppressive medications.

19. Chronic Rejection: Slow and progressive rejection of a transplanted organ that occurs over months or years, leading to gradual organ dysfunction and eventual organ failure.

20. Transplantation Team: A multidisciplinary team of healthcare professionals, including transplant surgeons, transplant nephrologists, transplant coordinators, social workers, and pharmacists, who work together to assess, manage, and follow up with transplant recipients.

21. Organ Allocation: The process of matching available organs with potential recipients based on various factors, such as blood type, HLA compatibility, medical urgency, and time spent on the transplant waiting list.

22. Transplantation Evaluation: The comprehensive assessment of potential transplant recipients to determine their suitability for transplantation, including medical, psychological, and social evaluations.

23. Transplantation Waiting List: A list maintained by transplant centers of patients who are awaiting organ transplantation, prioritized based on factors such as medical urgency and organ allocation policies.

24. Post-Transplant Care: The ongoing medical care and monitoring provided to transplant recipients after transplantation to ensure the long-term success of the transplant and manage any potential complications.

25. Organ Donor Registry: A database where individuals can register their decision to become organ donors after death, facilitating the organ donation process and increasing the availability of organs for transplantation.

Exercises for transcribing nephrology reports accurately

Exercise 1: Fill in the blanks

Transcribe the following sentence:

The patient has a history of __________ disease.

Answer:

The patient has a history of chronic kidney disease.

Exercise 2: True or False

Indicate whether the following statement is true or false:

Polycystic kidney disease is an inherited condition that causes the growth of fluid-filled cysts in the kidneys.

Answer:

True

Exercise 3: Fill in the blanks

Transcribe the following sentence:

The patient's creatinine level was _______ mg/dL.

Answer:

The patient's creatinine level was 1.5 mg/dL.

Exercise 4: Matching

Match the nephrology procedure with its description:

1. Hemodialysis

2. Kidney biopsy

3. Peritoneal dialysis

4. Nephrectomy

A. Filtering waste and excess fluid from the blood using a machine

B. Surgical removal of a kidney

C. Removing a small sample of kidney tissue for examination

D. Using the lining of the abdominal cavity to filter waste and excess fluid from the blood

Answer:

1. Hemodialysis

A. Filtering waste and excess fluid from the blood using a machine

2. Kidney biopsy

C. Removing a small sample of kidney tissue for examination

3. Peritoneal dialysis

D. Using the lining of the abdominal cavity to filter waste and excess fluid from the blood

4. Nephrectomy

B. Surgical removal of a kidney

Exercise 5: Fill in the blanks

Transcribe the following sentence:

The patient's urine output was _______ mL in the last 24 hours.

Answer:

The patient's urine output was 800 mL in the last 24 hours.

Exercise 6: True or False

Indicate whether the following statement is true or false:

Glomerulonephritis is an inflammation of the glomeruli, the filtering units of the kidneys.

Answer:

True

Exercise 7: Fill in the blanks

Transcribe the following sentence:

The patient is experiencing ________ edema.

Answer:

The patient is experiencing peripheral edema.

Exercise 8: Matching

Match the nephrology condition with its description:

1. Acute kidney injury

2. Glomerulonephritis

3. Polycystic kidney disease

4. Chronic kidney disease

A. Progressive loss of kidney function over time

B. Inflammation of the filtering units (glomeruli) in the kidneys

C. Inherited condition causing the growth of fluid-filled cysts in the kidneys

D. Sudden and temporary loss of kidney function

Answer:

1. Acute kidney injury

D. Sudden and temporary loss of kidney function

2. Glomerulonephritis

B. Inflammation of the filtering units (glomeruli) in the kidneys

3. Polycystic kidney disease

C. Inherited condition causing the growth of fluid-filled cysts in the kidneys

4. Chronic kidney disease

A. Progressive loss of kidney function over time

Exercise 9: True or False

Indicate whether the following statement is true or false:

Renal calculi are commonly known as kidney stones.

Answer:

True

Exercise 10: Fill in the blanks

Transcribe the following sentence:

The patient's estimated glomerular filtration rate (eGFR) is _______ mL/min/1.73m2.

Answer:

The patient's estimated glomerular filtration rate (eGFR) is 55 mL/min/1.73m2.

TYPES OF BONES

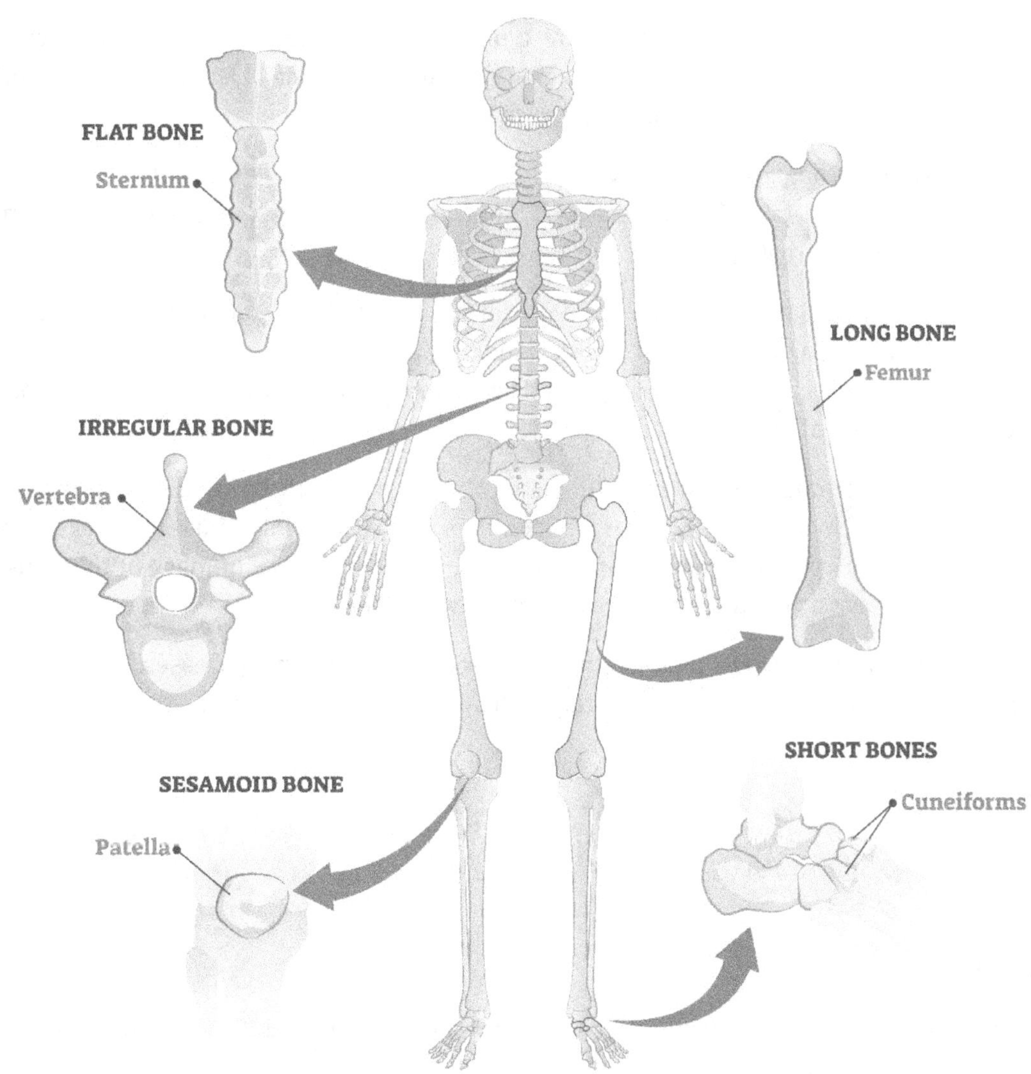

Overview of rheumatology and its specific terminology

Rheumatology is a sub-specialty in internal medicine and pediatrics that focuses on the diagnosis and therapy of rheumatic diseases. These are conditions characterized by inflammation and pain in the joints, muscles, and fibrous tissue, often affecting the immune system.

Here are some key points to understand as a beginner in this field:

1. Rheumatic Diseases: Rheumatologists treat more than 100 types of rheumatic diseases, some of which are very common, and others that are rare. These include arthritis, gout, lupus, osteoarthritis, rheumatoid arthritis, and certain auto-immune diseases, musculoskeletal pain disorders, and osteoporosis, among others.

2. Common Conditions: Rheumatic conditions are typically characterized by symptoms affecting the joints and muscles, such as pain, swelling, stiffness, and deformity. They can also have systemic effects, impacting organs including the kidneys, lungs, heart, and skin.

3. Diagnostic Tools: Rheumatologists use a variety of tools to diagnose these conditions. These can include patient history, physical exams, and specialized blood and imaging tests that look for inflammation or damage to the joints or internal organs.

4. Treatment Approaches: Treatment in rheumatology aims to alleviate symptoms and improve function. It often involves a combination of medication, physical therapy, and sometimes surgery. Medications can include pain relievers, anti-inflammatory drugs, and disease-modifying antirheumatic drugs (DMARDs), which can slow the progress of the disease.

5. Autoimmune and Inflammatory Diseases: Rheumatologists deal with both autoimmune diseases, where the immune system mistakenly attacks the body's own tissues, and inflammatory diseases, where the body's immune system leads to unneeded inflammation. While the cause of many of these diseases is unknown, they often have a genetic component and can run in families.

6. Multidisciplinary Approach: Given the systemic nature of many rheumatic diseases, rheumatologists often work in a multidisciplinary context, cooperating with other specialists to provide comprehensive care for their patients.

Rheumatic diseases, joint disorders, and treatment approaches

I. Rheumatic Diseases:

1. Rheumatic Diseases: A group of conditions characterized by inflammation, pain, and stiffness in the joints, muscles, and other tissues.

2. Rheumatoid Arthritis: An autoimmune disease causing chronic inflammation of the joints, leading to pain, swelling, and joint deformity.

3. Osteoarthritis: A degenerative joint disease characterized by the breakdown of cartilage and the development of bony growths, resulting in joint pain and stiffness.

4. Systemic Lupus Erythematosus (SLE): An autoimmune disease that affects multiple organs, including joints, skin, kidneys, and heart, causing inflammation and a range of symptoms.

5. Sjögren's Syndrome: An autoimmune disease primarily affecting the salivary and tear glands, leading to dry eyes and mouth.

6. Psoriatic Arthritis: A form of arthritis that occurs in individuals with psoriasis, causing joint pain, stiffness, and skin changes.

7. Ankylosing Spondylitis: An inflammatory arthritis primarily affecting the spine and sacroiliac joints, leading to stiffness and fusion of the joints.

8. Juvenile Idiopathic Arthritis: Arthritis that develops in children under the age of 16 and can affect one or multiple joints, causing pain, swelling, and stiffness.

9. Gout: A form of arthritis caused by the buildup of uric acid crystals in the joints, leading to sudden and severe joint pain and inflammation.

10. Polymyalgia Rheumatica: A condition characterized by pain and stiffness in the shoulders, neck, and hips, primarily affecting individuals over the age of 50.

11. Fibromyalgia: A chronic disorder characterized by widespread musculoskeletal pain, fatigue, and tenderness at specific points on the body.

12. Giant Cell Arteritis: A condition characterized by inflammation of the blood vessels, primarily affecting the arteries of the head and neck, causing headaches, jaw pain, and vision problems.

13. Reactive Arthritis: Arthritis that develops following an infection in another part of the body, typically causing joint pain, swelling, and inflammation.

14. Raynaud's Phenomenon: A condition characterized by spasms in the small blood vessels of the fingers and toes, leading to color changes, numbness, and coldness in the affected areas.

15. Polymyositis: An inflammatory disease that affects the muscles, causing muscle weakness, pain, and difficulty in performing daily activities.

16. Dermatomyositis: A condition similar to polymyositis but also involving skin inflammation, resulting in a distinctive rash.

17. Vasculitis: Inflammation of the blood vessels, which can affect various organs and tissues, causing a range of symptoms depending on the affected area.

18. Bursitis: Inflammation of the bursae, small fluid-filled sacs that cushion the joints, leading to joint pain and swelling.

19. Tendinitis: Inflammation of the tendons, the thick cords that attach muscles to bones, causing pain and tenderness in the affected area.

20. Myositis: Inflammation of the muscles, leading to muscle weakness, pain, and fatigue.

21. Behcet's Disease: A rare autoimmune disorder that causes inflammation in blood vessels throughout the body, leading to various symptoms, including mouth ulcers, genital sores, and joint pain.

22. Mixed Connective Tissue Disease (MCTD): An autoimmune disease characterized by a combination of symptoms seen in lupus, scleroderma, and polymyositis, such as joint pain, muscle weakness, and skin changes.

23. Antiphospholipid Syndrome (APS): An autoimmune disorder characterized by the presence of specific antibodies that increase the risk of blood clots, pregnancy complications, and organ damage.

24. Reactive Arthritis: Arthritis that develops following an infection in another part of the body, typically causing joint pain, swelling, and inflammation.

25. Rheumatic Fever: A complication of untreated strep throat infection that can affect the heart, joints, skin, and brain, leading to symptoms such as joint pain, fever, and rash.

II. Joint Disorders:

1. Osteoarthritis: A degenerative joint disease characterized by the breakdown of cartilage, leading to joint pain, stiffness, and reduced mobility.

2. Rheumatoid Arthritis: An autoimmune disease that causes chronic inflammation in the joints, resulting in pain, swelling, and joint deformity.

3. Psoriatic Arthritis: A form of arthritis that occurs in some individuals with psoriasis, causing joint pain, stiffness, and skin manifestations.

4. Juvenile Idiopathic Arthritis: A group of chronic arthritis conditions that occur in children under the age of 16, causing joint pain, swelling, and stiffness.

5. Ankylosing Spondylitis: An inflammatory arthritis that primarily affects the spine and sacroiliac joints, leading to pain, stiffness, and limited mobility.

6. Reactive Arthritis: Joint inflammation that develops in response to an infection in another part of the body, often affecting the joints, eyes, and urinary tract.

7. Gout: A form of arthritis caused by the accumulation of uric acid crystals in the joints, leading to sudden and severe joint pain, swelling, and inflammation.

8. Bursitis: Inflammation of the fluid-filled sacs (bursae) that cushion the joints, commonly affecting the shoulder, elbow, or knee, causing pain and limited range of motion.

9. Tendinitis: Inflammation of a tendon, often resulting from overuse or repetitive motion, leading to pain, swelling, and difficulty with joint movement.

10. Carpal Tunnel Syndrome: Compression of the median nerve in the wrist, causing numbness, tingling, and weakness in the hand and fingers.

11. Osteoporosis: A condition characterized by decreased bone density and increased risk of fractures, commonly affecting the spine, hips, and wrists.

12. Dupuytren's Contracture: A condition in which the fingers gradually bend inward due to the thickening and tightening of the connective tissue in the palm.

13. Frozen Shoulder: Also known as adhesive capsulitis, it causes pain and stiffness in the shoulder joint, limiting its range of motion.

14. TMJ Disorders: Dysfunction of the temporomandibular joint, causing jaw pain, clicking sounds, and difficulty with chewing and speaking.

15. Rotator Cuff Tear: A tear in the tendons of the shoulder's rotator cuff, leading to shoulder pain, weakness, and limited arm movement.

16. Meniscus Tear: A tear in the rubbery, C-shaped disc in the knee joint, causing pain, swelling, and difficulty with knee movement.

17. Plantar Fasciitis: Inflammation of the thick band of tissue (plantar fascia) that connects the heel bone to the toes, resulting in heel pain and stiffness.

18. Tennis Elbow: Pain and inflammation on the outside of the elbow, typically caused by overuse or repetitive motions of the forearm muscles.

19. Osteochondritis Dissecans: A condition in which a piece of cartilage and underlying bone separate from the joint surface, causing pain, swelling, and possible joint locking.

20. Scoliosis: Abnormal sideways curvature of the spine, which can cause back pain, uneven shoulders, and an uneven waistline.

21. Patellofemoral Pain Syndrome: Also known as runner's knee, it causes pain around the kneecap, especially during activities that involve bending the knee.

22. Septic Arthritis: Joint infection caused by bacteria, viruses, or fungi, leading to joint pain, swelling, and decreased range of motion.

23. Osteonecrosis: Death of bone tissue due to a lack of blood supply, resulting in joint pain and limited mobility.

24. Reactive Arthritis: Joint inflammation that develops in response to an infection in another part of the body, often affecting the joints, eyes, and urinary tract.

25. Hemarthrosis: Joint bleeding caused by injury or a bleeding disorder, leading to pain, swelling, and limited joint movement.

III. Treatment Approaches:

1. Medications: Nonsteroidal anti-inflammatory drugs (NSAIDs), corticosteroids, and disease-modifying antirheumatic drugs (DMARDs) are commonly prescribed to manage pain, reduce inflammation, and slow down disease progression.

2. Physical Therapy: Exercises, stretches, and manual techniques prescribed by a physical therapist to improve joint mobility, strength, and function.

3. Occupational Therapy: Helps individuals with joint disorders develop strategies and techniques to manage daily activities, maximize independence, and protect joints from further damage.

4. Assistive Devices: Joint supports, braces, splints, or orthotics may be recommended to provide stability, alleviate pain, and improve joint alignment.

5. Weight Management: Maintaining a healthy weight can reduce stress on weight-bearing joints and improve overall joint health.

6. Joint Injections: Corticosteroid or hyaluronic acid injections into the joint can provide temporary pain relief and reduce inflammation.

7. Joint Aspiration: The removal of excess fluid from the joint to alleviate pain and swelling.

8. Regenerative Medicine: Therapies such as platelet-rich plasma (PRP) or stem cell injections that promote tissue healing and regeneration.

9. Heat and Cold Therapy: The application of heat or cold packs to reduce pain and inflammation or improve joint flexibility.

10. Transcutaneous Electrical Nerve Stimulation (TENS): Electrical stimulation applied to the skin to relieve joint pain by blocking pain signals.

11. Acupuncture: The insertion of thin needles into specific points on the body to promote pain relief and improve joint function.

12. Massage Therapy: Manipulation of soft tissues to relieve muscle tension, reduce pain, and improve circulation around the affected joint.

13. Dietary Modifications: Certain foods, such as omega-3 fatty acids, antioxidants, and anti-inflammatory foods, may help reduce joint inflammation and improve symptoms.

14. Patient Education: Providing information and resources to help individuals understand their joint condition, make informed decisions, and manage their symptoms effectively.

15. Stress Reduction Techniques: Stress management techniques, such as mindfulness, meditation, or relaxation exercises, may help reduce joint pain associated with stress.

16. Joint Protection Strategies: Teaching individuals how to modify their movements and activities to minimize stress on the affected joints.

17. Aquatic Therapy: Exercises and movements performed in a pool environment to reduce joint impact and improve joint flexibility and strength.

18. Complementary and Alternative Medicine: Approaches like herbal supplements, homeopathy, or Ayurvedic medicine that may be used as adjunctive treatments for joint disorders.

19. Cognitive-Behavioral Therapy (CBT): Psychological therapy aimed at helping individuals cope with pain, manage stress, and improve overall well-being.

20. Surgical Intervention: In severe cases where conservative treatments fail, surgical procedures such as joint replacement, arthroscopy, or joint fusion may be considered.

21. Education and Self-Management Programs: Programs that provide information, skills, and support to empower individuals to actively participate in managing their joint disorder.

22. Assistive Technology: Use of devices like walking aids, adaptive tools, or joint protection aids to assist with mobility and daily activities.

23. Exercise Programs: Customized exercise regimens that include strength training, aerobic exercises, and flexibility exercises to improve joint function and overall fitness.

24. Pain Management Techniques: Strategies such as mindfulness, relaxation techniques, or distraction methods to manage and cope with joint pain.

25. Supportive Care: Access to support groups, counseling, or online communities where individuals with joint disorders can connect, share experiences, and find emotional support.

Practice activities for transcribing rheumatology reports effectively

Exercise 1: Fill in the blanks

Transcribe the following sentence:

The patient presents with joint pain and swelling consistent with __________.

Answer:

The patient presents with joint pain and swelling consistent with rheumatoid arthritis.

Exercise 2: True or False

Indicate whether the following statement is true or false:

Systemic lupus erythematosus (SLE) is an autoimmune disease that primarily affects the joints.

Answer:

False

Exercise 3: Fill in the blanks

Transcribe the following sentence:

The patient has a positive __________ test for rheumatoid factor.

Answer:

The patient has a positive serologic test for rheumatoid factor.

Exercise 4: Matching

Match the rheumatology procedure with its description:

1. Joint aspiration

2. Synovial biopsy

3. Magnetic resonance imaging (MRI)

4. Electromyography (EMG)

A. Inserting a needle into a joint to withdraw fluid for analysis

B. Surgical removal of a small piece of synovial tissue for examination

C. Imaging technique that uses magnetic fields and radio waves to visualize joint structures

D. Nerve conduction study to evaluate muscle and nerve function

Answer:

1. Joint aspiration

A. Inserting a needle into a joint to withdraw fluid for analysis

2. Synovial biopsy

B. Surgical removal of a small piece of synovial tissue for examination

3. Magnetic resonance imaging (MRI)

C. Imaging technique that uses magnetic fields and radio waves to visualize joint structures

4. Electromyography (EMG)

D. Nerve conduction study to evaluate muscle and nerve function

Exercise 5: Fill in the blanks

Transcribe the following sentence:

The patient reports morning stiffness lasting more than ________.

Answer:

The patient reports morning stiffness lasting more than one hour.

Exercise 6: True or False

Indicate whether the following statement is true or false:

Gout is a type of arthritis caused by the accumulation of uric acid crystals in the joints.

Answer:

True

Exercise 7: Fill in the blanks

Transcribe the following sentence:

The patient has a history of ________ spondylitis.

Answer:

The patient has a history of ankylosing spondylitis.

Exercise 8: Matching

Match the rheumatology condition with its description:

1. Osteoarthritis

2. Rheumatoid arthritis

3. Psoriatic arthritis

4. Ankylosing spondylitis

A. Chronic inflammatory disease primarily affecting the spine and sacroiliac joints

B. Degenerative joint disease characterized by the breakdown of cartilage and bone

C. Inflammatory arthritis associated with psoriasis

D. Systemic autoimmune disease affecting multiple joints

Answer:

1. Osteoarthritis

B. Degenerative joint disease characterized by the breakdown of cartilage and bone

2. Rheumatoid arthritis

D. Systemic autoimmune disease affecting multiple joints

3. Psoriatic arthritis

C. Inflammatory arthritis associated with psoriasis

4. Ankylosing spondylitis

A. Chronic inflammatory disease primarily affecting the spine and sacroiliac joints

Exercise 9: True or False

Indicate whether the following statement is true or false:

Fibromyalgia is a rheumatic condition characterized by widespread muscle pain and tenderness.

Answer:

True

Exercise 10: Fill in the blanks

Transcribe the following sentence:

The patient's erythrocyte sedimentation rate (ESR) is _________ mm/h.

Answer:

The patient's erythrocyte sedimentation rate (ESR) is 30 mm/h.

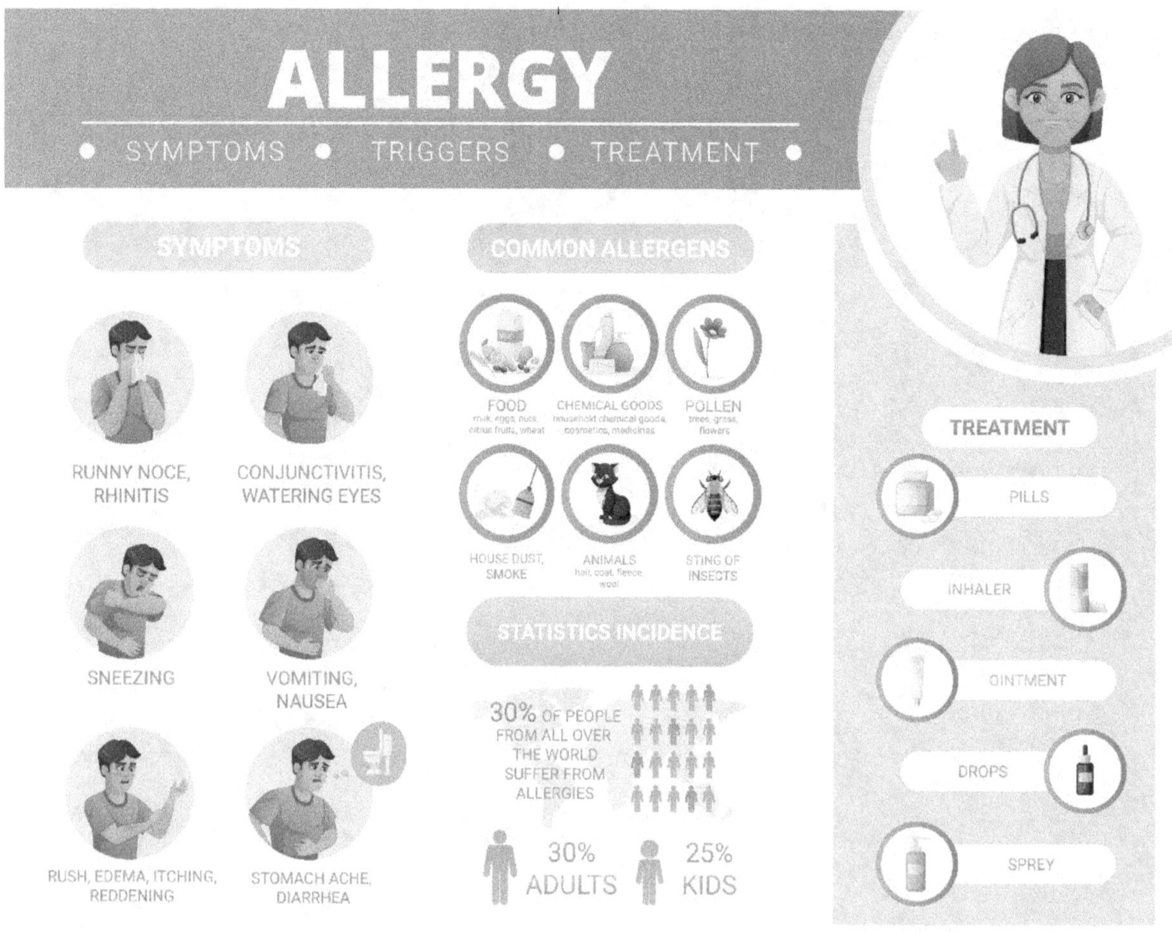

Introduction to allergy and immunology and their unique terminology

Allergy and Immunology, also known as Allergology, is a medical specialty focused on the diagnosis and treatment of allergies, asthma, and disorders of the immune system. These can involve different parts of the body and can be either acute or chronic.

Here are some key points to understand as a beginner in this field:

1. Allergies and Immune Disorders: Allergists/Immunologists are trained to determine the causes of allergies, whether they're environmental, food, or drug-related, as well as to diagnose and manage diseases of the immune system.

2. Common Conditions: These specialists deal with conditions such as hay fever (allergic rhinitis), food allergies, atopic dermatitis (eczema), anaphylaxis (a severe, potentially life-threatening allergic reaction), asthma, and immune deficiencies.

3. Diagnostic Tools: Diagnostic tools in this field include allergy testing, such as skin tests or blood tests to identify specific allergens. Pulmonary function tests may be used in the case of asthma. In the case of suspected immune deficiencies, additional specialized testing of the immune system may be required.

4. Treatment Approaches: Treatment strategies in allergy and immunology include avoiding identified allergens, medications to reduce symptoms, and immunotherapy (allergy shots or sublingual tablets) to desensitize the patient to allergenic substances. For certain immune deficiencies, treatment may include replacement of specific immune components.

5. Subspecialties: Subspecialties within this field can include pediatric allergy and immunology, focusing specifically on these disorders in children.

6. Asthma Management: A significant aspect of this specialty is the management of asthma, a chronic condition that can cause coughing, wheezing, and shortness of breath. This involves the use of medications, including inhalers, and creating action plans for when asthma symptoms worsen.

Allergic conditions, immune system disorders, and immunotherapy

I. Allergic Conditions:

1. Allergic Rhinitis: Also known as hay fever, it is an allergic reaction that occurs when the immune system overreacts to allergens in the environment, such as pollen, dust mites, or pet dander. Symptoms include sneezing, itching, nasal congestion, and watery eyes.

2. Asthma: A chronic respiratory condition characterized by inflammation and narrowing of the airways, leading to symptoms like wheezing, coughing, shortness of breath, and chest tightness. Allergens, such as pollen, dust mites, or pet dander, can trigger asthma attacks.

3. Atopic Dermatitis: Also known as eczema, it is a chronic skin condition characterized by dry, itchy, and inflamed skin. Allergens, irritants, or genetic factors can contribute to the development of atopic dermatitis.

4. Food Allergies: Allergic reactions to certain foods, such as peanuts, tree nuts, milk, eggs, shellfish, or wheat. Ingesting or even coming into contact with the allergenic food can trigger symptoms ranging from mild itching to severe allergic reactions.

5. Drug Allergies: Allergic reactions to medications, such as antibiotics, nonsteroidal anti-inflammatory drugs (NSAIDs), or certain vaccines. Symptoms can range from mild skin rashes to severe reactions like anaphylaxis.

6. Insect Sting Allergies: Allergic reactions to insect stings, such as those from bees, wasps, hornets, or fire ants. Some individuals may experience localized reactions, while others may develop severe systemic reactions.

7. Allergic Conjunctivitis: Inflammation of the conjunctiva (the thin membrane covering the white part of the eye and the inner surface of the eyelids) due to allergens like pollen, dust mites, or pet dander. Symptoms include redness, itching, watering, and swollen eyelids.

8. Allergic Contact Dermatitis: A skin reaction that occurs when the skin comes into direct contact with allergens or irritants, leading to symptoms like redness, itching, and rash.

9. Allergic Asthma: A type of asthma triggered by exposure to specific allergens, such as pollen, mold spores, or pet dander. It causes airway inflammation and can lead to asthma symptoms.

10. Allergic Sinusitis: Inflammation of the sinuses caused by an allergic reaction to allergens like pollen, dust mites, or mold spores. Symptoms include facial pain, nasal congestion, and postnasal drip.

11. Allergic Conjunctivitis: Inflammation of the conjunctiva (the thin membrane covering the white part of the eye and the inner surface of the eyelids) due to allergens like pollen, dust mites, or pet dander. Symptoms include redness, itching, watering, and swollen eyelids.

12. Allergic Contact Dermatitis: A skin reaction that occurs when the skin comes into direct contact with allergens or irritants, leading to symptoms like redness, itching, and rash.

13. Allergic Asthma: A type of asthma triggered by exposure to specific allergens, such as pollen, mold spores, or pet dander. It causes airway inflammation and can lead to asthma symptoms.

14. Allergic Sinusitis: Inflammation of the sinuses caused by an allergic reaction to allergens like pollen, dust mites, or mold spores. Symptoms include facial pain, nasal congestion, and postnasal drip.

15. Anaphylaxis: A severe, life-threatening allergic reaction that can occur within seconds or minutes after exposure to allergens. It can cause symptoms like difficulty breathing, swelling of the face and throat, rapid heartbeat, and drop in blood pressure.

16. Patch Testing: A diagnostic test performed to identify allergens causing allergic contact dermatitis. Small amounts of potential allergens are applied to the skin using patches, and reactions are evaluated after a specific period.

17. Skin Prick Test: A diagnostic test that involves pricking the skin with small amounts of allergens to identify specific allergies. Reactions, such as redness or swelling, indicate sensitization to the allergen.

18. Immunotherapy: Also known as allergy shots or allergen immunotherapy, it involves gradually exposing individuals to increasing amounts of allergens to build tolerance and reduce allergic reactions over time.

19. Antihistamines: Medications that block the effects of histamine, a chemical released during an allergic reaction, to relieve symptoms like itching, sneezing, and runny nose.

20. Nasal Corticosteroids: Medications that reduce inflammation in the nasal passages to alleviate symptoms of allergic rhinitis, such as nasal congestion, itching, and sneezing.

21. Decongestants: Medications that constrict blood vessels in the nasal passages to relieve nasal congestion associated with allergies or the common cold.

22. Leukotriene Inhibitors: Medications that block the action of leukotrienes, substances involved in the inflammatory response, to manage symptoms of allergic asthma and allergic rhinitis.

23. Avoidance of Allergens: Identifying and avoiding triggers and allergens that cause allergic reactions can help prevent or minimize symptoms.

24. Sublingual Immunotherapy: A form of immunotherapy where allergen extracts are placed under the tongue to induce tolerance and reduce allergic symptoms.

25. Allergen-Proofing Measures: Taking steps to minimize exposure to allergens, such as using allergen-proof bedding covers, regular cleaning, and air purifiers, to create a more allergen-free environment.

II. Immune System Disorders:

1. Rheumatoid Arthritis: An autoimmune disease characterized by chronic inflammation of the joints, causing pain, stiffness, and swelling. The immune system mistakenly attacks the body's own tissues, primarily affecting the joints but can also impact other organs.

2. Systemic Lupus Erythematosus (SLE): A chronic autoimmune disease that can affect multiple organs and tissues, including the skin, joints, kidneys, heart, and lungs. It can cause a range of symptoms, such as joint pain, fatigue, rash, and organ damage.

3. Multiple Sclerosis (MS): An autoimmune disease that affects the central nervous system, causing damage to the protective covering of nerve fibers. This can lead to various neurological symptoms, including muscle weakness, coordination difficulties, and cognitive impairment.

4. Type 1 Diabetes: An autoimmune condition in which the immune system attacks and destroys the insulin-producing cells in the pancreas. This leads to an inability to regulate blood sugar levels, requiring lifelong insulin treatment.

5. Celiac Disease: An autoimmune disorder triggered by the ingestion of gluten, a protein found in wheat, barley, and rye. It damages the lining of the small intestine, leading to digestive issues, malabsorption, and various systemic symptoms.

6. Psoriasis: A chronic inflammatory skin condition characterized by red, scaly patches on the skin. It occurs when the immune system mistakenly attacks healthy skin cells, causing rapid cell turnover and the formation of plaques.

7. Graves' Disease: An autoimmune disorder that affects the thyroid gland, leading to the overproduction of thyroid hormones. It can cause symptoms like weight loss, rapid heartbeat, anxiety, and heat intolerance.

8. Hashimoto's Thyroiditis: An autoimmune condition that causes chronic inflammation of the thyroid gland, leading to decreased thyroid hormone production. It can result in symptoms such as fatigue, weight gain, and depression.

9. Sjögren's Syndrome: An autoimmune disease that primarily affects the salivary and tear glands, resulting in dry eyes and dry mouth. It can also affect other organs and cause fatigue, joint pain, and systemic symptoms.

10. Guillain-Barré Syndrome: A rare neurological disorder in which the immune system mistakenly attacks the peripheral nerves, leading to muscle weakness, numbness, and in severe cases, paralysis.

11. Crohn's Disease: An inflammatory bowel disease characterized by chronic inflammation of the digestive tract. It can cause abdominal pain, diarrhea, fatigue, and nutrient deficiencies due to impaired nutrient absorption.

12. Ulcerative Colitis: Another form of inflammatory bowel disease that causes inflammation and ulcers in the lining of the colon and rectum. It leads to symptoms such as bloody diarrhea, abdominal pain, and urgency to have a bowel movement.

13. Myasthenia Gravis: A neuromuscular disorder in which the immune system attacks the connection between nerves and muscles, resulting in muscle weakness and fatigue.

14. Pernicious Anemia: An autoimmune condition in which the immune system attacks the cells in the stomach that produce a protein called intrinsic factor. This leads to vitamin B12 deficiency and anemia.

15. Goodpasture Syndrome: A rare autoimmune disease characterized by the immune system attacking the kidneys and lungs, leading to kidney damage and lung bleeding.

16. Vitiligo: A condition in which the immune system attacks and destroys the melanocytes, causing depigmentation of the skin and the appearance of white patches.

17. Ankylosing Spondylitis: An inflammatory arthritis that primarily affects the spine, causing pain, stiffness, and reduced mobility. It is associated with chronic inflammation and structural changes in the spine and other joints.

18. Wegener's Granulomatosis: An autoimmune vasculitis that primarily affects the respiratory tract and kidneys, leading to inflammation and damage to blood vessels.

19. Polymyalgia Rheumatica: An inflammatory disorder characterized by pain and stiffness in the muscles, especially in the shoulders and hips. It typically affects older adults and can be associated with giant cell arteritis.

20. Dermatomyositis: An inflammatory disease that causes muscle weakness and skin rashes. It is characterized by inflammation of the muscles and blood vessels.

21. Addison's Disease: An autoimmune condition that affects the adrenal glands, leading to insufficient production of hormones like cortisol and aldosterone. It can cause fatigue, weight loss, low blood pressure, and electrolyte imbalances.

22. Antiphospholipid Syndrome: An autoimmune disorder that increases the risk of abnormal blood clotting. It can lead to complications such as deep vein thrombosis, stroke, and recurrent miscarriages.

23. Vasculitis: A group of disorders characterized by inflammation of blood vessels, which can affect various organs and tissues. Symptoms depend on the organs involved but can include fever, fatigue, joint pain, and organ dysfunction.

24. Mixed Connective Tissue Disease: An autoimmune disease with overlapping features of different connective tissue disorders, including symptoms of lupus, scleroderma, and polymyositis.

25. Eosinophilic Esophagitis: An immune-mediated disorder characterized by inflammation of the esophagus, leading to swallowing difficulties, food impaction, and symptoms similar to gastroesophageal reflux disease (GERD).

III. Immunotherapy:

1. Monoclonal Antibodies: Monoclonal antibodies are laboratory-produced molecules that can target specific proteins on cancer cells, stimulating the immune system to attack and destroy those cells.

2. Checkpoint Inhibitors: Checkpoint inhibitors are drugs that block proteins on immune cells or cancer cells, releasing the brakes on the immune system and allowing it to recognize and attack cancer cells more effectively.

3. CAR-T Cell Therapy: CAR-T cell therapy involves collecting a patient's T cells, modifying them in the laboratory to express chimeric antigen receptors (CARs), and then reinfusing them into the patient. CAR-T cells can recognize and kill cancer cells more efficiently.

4. Immune Checkpoint Blockade: Immune checkpoint blockade refers to the use of drugs that target specific immune checkpoints, such as PD-1 or CTLA-4, to enhance the immune system's response against cancer cells.

5. Vaccines: Cancer vaccines are designed to stimulate the immune system to recognize and destroy cancer cells. They can be preventive vaccines or therapeutic vaccines targeting existing cancers.

6. Interferons: Interferons are naturally occurring proteins that can stimulate the immune system to enhance its anti-cancer activity. They can be used as a form of immunotherapy for certain cancers.

7. Interleukin Therapy: Interleukins are signaling molecules that play a crucial role in immune system regulation. Interleukin therapy involves the administration of specific interleukins to modulate immune responses and target cancer cells.

8. Adoptive Cell Transfer: Adoptive cell transfer involves isolating T cells from a patient, expanding and enhancing them in the laboratory, and then reinfusing them back into the patient to target and kill cancer cells.

9. Immune Stimulants: Immune stimulants, such as cytokines or other immune-modulating molecules, are used to activate the immune system and enhance its response against cancer cells.

10. Oncolytic Viruses: Oncolytic viruses are viruses that can selectively infect and destroy cancer cells. They can be used as a form of immunotherapy to stimulate an immune response against cancer.

11. Antibody-Drug Conjugates: Antibody-drug conjugates combine monoclonal antibodies with cytotoxic drugs. The antibodies target cancer cells, delivering the drug specifically to those cells to destroy them while minimizing damage to healthy cells.

12. Tumor-Infiltrating Lymphocyte Therapy: Tumor-infiltrating lymphocyte therapy involves isolating T cells from a patient's tumor, expanding them in the laboratory, and reinfusing them back into the patient to target and kill cancer cells.

13. Dendritic Cell Vaccines: Dendritic cells are a type of immune cell that plays a crucial role in activating T cells. Dendritic cell vaccines involve isolating dendritic cells from a patient, loading them with cancer-specific antigens, and reinfusing them back into the patient to stimulate an immune response against cancer.

14. Bispecific Antibodies: Bispecific antibodies are engineered molecules that can simultaneously bind to cancer cells and immune cells, bridging them together to enhance the immune system's ability to target cancer cells.

15. Immune Cell Therapy: Immune cell therapy involves using various immune cells, such as natural killer (NK) cells or macrophages, to target and kill cancer cells.

16. Cytokine Therapy: Cytokines are signaling molecules that play a crucial role in immune system regulation. Cytokine therapy involves the administration of specific cytokines to enhance immune responses against cancer cells.

17. Immunomodulatory Drugs: Immunomodulatory drugs, such as thalidomide or lenalidomide, can modulate the immune system's response against cancer cells and improve immune function.

18. Immune Priming: Immune priming involves the administration of substances or agents that can enhance the immune system's response against cancer cells, preparing it to better recognize and target cancer cells.

19. Combination Therapy: Combination therapy refers to the use of multiple immunotherapy agents or combining immunotherapy with other treatment modalities, such as chemotherapy or radiation therapy, to enhance the overall anti-cancer response.

20. Personalized Immunotherapy: Personalized immunotherapy involves tailoring treatment based on an individual's specific tumor characteristics, immune profile, and genetic makeup to optimize the immune response against cancer cells.

21. Immune Modulators: Immune modulators are drugs that can regulate immune responses and balance immune function to improve the body's ability to target and destroy cancer cells.

22. Immune Cell Engineering: Immune cell engineering techniques involve genetically modifying immune cells, such as T cells, to enhance their anti-cancer activity and improve their ability to recognize and kill cancer cells.

23. Immune System Training: Immune system training approaches aim to educate and train the immune system to recognize and attack cancer cells more effectively, enhancing its overall anti-cancer response.

24. Antibody Therapy: Antibody therapy involves the administration of antibodies that specifically target and bind to cancer cells, marking them for destruction by the immune system or delivering therapeutic agents directly to cancer cells.

25. Immune Surveillance: Immune surveillance is the natural ability of the immune system to detect and eliminate cancer cells. Immunotherapy aims to enhance immune surveillance and boost the immune system's ability to identify and destroy cancer cells.

Exercise 1: Fill in the blanks

Transcribe the following sentence:

The patient presents with symptoms of _________ to various environmental allergens.

Answer:

The patient presents with symptoms of allergic rhinitis to various environmental allergens.

Exercise 2: True or False

Indicate whether the following statement is true or false:

Anaphylaxis is a severe, life-threatening allergic reaction that can involve multiple organ systems.

Answer:

True

Exercise 3: Fill in the blanks

Transcribe the following sentence:

The patient has a history of _________ asthma triggered by pet dander.

Answer:

The patient has a history of allergic asthma triggered by pet dander.

Exercise 4: Matching

Match the immunological test with its description:

1. Skin prick test

2. IgE blood test

3. Patch test

4. Challenge test

A. Injection of a small amount of allergen into the skin to measure the allergic response

B. Blood test to measure the levels of immunoglobulin E, an antibody associated with allergies

C. Application of allergens to the skin under occlusion to detect delayed hypersensitivity reactions

D. Controlled exposure to a suspected allergen to confirm or rule out an allergic reaction

Answer:

1. Skin prick test

A. Injection of a small amount of allergen into the skin to measure the allergic response

2. IgE blood test

B. Blood test to measure the levels of immunoglobulin E, an antibody associated with allergies

3. Patch test

C. Application of allergens to the skin under occlusion to detect delayed hypersensitivity reactions

4. Challenge test

D. Controlled exposure to a suspected allergen to confirm or rule out an allergic reaction

Exercise 5: Fill in the blanks

Transcribe the following sentence:

The patient experiences _________ when exposed to peanuts.

Answer:

The patient experiences anaphylaxis when exposed to peanuts.

Exercise 6: True or False

Indicate whether the following statement is true or false:

Immunodeficiency disorders are characterized by a weakened or absent immune response, making individuals more susceptible to infections.

Answer:

True

Exercise 7: Fill in the blanks

Transcribe the following sentence:

The patient is advised to carry an _________ device in case of a severe allergic reaction.

Answer:

The patient is advised to carry an epinephrine autoinjector device in case of a severe allergic reaction.

Exercise 8: Matching

Match the allergy-related condition with its description:

1. Allergic rhinitis

2. Atopic dermatitis

3. Allergic conjunctivitis

4. Contact dermatitis

A. Inflammation of the skin caused by contact with an allergen

B. Allergic reaction triggered by airborne allergens, leading to symptoms like sneezing and nasal congestion

C. Inflammatory skin condition characterized by dry, itchy, and inflamed patches

D. Allergic reaction affecting the eyes, causing redness, itching, and swelling

Answer:

1. Allergic rhinitis

B. Allergic reaction triggered by airborne allergens, leading to symptoms like sneezing and nasal congestion

2. Atopic dermatitis

C. Inflammatory skin condition characterized by dry, itchy, and inflamed patches

3. Allergic conjunctivitis

D. Allergic reaction affecting the eyes, causing redness, itching, and swelling

4. Contact dermatitis

A. Inflammation of the skin caused by contact with an allergen

Exercise 9: True or False

Indicate whether the following statement is true or false:

Immunotherapy, such as allergy shots, is a treatment option for allergies that aims to desensitize the immune system to specific allergens.

Answer:

True

Exercise 10: Fill in the blanks

Transcribe the following sentence:

The patient has a positive __________ test for dust mites.

Answer:

The patient has a positive skin prick test for dust mites.

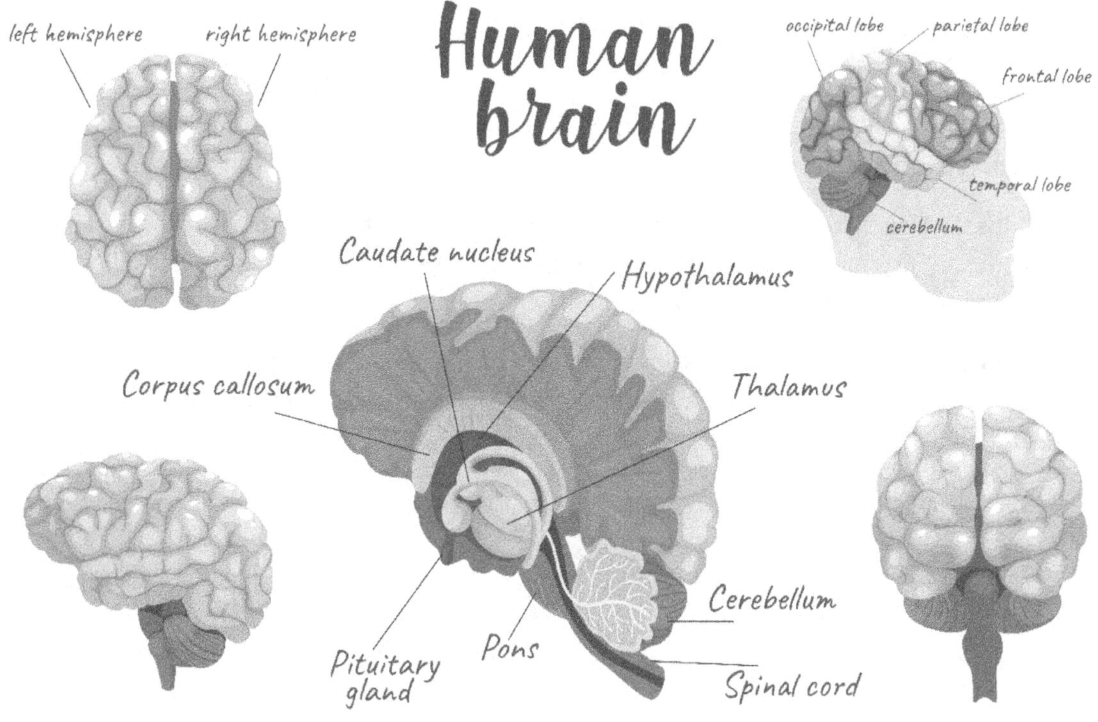

Understanding psychiatry and its specialized vocabulary

Psychiatry is a branch of medicine that focuses on the diagnosis, treatment, and prevention of mental, emotional, and behavioral disorders. Psychiatrists are medical doctors who are experts in mental health, including substance use disorders.

Here are some key points to understand as a beginner in this field:

1. Mental Health Disorders: Psychiatrists diagnose and treat a wide range of mental health conditions, such as depression, anxiety disorders, schizophrenia, bipolar disorder, eating disorders, addiction, and many others.

2. Diagnostic Tools: Psychiatry utilizes various tools for diagnosis, depending on the condition. These may include comprehensive psychiatric evaluation, psychological testing, and, in some cases, neuroimaging and blood tests.

3. Treatment Approaches: Treatment strategies in psychiatry are often individualized, based on the specific disorder and the needs of the patient. They often include psychotherapy (talking therapies), medications, psychiatric rehabilitation, and, less commonly, brain stimulation therapies like electroconvulsive therapy (ECT).

4. Psychotherapy: Psychiatrists are trained in different types of psychotherapy, such as cognitive-behavioral therapy (CBT), interpersonal therapy (IPT), psychodynamic therapy, and family therapy. These therapies can be used alone or in combination with medications.

5. Pharmacotherapy: As medical doctors, psychiatrists can prescribe medication. The specific drugs used will depend on the condition, and may include antidepressants, mood stabilizers, antipsychotic medications, stimulants, and anxiolytics.

6. Subspecialties: There are several subspecialties within psychiatry, including child and adolescent psychiatry, geriatric psychiatry, addiction psychiatry, forensic psychiatry, and consultation-liaison psychiatry (psychiatry in the general hospital setting).

7. Mind-Body Connection: Psychiatrists understand the complex relationship between physical and mental health. They often work in tandem with other physicians to ensure that all aspects of a person's health are addressed.

Mental health conditions, diagnostic criteria, and treatment modalities

I. Mental Health Conditions:

1. Depression: Depression is a mood disorder characterized by persistent feelings of sadness, loss of interest or pleasure, changes in appetite or sleep patterns, and difficulties in concentration and decision-making.

2. Anxiety Disorders: Anxiety disorders encompass a range of conditions, such as generalized anxiety disorder, panic disorder, social anxiety disorder, and specific phobias, characterized by excessive and persistent worry, fear, or anxiety that can interfere with daily functioning.

3. Bipolar Disorder: Bipolar disorder is a mental health condition characterized by alternating periods of mania (elevated mood, increased energy) and depression.

4. Schizophrenia: Schizophrenia is a chronic mental disorder characterized by disturbances in perception, thoughts, emotions, and behavior, often accompanied by hallucinations and delusions.

5. Obsessive-Compulsive Disorder (OCD): OCD is an anxiety disorder characterized by recurrent and intrusive thoughts (obsessions) and repetitive behaviors or mental acts (compulsions) that individuals feel driven to perform to alleviate anxiety.

6. Post-Traumatic Stress Disorder (PTSD): PTSD is a mental health condition that can develop after exposure to a traumatic event, characterized by symptoms such as intrusive memories, flashbacks, nightmares, hypervigilance, and avoidance of trauma-related triggers.

7. Attention-Deficit/Hyperactivity Disorder (ADHD): ADHD is a neurodevelopmental disorder characterized by persistent patterns of inattention, hyperactivity, and impulsivity that can interfere with daily functioning and social relationships.

8. Eating Disorders: Eating disorders, such as anorexia nervosa, bulimia nervosa, and binge-eating disorder, involve disturbances in eating behaviors and distorted body image, often leading to severe physical and psychological consequences.

9. Substance Use Disorders: Substance use disorders refer to a range of conditions characterized by the misuse or addiction to substances, such as alcohol, drugs, or medications, leading to significant impairment in daily functioning and adverse health effects.

10. Autism Spectrum Disorder (ASD): ASD is a developmental disorder characterized by difficulties in social interaction, communication challenges, and restricted and repetitive patterns of behavior, interests, or activities.

11. Borderline Personality Disorder (BPD): BPD is a mental health disorder characterized by unstable self-image, intense and unstable relationships, impulsivity, and emotional dysregulation.

12. Schizoaffective Disorder: Schizoaffective disorder is a mental health condition that combines symptoms of both schizophrenia (psychotic symptoms) and mood disorders (e.g., depression or mania).

13. Dissociative Disorders: Dissociative disorders involve disruptions in consciousness, memory, identity, or perception, often as a response to trauma or severe stress.

14. Major Depressive Disorder (MDD): MDD is a mood disorder characterized by persistent feelings of sadness, loss of interest, and a lack of pleasure in daily activities, lasting for at least two weeks.

15. Generalized Anxiety Disorder (GAD): GAD is an anxiety disorder characterized by excessive and uncontrollable worrying about various aspects of life, accompanied by physical symptoms such as restlessness, fatigue, and difficulty concentrating.

16. Panic Disorder: Panic disorder is characterized by recurrent and unexpected panic attacks, which are intense periods of extreme fear or discomfort, often accompanied by physical symptoms such as rapid heartbeat, shortness of breath, and chest pain.

17. Social Anxiety Disorder: Social anxiety disorder, also known as social phobia, is an anxiety disorder characterized by intense fear or anxiety in social situations, leading to avoidance or extreme distress.

18. Postpartum Depression: Postpartum depression is a type of depression that occurs in women after childbirth, characterized by feelings of sadness, exhaustion, and a lack of bonding with the newborn.

19. Seasonal Affective Disorder (SAD): SAD is a subtype of depression that occurs during specific seasons, typically during the winter months, and is related to changes in light exposure.

20. Specific Phobias: Specific phobias are intense and irrational fears of specific objects, situations, or activities, leading to avoidance behaviors and significant distress.

21. Body Dysmorphic Disorder (BDD): BDD is a mental health disorder characterized by obsessive preoccupation with perceived flaws or defects in one's appearance, leading to significant distress and impaired functioning.

22. Substance-Induced Disorders: Substance-induced disorders refer to mental health conditions that develop as a result of substance abuse or withdrawal, such as substance-induced psychosis or substance-induced mood disorders.

23. Conduct Disorder: Conduct disorder is a childhood-onset disorder characterized by persistent patterns of behavior that violate societal norms and the rights of others, such as aggression, theft, or destruction of property.

24. Intellectual Disability: Intellectual disability is a developmental disorder characterized by limitations in intellectual functioning and adaptive behavior, leading to difficulties in learning, communication, and daily living skills.

25. Adjustment Disorders: Adjustment disorders occur in response to significant life stressors and involve emotional or behavioral symptoms that exceed what is considered a typical response, causing significant distress or impairment in functioning.

II. Diagnostic Criteria:

1. Depressive Episode: A period of at least two weeks with persistent low mood, loss of interest or pleasure, and other symptoms such as changes in appetite, sleep, energy, concentration, or suicidal thoughts.

2. Generalized Anxiety Disorder (GAD): Excessive worry and anxiety about various aspects of life, occurring more days than not for at least six months, accompanied by physical symptoms such as restlessness, fatigue, irritability, muscle tension, and sleep disturbances.

3. Panic Attack: A sudden episode of intense fear or discomfort, typically reaching its peak within minutes, accompanied by physical symptoms such as palpitations, sweating, trembling, shortness of breath, chest pain, or fear of losing control or dying.

4. Social Anxiety Disorder: Persistent and intense fear or anxiety in social situations, leading to avoidance or distress, often accompanied by physical symptoms such as blushing, trembling, sweating, or fear of being embarrassed or humiliated.

5. Obsessive-Compulsive Disorder (OCD): Presence of obsessions (intrusive thoughts, images, or urges) and/or compulsions (repetitive behaviors or mental acts) that are time-consuming, cause distress, and significantly interfere with daily functioning.

6. Post-Traumatic Stress Disorder (PTSD): Exposure to a traumatic event followed by the presence of intrusive memories, nightmares, flashbacks, avoidance of trauma-related stimuli, negative mood, changes in arousal or reactivity, and disturbances in cognition or mood lasting more than one month.

7. Autism Spectrum Disorder (ASD): Persistent deficits in social communication and interaction, along with restricted and repetitive patterns of behavior, interests, or activities, manifested early in development and causing significant impairment in functioning.

8. Attention-Deficit/Hyperactivity Disorder (ADHD): Persistent patterns of inattention, hyperactivity, and impulsivity that are inconsistent with developmental level and interfere with functioning in multiple settings.

9. Borderline Personality Disorder (BPD): Enduring patterns of instability in interpersonal relationships, self-image, and affects, along with impulsivity and marked fear of abandonment, often leading to self-harm behaviors or suicidal ideation.

10. Schizophrenia: Presence of two or more characteristic symptoms, such as delusions, hallucinations, disorganized speech, grossly disorganized or catatonic behavior, or negative symptoms, persisting for a significant portion of time during a one-month period.

11. Major Depressive Disorder (MDD): Presence of at least one major depressive episode characterized by depressed mood, loss of interest or pleasure, and other symptoms such as changes in appetite, sleep, energy, concentration, or suicidal thoughts, lasting for at least two weeks.

12. Specific Phobia: Marked fear or anxiety about a specific object or situation, leading to avoidance or distress, out of proportion to the actual threat, and persisting for at least six months.

13. Bipolar Disorder: Presence of at least one manic or hypomanic episode characterized by elevated mood, increased energy, grandiosity, decreased need for sleep, racing thoughts, or excessive involvement in pleasurable activities, along with periods of depressive episodes.

14. Schizoaffective Disorder: Presence of a major mood episode (depressive or manic) concurrent with symptoms of schizophrenia, including hallucinations, delusions, disorganized speech, or negative symptoms.

15. Substance Use Disorder: A problematic pattern of substance use leading to clinically significant impairment or distress, characterized by impaired control, social impairment, risky use, tolerance, or withdrawal symptoms.

16. Eating Disorders: Persistent disturbance in eating patterns, body image, and weight management, such as anorexia nervosa, bulimia nervosa, or binge-eating disorder.

17. Dissociative Identity Disorder (DID): Disruption of identity characterized by the presence of two or more distinct personality states or experiences of possession, along with recurrent gaps in memory.

18. Oppositional Defiant Disorder (ODD): Enduring pattern of angry/irritable mood, argumentative/defiant behavior, or vindictiveness, often directed towards authority figures, causing significant impairment in functioning.

19. Substance Withdrawal: Development of a substance-specific syndrome due to the cessation or reduction in heavy or prolonged substance use, resulting in physical and psychological symptoms.

20. Conduct Disorder: Persistent patterns of behavior that violate the rights of others or societal norms, such as aggression towards people or animals, destruction of property, or theft, causing significant impairment in functioning.

21. Gender Dysphoria: Incongruence between one's experienced gender and assigned gender at birth, characterized by significant distress or impairment in social, occupational, or other areas of functioning.

22. Intellectual Disability: Deficits in intellectual functioning (IQ below a certain threshold) and adaptive functioning in areas such as communication, self-care, and social skills, resulting in significant limitations in functioning.

23. Hoarding Disorder: Persistent difficulty discarding or parting with possessions, regardless of their actual value, due to a perceived need to save them, leading to significant clutter and impairment in living spaces.

24. Schizotypal Personality Disorder: Pervasive pattern of social and interpersonal deficits, along with cognitive or perceptual distortions, eccentric behavior, and odd beliefs or magical thinking.

25. Sleep Disorders: Disruptions in the sleep-wake cycle, including insomnia, hypersomnia, sleep-related breathing disorders, parasomnias, or circadian rhythm disorders, causing significant distress or impairment in daily functioning.

III. Treatment Modalities:

1. Psychotherapy: Also known as talk therapy, it involves a therapeutic relationship between a mental health professional and an individual or group, aimed at addressing emotional and psychological challenges.

2. Cognitive Behavioral Therapy (CBT): A goal-oriented therapy that focuses on identifying and modifying negative thoughts and behaviors to improve mental health and well-being.

3. Medication Management: The use of prescribed medications, such as antidepressants, antipsychotics, or mood stabilizers, to alleviate symptoms of mental health disorders.

4. Dialectical Behavior Therapy (DBT): A type of therapy that combines elements of CBT with skills training in emotional regulation, distress tolerance, interpersonal effectiveness, and mindfulness.

5. Supportive Therapy: Providing emotional support, empathy, and guidance to individuals facing challenges, helping them develop coping mechanisms and improve overall well-being.

6. Psychodynamic Therapy: Exploring unconscious processes and early life experiences to gain insight into current emotional and relational patterns, fostering personal growth and healing.

7. Group Therapy: Therapy conducted in a group setting, allowing individuals to share experiences, learn from others, and receive support from peers facing similar challenges.

8. Family Therapy: Involving the entire family system to address relational dynamics, communication issues, and conflicts that may contribute to mental health concerns.

9. Mindfulness-Based Interventions: Techniques that cultivate present-moment awareness, such as mindfulness meditation, to reduce stress, enhance self-compassion, and improve overall mental well-being.

10. Art Therapy: Utilizing creative processes, such as painting, drawing, or sculpting, to promote self-expression, emotional healing, and self-discovery.

11. Music Therapy: Using music-based interventions, such as listening, singing, or playing instruments, to enhance emotional expression, communication, and overall well-being.

12. Occupational Therapy: Assisting individuals in developing and maintaining meaningful daily activities and routines to improve overall mental health and quality of life.

13. Play Therapy: A therapeutic approach that uses play as a means of communication, allowing children to express emotions, resolve conflicts, and develop coping skills.

14. Electroconvulsive Therapy (ECT): A medical procedure that induces controlled seizures to treat severe depression, mania, or certain psychiatric conditions when other interventions have been ineffective.

15. Transcranial Magnetic Stimulation (TMS): Non-invasive brain stimulation technique that uses magnetic fields to target specific regions of the brain for the treatment of depression and other mental health disorders.

16. Eye Movement Desensitization and Reprocessing (EMDR): A therapy modality used to process traumatic memories and alleviate associated distress through bilateral stimulation techniques.

17. Pharmacotherapy: The use of medications to manage symptoms of mental health disorders, such as antidepressants, anxiolytics, or mood stabilizers.

18. Rehabilitation Programs: Comprehensive programs that provide support and skills training to individuals with mental health conditions to enhance independence, social functioning, and vocational skills.

19. Expressive Therapy: Therapeutic interventions that promote self-expression and emotional release through various creative mediums, such as dance, drama, or poetry.

20. Integrative Therapy: An approach that combines multiple therapeutic modalities, tailoring treatment to individual needs, and incorporating a holistic perspective.

21. Crisis Intervention: Providing immediate support and intervention in times of acute mental health crisis or emotional distress to ensure safety and stabilization.

22. Self-Help and Support Groups: Participating in peer-led groups focused on shared experiences, encouragement, and mutual support for individuals with similar mental health concerns.

23. Psychoeducation: Providing individuals and their families with information and education about mental health conditions, treatment options, and coping strategies.

24. Teletherapy: Delivery of therapy services through video conferencing or telephone, providing access to mental health support remotely.

25. Case Management: Coordinating and connecting individuals with mental health services, resources, and community supports to optimize treatment outcomes and overall well-being.

Practice activities for transcribing psychiatry reports effectively

Exercise 1: Fill in the blanks

Transcribe the following sentence:

The patient reports feeling ________ most of the day for at least two weeks.

Answer:

The patient reports feeling depressed most of the day for at least two weeks.

Exercise 2: True or False

Indicate whether the following statement is true or false:

Anxiety disorders are characterized by excessive worry, fear, or unease that interferes with daily functioning.

Answer:

True

Exercise 3: Fill in the blanks

Transcribe the following sentence:

The patient has a history of ________ disorder characterized by recurring, intrusive thoughts and repetitive behaviors.

Answer:

The patient has a history of obsessive-compulsive disorder characterized by recurring, intrusive thoughts and repetitive behaviors.

Exercise 4: Matching

Match the psychiatric assessment tool with its description:

1. Beck Depression Inventory (BDI)

2. Hamilton Rating Scale for Depression (HAM-D)

3. Generalized Anxiety Disorder 7-item Scale (GAD-7)

4. Mini-Mental State Examination (MMSE)

A. Measures severity of anxiety symptoms

B. Assesses the presence and severity of depressive symptoms

C. Evaluates symptoms and severity of depression

D. Screens for cognitive impairment and assesses orientation, memory, and attention

Answer:

1. Beck Depression Inventory (BDI)

B. Assesses the presence and severity of depressive symptoms

2. Hamilton Rating Scale for Depression (HAM-D)

C. Evaluates symptoms and severity of depression

3. Generalized Anxiety Disorder 7-item Scale (GAD-7)

A. Measures severity of anxiety symptoms

4. Mini-Mental State Examination (MMSE)

D. Screens for cognitive impairment and assesses orientation, memory, and attention

Exercise 5: Fill in the blanks

Transcribe the following sentence:

The patient exhibits __________ behavior, showing little interest in social interactions and preferring solitary activities.

Answer:

The patient exhibits withdrawn behavior, showing little interest in social interactions and preferring solitary activities.

Exercise 6: True or False

Indicate whether the following statement is true or false:

Schizophrenia is a chronic psychiatric disorder characterized by disturbances in perception, thoughts, emotions, and behavior.

Answer:

True

Exercise 7: Fill in the blanks

Transcribe the following sentence:

The patient has a history of _________ disorder, experiencing extreme mood swings ranging from depressive episodes to manic episodes.

Answer:

The patient has a history of bipolar disorder, experiencing extreme mood swings ranging from depressive episodes to manic episodes.

Exercise 8: Matching

Match the psychiatric medication with its description:

1. Selective Serotonin Reuptake Inhibitors (SSRIs)

2. Benzodiazepines

3. Mood Stabilizers

4. Antipsychotics

A. Antipsychotic medication used to treat schizophrenia and other psychotic disorders

B. Medication used to relieve symptoms of anxiety and promote relaxation

C. Medication used to treat depression by increasing the availability of serotonin in the brain

D. Medication used to stabilize mood and prevent or reduce manic or depressive episodes in bipolar disorder

Answer:

1. Selective Serotonin Reuptake Inhibitors (SSRIs)

C. Medication used to treat depression by increasing the availability of serotonin in the brain

2. Benzodiazepines

B. Medication used to relieve symptoms of anxiety and promote relaxation

3. Mood Stabilizers

D. Medication used to stabilize mood and prevent or reduce manic or depressive episodes in bipolar disorder

4. Antipsychotics

A. Antipsychotic medication used to treat schizophrenia and other psychotic disorders

Exercise 9: True or False

Indicate whether the following statement is true or false:

Cognitive-behavioral therapy (CBT) is a common psychotherapy approach that focuses on changing negative thoughts and behaviors to improve mental health.

Answer:

True

Exercise 10: Fill in the blanks

Transcribe the following sentence:

The patient exhibits __________ symptoms, including hallucinations and delusions.

Answer:

The patient exhibits psychotic symptoms, including hallucinations and delusions.

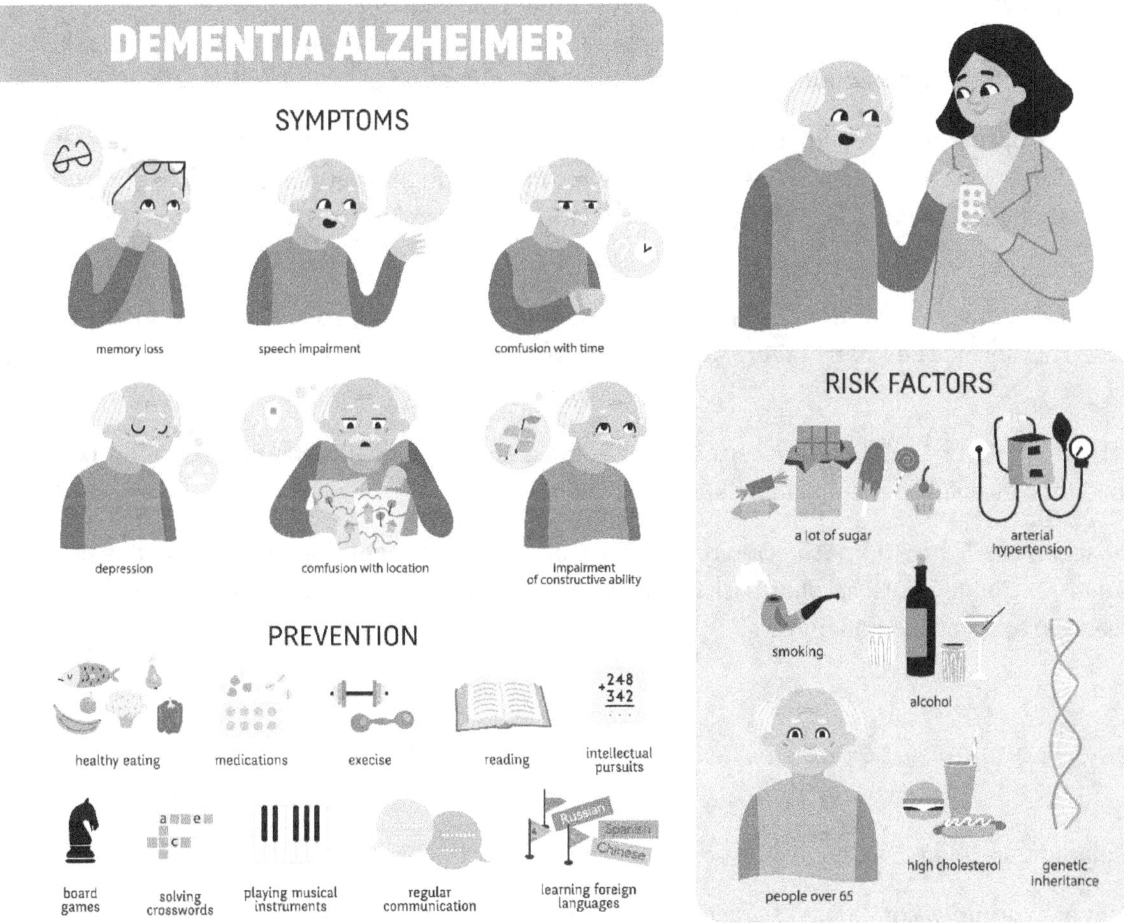

Overview of geriatrics and its specific terminology

Geriatrics is a branch of medicine that focuses on the health care of elderly people. It aims to promote health by preventing and treating diseases and disabilities in older adults, focusing not only on the medical aspects of aging but also on the psychological, social, and functional aspects.

Here are some key points to understand as a beginner in this field:

1. Aging Population: Geriatricians manage the health of older adults, a rapidly growing population. They are specialized in managing the unique healthcare needs and treatment preferences of older people.

2. Common Conditions: Geriatricians often manage several chronic conditions in an individual patient, such as heart disease, hypertension, diabetes, arthritis, dementia, osteoporosis, and Alzheimer's disease. They also deal with issues related to frailty, falls, incontinence, and functional losses.

3. Comprehensive Geriatric Assessment (CGA): This multidimensional and multidisciplinary diagnostic process focuses on determining a frail elderly person's medical, functional, and psychosocial capabilities and problems, with the aim of developing a coordinated and integrated plan for treatment and follow-up.

4. Treatment Approaches: Geriatricians aim to maintain the well-being and functional independence of older adults for as long as possible. This may involve a combination of treatments, including medication management, physical therapy, and lifestyle modifications. They also focus on palliative care and end-of-life issues.

5. Geriatric Syndromes: These are clinical conditions in older persons that do not fit into discrete disease categories. They include delirium, frailty, cognitive impairment, dizziness, syncope, and mobility disorders like falls.

6. Geriatric Psychiatry: This is a subspecialty that addresses mental health and emotional problems in elderly patients, including dementia and depression.

7. Interdisciplinary Team Approach: Geriatric practice often involves coordinating a team of health care professionals including nurses, pharmacists, physical therapists, and social workers to provide a comprehensive approach to patient care.

Age-related conditions, geriatric assessments, and care management

I. Age-Related Conditions:

1. Dementia: A group of conditions characterized by cognitive decline, memory loss, and difficulties with thinking, problem-solving, and language.

2. Alzheimer's Disease: The most common form of dementia, characterized by progressive memory loss, cognitive decline, and changes in behavior and personality.

3. Osteoporosis: A condition in which the bones become weak and brittle, increasing the risk of fractures, commonly associated with aging.

4. Arthritis: Inflammation of the joints, resulting in pain, stiffness, and reduced mobility, commonly seen in older adults.

5. Cataracts: Clouding of the lens in the eye, leading to blurry vision and decreased visual acuity, often associated with aging.

6. Macular Degeneration: A progressive eye disease that affects the central part of the retina, leading to loss of central vision and difficulty seeing fine details.

7. Hearing Loss: Gradual or sudden loss of hearing ability, often associated with age-related changes in the inner ear.

8. Cardiovascular Disease: Various conditions affecting the heart and blood vessels, including hypertension, coronary artery disease, and heart failure, which become more common with age.

9. Diabetes: A metabolic disorder characterized by high blood sugar levels, which can develop or become more prevalent in older adults.

10. Stroke: A sudden interruption of blood flow to the brain, resulting in neurological deficits and potentially long-term disability, more common in older age groups.

11. Osteoarthritis: A degenerative joint disease characterized by the breakdown of cartilage, causing pain, swelling, and stiffness in the joints.

12. Chronic Obstructive Pulmonary Disease (COPD): A progressive lung disease that causes breathing difficulties, often associated with smoking and long-term exposure to lung irritants.

13. Parkinson's Disease: A neurodegenerative disorder that affects movement and coordination, characterized by tremors, muscle stiffness, and difficulty with balance.

14. Urinary Incontinence: The involuntary leakage of urine, often associated with weakened pelvic floor muscles and changes in bladder control that can occur with aging.

15. Hypertension: High blood pressure, a condition that becomes more common as individuals age and can increase the risk of cardiovascular problems.

16. Depression: A mood disorder characterized by persistent feelings of sadness, loss of interest, and decreased energy, which can be more prevalent in older adults.

17. Frailty: A syndrome characterized by weakness, decreased physical function, and increased vulnerability to adverse health outcomes, commonly seen in older adults.

18. Sarcopenia: Age-related loss of muscle mass and strength, leading to reduced mobility and functional decline.

19. Osteoarthritis: A degenerative joint disease characterized by the breakdown of cartilage, causing pain, swelling, and stiffness in the joints.

20. Falls and Fall-Related Injuries: The increased risk of falls and subsequent injuries due to age-related changes in balance, strength, and mobility.

21. Visual Impairment: Age-related changes in vision, such as presbyopia (difficulty focusing on close objects) or age-related macular degeneration, leading to visual limitations.

22. Delirium: An acute confusional state characterized by sudden changes in mental function, attention, and cognition, often seen in older adults with underlying medical conditions.

23. Sleep Disorders: Age-related changes in sleep patterns, including insomnia, sleep apnea, or restless legs syndrome, affecting the quality and duration of sleep.

24. Malnutrition: Nutritional deficiencies or inadequate nutrient intake, which can be more common in older adults due to reduced appetite, dental problems, or medication side effects.

25. Polypharmacy: The use of multiple medications concurrently, which can increase the risk of adverse drug reactions, drug interactions, and medication errors, particularly in older adults.

II. Geriatric Assessments:

1. Mini Mental State Examination (MMSE): A cognitive screening tool used to assess mental status, memory, and orientation in older adults.

2. Geriatric Depression Scale (GDS): A questionnaire to assess and screen for depressive symptoms in older adults.

3. Activities of Daily Living (ADL) Assessment: Evaluation of an individual's ability to independently perform essential self-care activities such as bathing, dressing, eating, and toileting.

4. Instrumental Activities of Daily Living (IADL) Assessment: Assessment of an individual's ability to perform complex tasks necessary for independent living, such as managing finances, shopping, cooking, and using transportation.

5. Timed Up and Go Test (TUG): A measure of mobility and balance that assesses the time it takes an individual to stand up, walk a short distance, turn around, and return to sitting.

6. Falls Risk Assessment: Evaluation of an individual's risk factors for falls, including history of falls, balance impairments, gait abnormalities, and environmental hazards.

7. Geriatric Nutritional Risk Index (GNRI): A screening tool to assess the nutritional status of older adults based on their body weight, serum albumin levels, and recent weight loss.

8. Geriatric Syndromes Assessment: Evaluation of common geriatric syndromes such as frailty, cognitive impairment, urinary incontinence, polypharmacy, and functional decline.

9. Pain Assessment: Evaluation of an individual's pain intensity, location, and impact on daily activities using standardized pain assessment tools, such as the Numeric Rating Scale or the Wong-Baker FACES Pain Rating Scale.

10. Geriatric Assessment for Polypharmacy: Evaluation of an individual's medication regimen, including medication list review, assessment of potential drug interactions, and identification of inappropriate medications.

11. Delirium Assessment: Evaluation of an individual's cognitive function and presence of delirium symptoms, such as acute onset confusion, disorientation, and changes in attention and awareness.

12. Functional Mobility Assessment: Assessment of an individual's ability to move safely and independently, including tasks such as transferring from bed to chair, walking, and navigating stairs.

13. Pressure Ulcer Risk Assessment: Evaluation of an individual's risk factors for developing pressure ulcers, including immobility, malnutrition, sensory impairment, and moisture exposure.

14. Medication Reconciliation: A process of comparing a patient's current medication regimen to previous regimens during care transitions to identify discrepancies, potential interactions, and optimize medication management.

15. Palliative Care Assessment: Evaluation of an individual's physical, psychological, and spiritual needs in the context of serious illness, with a focus on improving quality of life and symptom management.

16. Functional Capacity Evaluation: Assessment of an individual's physical abilities and limitations related to work tasks and activities, often performed in the context of disability evaluations or occupational therapy.

17. Geriatric Assessment for Fall Prevention: Comprehensive evaluation of an individual's fall risk factors, including gait and balance assessment, vision assessment, home safety assessment, and review of medications.

18. Geriatric Assessment for Dementia: Evaluation of cognitive function, memory, and behavior to assess for possible dementia or cognitive impairment.

19. Geriatric Assessment for Urinary Incontinence: Assessment of urinary symptoms, fluid intake, bladder habits, and related factors to identify the cause and develop a management plan for urinary incontinence.

20. Geriatric Assessment for Frailty: Evaluation of an individual's overall health status, functional abilities, and physiological reserve to determine their level of frailty and risk of adverse health outcomes.

21. Advanced Care Planning Assessment: Discussion and documentation of an individual's preferences for future medical care, including decisions about life-sustaining treatments and end-of-life care.

22. Geriatric Assessment for Polypharmacy: Evaluation of an older adult's medication regimen to identify potential drug interactions, side effects, and opportunities for deprescribing or optimizing medication use.

23. Geriatric Assessment for Elder Abuse: Assessment of an older adult's physical, psychological, or financial well-being to identify signs of abuse, neglect, or exploitation.

24. Geriatric Assessment for Driving Safety: Evaluation of an older adult's physical and cognitive abilities related to driving, including vision, reaction time, and decision-making skills.

25. Geriatric Assessment for Geriatric Syndromes: Comprehensive evaluation of common geriatric syndromes such as falls, incontinence, cognitive impairment, and malnutrition to identify contributing factors and develop appropriate management plans.

III. Care Management:

1. Comprehensive Geriatric Assessment (CGA): A systematic evaluation of an older adult's medical, functional, cognitive, and psychosocial status to guide care planning and management.

2. Care Coordination: The process of organizing and integrating healthcare services across multiple providers and settings to ensure seamless and efficient care delivery for older adults.

3. Medication Management: The review, reconciliation, and optimization of medication regimens to ensure the safe and effective use of medications by older adults.

4. Chronic Disease Management: The ongoing monitoring, treatment, and support for older adults with chronic conditions such as diabetes, hypertension, or heart disease to optimize their health outcomes.

5. Caregiver Support and Education: Providing guidance, resources, and education to family caregivers who play a crucial role in supporting the well-being of older adults.

6. Advance Care Planning: Discussions and documentation of an older adult's preferences for future healthcare decisions, including the designation of a healthcare proxy and the creation of advance directives.

7. Transitional Care: Coordinating and managing the safe and smooth transition of older adults between different care settings, such as hospitals, rehabilitation facilities, and home.

8. Palliative Care: Specialized medical care that focuses on relieving symptoms, managing pain, and improving the quality of life for older adults with serious or life-limiting illnesses.

9. Caregiver Training: Providing education and skills training to family caregivers on topics such as safe transfers, medication administration, and managing behavioral symptoms in older adults.

10. Caregiver Respite Services: Offering temporary relief and support to family caregivers through the provision of respite care services, allowing them time to recharge and attend to their own needs.

11. Home Safety Assessments: Evaluating the home environment of older adults to identify potential hazards and recommending modifications or assistive devices to enhance safety and independence.

12. Nutrition Counseling: Providing dietary guidance and education to older adults to support healthy eating habits and manage nutrition-related conditions.

13. Social Support Services: Connecting older adults with community resources, support groups, and social activities to combat isolation and promote social engagement.

14. Mental Health Support: Assessing and addressing the mental health needs of older adults through counseling, therapy, and appropriate referral to specialists.

15. Functional Rehabilitation: Developing personalized rehabilitation programs to improve physical functioning, mobility, and activities of daily living in older adults.

16. Cognitive Stimulation: Engaging older adults in activities, exercises, and therapies to enhance cognitive function, memory, and overall brain health.

17. Home Health Services: Arranging and coordinating skilled nursing, therapy, and support services provided at home to meet the healthcare needs of older adults who may have difficulty accessing traditional healthcare settings.

18. Assistive Devices and Technologies: Assessing and recommending appropriate assistive devices, such as walking aids or hearing aids, to enhance independence and quality of life for older adults.

19. Care Transitions Coaching: Providing education and coaching to older adults and their caregivers to navigate healthcare transitions successfully and avoid potential pitfalls.

20. Disease Prevention and Health Promotion: Offering preventive services, health screenings, vaccinations, and health education programs to promote wellness and prevent illnesses in older adults.

21. Chronic Pain Management: Developing individualized pain management plans to address chronic pain issues in older adults, combining pharmacological, physical, and psychological interventions.

22. End-of-Life Care Planning: Assisting older adults and their families in making decisions and planning for end-of-life care, including hospice care and advance care directives.

23. Community Integration: Facilitating the integration of older adults into the community through engagement in local activities, volunteer opportunities, and social support networks.

24. Financial Assistance and Benefits: Providing information and assistance with accessing financial resources, such as insurance programs, Medicare, Medicaid, and other benefits available to older adults.

25. Quality Assurance and Outcomes Monitoring: Implementing processes to ensure the quality of care provided to older adults, including monitoring outcomes, conducting satisfaction surveys, and making improvements based on feedback.

Exercises for transcribing geriatrics reports accurately

Exercise 1: Fill in the blanks

Transcribe the following sentence:

The patient presents with _________ and _________ gait, requiring assistance with walking.

Answer:

The patient presents with unsteady and shuffling gait, requiring assistance with walking.

Exercise 2: True or False

Indicate whether the following statement is true or false:

Polypharmacy refers to the use of multiple medications by a patient, typically taking five or more medications concurrently.

Answer:

True

Exercise 3: Fill in the blanks

Transcribe the following sentence:

The patient has a history of _________ disease, characterized by a gradual loss of memory, cognitive decline, and impaired functioning.

Answer:

The patient has a history of Alzheimer's disease, characterized by a gradual loss of memory, cognitive decline, and impaired functioning.

Exercise 4: Matching

Match the geriatric assessment tool with its description:

1. Mini-Cog Assessment

2. Geriatric Depression Scale (GDS)

3. Timed Up and Go (TUG) Test

4. Activities of Daily Living (ADL) Scale

A. Screens for depression symptoms and assesses their severity

B. Assesses cognitive function and memory recall

C. Evaluates functional mobility and fall risk

D. Measures independence in performing daily self-care activities

Answer:

1. Mini-Cog Assessment

B. Assesses cognitive function and memory recall

2. Geriatric Depression Scale (GDS)

A. Screens for depression symptoms and assesses their severity

3. Timed Up and Go (TUG) Test

C. Evaluates functional mobility and fall risk

4. Activities of Daily Living (ADL) Scale

D. Measures independence in performing daily self-care activities

Exercise 5: Fill in the blanks

Transcribe the following sentence:

The patient has _________ impairments, experiencing difficulty with memory, attention, and decision-making.

Answer:

The patient has cognitive impairments, experiencing difficulty with memory, attention, and decision-making.

Exercise 6: True or False

Indicate whether the following statement is true or false:

Frailty is a clinical syndrome characterized by decreased physiological reserve and increased vulnerability to stressors.

Answer:

True

Exercise 7: Fill in the blanks

Transcribe the following sentence:

The patient has ________ syndrome, presenting with symptoms such as muscle weakness, fatigue, and decreased physical performance.

Answer:

The patient has frailty syndrome, presenting with symptoms such as muscle weakness, fatigue, and decreased physical performance.

Exercise 8: Matching

Match the geriatric condition with its description:

1. Osteoporosis

2. Arthritis

3. Chronic Obstructive Pulmonary Disease (COPD)

4. Hearing Loss

A. Chronic pain and inflammation in the joints, commonly affecting the hands, knees, and hips

B. Loss of bone density, leading to increased risk of fractures

C. Progressive lung disease that causes difficulty breathing and reduced lung function

D. Gradual deterioration of hearing ability, affecting communication and quality of life

Answer:

1. Osteoporosis

B. Loss of bone density, leading to increased risk of fractures

2. Arthritis

A. Chronic pain and inflammation in the joints, commonly affecting the hands, knees, and hips

3. Chronic Obstructive Pulmonary Disease (COPD)

C. Progressive lung disease that causes difficulty breathing and reduced lung function

4. Hearing Loss

D. Gradual deterioration of hearing ability, affecting communication and quality of life

Exercise 9: True or False

Indicate whether the following statement is true or false:

Advance directives are legal documents that outline a person's preferences for medical treatment in the event they are unable to make decisions for themselves.

Answer:

True

Exercise 10: Fill in the blanks

Transcribe the following sentence:

The patient requires __________ care services to assist with activities such as bathing, dressing, and meal preparation.

Answer:

The patient requires home care services to assist with activities such as bathing, dressing, and meal preparation.

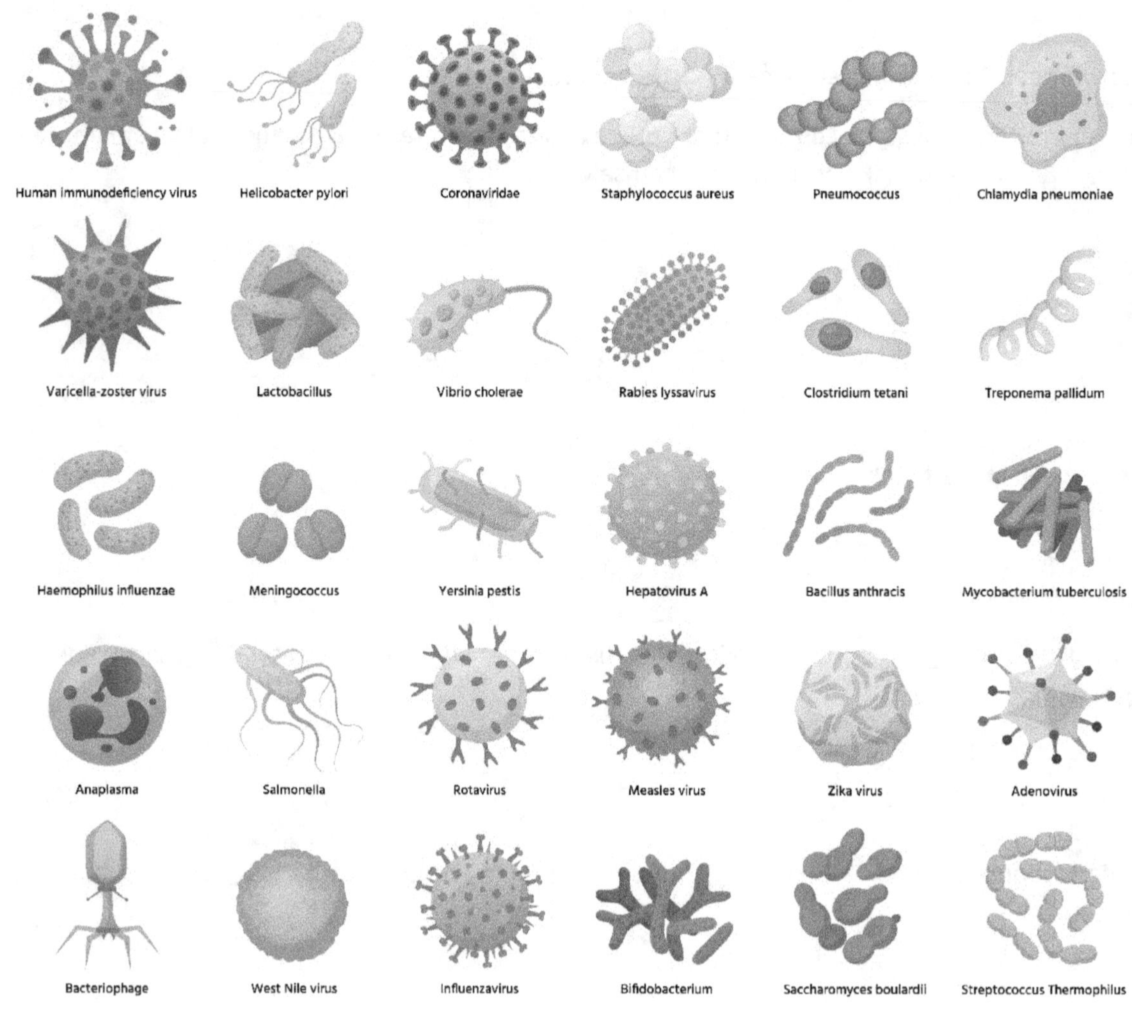

Introduction to infectious diseases and their unique terminology

Infectious Diseases is a branch of medicine that focuses on diagnosing, managing, and treating infections. This specialty includes diseases caused by bacteria, viruses, fungi, and parasites. Infectious disease specialists often serve as consultants to other physicians in cases of complex infections, and manage patients with novel, emerging, or chronic infections.

Here are some key points to understand as a beginner in this field:

1. Diverse Pathogens: Infectious diseases are caused by a wide range of organisms, including bacteria, viruses, fungi, and parasites. The infectious disease specialist must have a broad knowledge base to identify and treat these various pathogens.

2. Common Conditions: These specialists treat a variety of diseases, including pneumonia, tuberculosis, HIV/AIDS, malaria, and infections that can occur in those with weakened immune systems.

3. Diagnostic Tools: Diagnosis of infectious diseases often involves microbiological studies to identify the pathogen, such as cultures, serology, microscopy, and increasingly, molecular diagnostic tests. Advanced imaging techniques may also be used in some cases.

4. Treatment Approaches: Treatments can include antibiotics for bacterial infections, antiviral drugs for viral infections, antifungal medications for fungal infections, and antiparasitic treatments for parasitic infections. Preventive measures, such as vaccinations, are also a major part of infectious disease medicine.

5. Antibiotic Stewardship: Given the rise of antibiotic resistance, infectious disease specialists are deeply involved in antibiotic stewardship – the proper use of antibiotics to minimize resistance and ensure the effectiveness of these important drugs.

6. Infection Control: Infectious disease specialists also play a key role in hospital infection control, helping to prevent healthcare-associated infections and contain outbreaks when they occur.

7. Global Health: The field of infectious diseases is closely tied to global health, given that many infections spread across borders. Infectious disease specialists may work on global challenges such as HIV/AIDS, tuberculosis, malaria, and emerging infectious diseases like COVID-19.

8. Research and Emerging Diseases: Many infectious disease specialists are also involved in research, studying new ways to diagnose, treat, and prevent infections. They are on the front lines in the fight against emerging infectious diseases.

Common infections, diagnostic tests, and antimicrobial therapies

I. Common Infections:

1. Upper Respiratory Tract Infection (URTI): An infection primarily affecting the nose, throat, and sinuses, often caused by viruses like the common cold or influenza.

2. Urinary Tract Infection (UTI): An infection in any part of the urinary system, such as the bladder or urethra, commonly caused by bacteria entering the urinary tract.

3. Pneumonia: An infection that inflames the air sacs in one or both lungs, typically caused by bacteria, viruses, or fungi.

4. Influenza (Flu): A highly contagious viral infection that affects the respiratory system and can cause fever, body aches, cough, and fatigue.

5. Gastroenteritis: An inflammation of the stomach and intestines, often caused by viruses or bacteria, resulting in symptoms like diarrhea, vomiting, and abdominal pain.

6. Skin Infections: Various infections affecting the skin, such as cellulitis (bacterial infection of the skin and underlying tissues), impetigo (bacterial skin infection), or fungal infections like athlete's foot or ringworm.

7. Sinusitis: Inflammation of the sinuses, commonly caused by a viral or bacterial infection, leading to symptoms such as facial pain, headache, and nasal congestion.

8. Strep Throat: An infection caused by the group A Streptococcus bacteria, resulting in a sore throat, difficulty swallowing, and swollen tonsils.

9. Bronchitis: Inflammation of the bronchial tubes, often due to a viral infection, causing cough, chest discomfort, and production of mucus.

10. Conjunctivitis (Pink Eye): Inflammation of the conjunctiva, the thin tissue covering the white part of the eye and the inside of the eyelids, typically caused by viruses, bacteria, or allergies.

11. Ear Infections: Infections affecting the middle ear, such as acute otitis media (infection of the middle ear) or otitis externa (infection of the outer ear canal).

12. Dental Infections: Infections of the teeth, gums, or oral tissues, commonly caused by bacteria, resulting in tooth decay, gum disease, or abscesses.

13. Sexually Transmitted Infections (STIs): Infections transmitted through sexual contact, including chlamydia, gonorrhea, syphilis, herpes, and human immunodeficiency virus (HIV).

14. Tuberculosis (TB): A bacterial infection caused by Mycobacterium tuberculosis, primarily affecting the lungs but can also affect other organs, leading to persistent cough, fever, and weight loss.

15. Lyme Disease: An infectious disease transmitted through tick bites, caused by the bacterium Borrelia burgdorferi, resulting in symptoms such as rash, fatigue, and joint pain.

16. Meningitis: Inflammation of the membranes surrounding the brain and spinal cord, often caused by bacteria or viruses, leading to symptoms like headache, fever, and stiff neck.

17. Hepatitis: Inflammation of the liver, typically caused by viral infections (hepatitis A, B, C, etc.), resulting in liver dysfunction and various symptoms depending on the type of hepatitis.

18. Dental Caries (Tooth Decay): Bacterial infection that causes tooth decay and cavities, often resulting from poor oral hygiene and dietary factors.

19. Shingles (Herpes Zoster): A viral infection caused by the varicella-zoster virus, leading to a painful rash and blisters, usually occurring in people who had chickenpox earlier in life.

20. Yeast Infections: Infections caused by an overgrowth of yeast (Candida) in various parts of the body, such as the mouth (thrush), genital area, or skin folds.

21. Gastrointestinal Parasitic Infections: Infections caused by various parasites, such as Giardia, Cryptosporidium, or roundworms, resulting in symptoms like diarrhea, abdominal pain, and weight loss.

22. Malaria: A mosquito-borne parasitic infection caused by Plasmodium parasites, leading to recurring fever, chills, and flu-like symptoms.

23. Urinary Tract Stones: The formation of hardened mineral deposits in the urinary tract, which can lead to pain, urinary tract infections, and obstruction of urine flow.

24. Helicobacter pylori Infection: A bacterial infection that affects the stomach, often leading to peptic ulcers and gastritis.

25. Respiratory Syncytial Virus (RSV): A common viral infection that primarily affects the respiratory system, especially in infants and young children, causing symptoms similar to the common cold.

II. Diagnostic Tests:

1. Blood Tests: Laboratory tests that analyze various components of the blood, such as complete blood count (CBC), blood glucose levels, cholesterol levels, or specific markers indicating infection or inflammation.

2. X-rays: Imaging tests that use electromagnetic radiation to produce images of the internal structures of the body, primarily bones and some organs.

3. Ultrasound: A diagnostic imaging technique that uses high-frequency sound waves to create images of organs, tissues, and blood flow in real-time.

4. Magnetic Resonance Imaging (MRI): An imaging technique that uses a magnetic field and radio waves to create detailed images of the body's structures, providing information about organs, soft tissues, and blood vessels.

5. Computed Tomography (CT) Scan: A diagnostic imaging test that uses a combination of X-rays and computer technology to produce cross-sectional images of the body.

6. Electrocardiogram (ECG or EKG): A test that records the electrical activity of the heart to evaluate heart rhythm, identify abnormalities, and diagnose conditions such as heart attacks or arrhythmias.

7. Electroencephalogram (EEG): A test that records the electrical activity of the brain, helping to diagnose conditions such as epilepsy, sleep disorders, or brain abnormalities.

8. Spirometry: A pulmonary function test that measures lung function by assessing the volume of air inhaled and exhaled and how efficiently the lungs exchange gases.

9. Colonoscopy: A procedure that uses a flexible tube with a camera (endoscope) to visualize the inner lining of the colon and rectum, aiding in the diagnosis of conditions like colorectal cancer or inflammatory bowel disease.

10. Biopsy: A procedure in which a small sample of tissue is removed from the body and examined under a microscope to diagnose diseases such as cancer or infections.

11. Pap Smear: A screening test for cervical cancer that involves collecting cells from the cervix to detect any abnormal changes or precancerous conditions.

12. Mammogram: An X-ray of the breast used for screening or diagnosing breast cancer, capturing images of breast tissue to detect any abnormalities or tumors.

13. Bone Density Scan: A test that measures bone mineral density to assess bone health and diagnose conditions such as osteoporosis or osteopenia.

14. Genetic Testing: Analysis of DNA or genetic material to identify genetic mutations or variations associated with inherited disorders or the risk of developing certain conditions.

15. Urine Analysis: Laboratory examination of a urine sample to evaluate kidney function, detect infections, or identify abnormal substances.

16. Stool Analysis: Laboratory testing of a stool sample to detect abnormalities, parasites, or signs of digestive disorders or infections.

17. Skin Biopsy: A procedure that involves removing a small piece of skin for microscopic examination to diagnose skin conditions, such as skin cancer or rashes.

18. Lumbar Puncture (Spinal Tap): A procedure in which a needle is inserted into the lower back to collect cerebrospinal fluid for analysis, helping diagnose conditions like meningitis or neurological disorders.

19. Endoscopy: A procedure that uses a flexible tube with a camera (endoscope) to visualize and examine internal organs or structures, such as the gastrointestinal tract or airways.

20. Allergy Testing: Diagnostic tests, such as skin prick tests or blood tests, to identify specific allergens triggering allergic reactions in individuals.

21. Papillary Muscle Stress Test: A cardiac stress test that evaluates the function of the papillary muscles, which help control the movement of the heart valves.

22. Audiometry: A test that measures hearing ability by assessing the individual's response to different sound frequencies and intensities.

23. Imaging-guided Biopsy: A biopsy procedure guided by imaging techniques to precisely target and sample suspicious areas in the body, aiding in the diagnosis of cancers or other conditions.

24. Hysterosalpingogram (HSG): A radiology procedure that uses contrast dye to evaluate the shape and function of the uterus and fallopian tubes, assisting in the diagnosis of infertility or other reproductive issues.

25. Sigmoidoscopy: A procedure that uses a flexible tube with a camera (endoscope) to examine the lower part of the large intestine (sigmoid colon) and rectum, often performed to detect signs of inflammation, polyps, or cancer.

III. Antimicrobial Therapies:

1. Antibiotics: Medications that target and kill bacteria or inhibit their growth, helping to treat bacterial infections.

2. Antivirals: Drugs that specifically target viruses and inhibit their replication, helping to treat viral infections such as influenza or herpes.

3. Antifungals: Medications that target and eliminate fungal infections, such as athlete's foot or yeast infections.

4. Antimalarials: Drugs used to prevent or treat malaria, a parasitic infection transmitted by mosquitoes in certain regions.

5. Antiretrovirals: Medications used to suppress the replication of the human immunodeficiency virus (HIV) and slow down the progression of acquired immunodeficiency syndrome (AIDS).

6. Antiparasitics: Medications used to treat various parasitic infections, including intestinal worms, lice, or scabies.

7. Antituberculosis Agents: Drugs used to treat tuberculosis (TB), a bacterial infection that primarily affects the lungs.

8. Antiseptics: Chemical substances that are applied to living tissue to prevent or inhibit the growth of microorganisms, typically used for wound care.

9. Disinfectants: Agents that are used to kill or eliminate microorganisms on surfaces or inanimate objects, commonly used in cleaning and sterilization procedures.

10. Antifungal Creams: Topical medications applied to the skin to treat fungal infections, such as ringworm or athlete's foot.

11. Antimicrobial Peptides: Naturally occurring peptides that possess antimicrobial properties, often used in the development of novel therapeutic agents.

12. Antimicrobial Mouthwashes: Oral rinses containing antimicrobial agents, used to help control oral infections or treat conditions like gingivitis.

13. Antihelminthics: Medications used to treat parasitic worm infections, including roundworms, tapeworms, and hookworms.

14. Antimicrobial Ointments: Topical formulations containing antimicrobial agents, applied to the skin to prevent or treat bacterial or fungal infections.

15. Antiviral Vaccines: Vaccines that stimulate the immune system to produce an immune response against specific viruses, providing protection against infection.

16. Antiseptic Wipes: Pre-moistened wipes or swabs containing antiseptic agents, used to cleanse the skin before medical procedures or to disinfect wounds.

17. Antifungal Nail Lacquers: Topical solutions applied to the nails to treat fungal infections, such as onychomycosis (nail fungus).

18. Broad-Spectrum Antibiotics: Antibiotics that are effective against a wide range of bacterial species, making them useful in treating infections when the specific causative agent is unknown.

19. Combination Therapy: The use of two or more antimicrobial agents together to enhance efficacy and prevent the development of resistance in the treatment of certain infections.

20. Antiviral Creams: Topical formulations containing antiviral agents, applied to the skin to treat viral infections like cold sores or genital herpes.

21. Prophylactic Antibiotics: Antibiotics administered before surgery or certain medical procedures to prevent infections.

22. Topical Antimicrobial Solutions: Liquid or gel formulations containing antimicrobial agents, applied to the skin to prevent or treat infections in specific areas.

23. Antifungal Powders: Powders containing antifungal agents, used to prevent or treat fungal infections, particularly in areas prone to moisture, such as between the toes or in the groin.

24. Antimicrobial Catheters: Catheters coated or impregnated with antimicrobial agents to reduce the risk of catheter-associated infections.

25. Antiviral Therapy for Hepatitis: Medications used to treat viral hepatitis infections, including hepatitis B and hepatitis C, to suppress viral replication and prevent disease progression.

Practice activities for transcribing infectious diseases reports effectively

Exercise 1: Fill in the blanks

Transcribe the following sentence:

The patient was diagnosed with __________, a contagious respiratory infection caused by a viral pathogen.

Answer:

The patient was diagnosed with influenza, a contagious respiratory infection caused by a viral pathogen.

Exercise 2: True or False

Indicate whether the following statement is true or false:

Meningitis is an inflammation of the brain and spinal cord membranes, usually caused by a bacterial or viral infection.

Answer:

True

Exercise 3: Fill in the blanks

Transcribe the following sentence:

The patient presented with symptoms of __________, including fever, cough, and sore throat, suggestive of a respiratory tract infection.

Answer:

The patient presented with symptoms of pharyngitis, including fever, cough, and sore throat, suggestive of a respiratory tract infection.

Exercise 4: Matching

Match the infectious disease with its causative agent:

1. Tuberculosis

2. Hepatitis B

3. Chickenpox

4. Pneumonia

A. Varicella-zoster virus

B. Streptococcus pneumoniae

C. Mycobacterium tuberculosis

D. Hepatitis B virus

Answer:

1. Tuberculosis

C. Mycobacterium tuberculosis

2. Hepatitis B

D. Hepatitis B virus

3. Chickenpox

A. Varicella-zoster virus

4. Pneumonia

B. Streptococcus pneumoniae

Exercise 5: Fill in the blanks

Transcribe the following sentence:

The patient was started on _________ therapy, a common antibiotic used to treat bacterial skin infections.

Answer:

The patient was started on cephalexin therapy, a common antibiotic used to treat bacterial skin infections.

Exercise 6: True or False

Indicate whether the following statement is true or false:

Human immunodeficiency virus (HIV) is a viral infection that attacks the immune system, leading to acquired immunodeficiency syndrome (AIDS).

Answer:

True

Exercise 7: Fill in the blanks

Transcribe the following sentence:

The patient's blood culture was positive for _________, indicating a bloodstream infection.

Answer:

The patient's blood culture was positive for Staphylococcus aureus, indicating a bloodstream infection.

Exercise 8: Matching

Match the symptom with the corresponding infectious disease:

1. Diarrhea

2. Rash

3. Fever

4. Headache

A. Malaria

B. Clostridium difficile infection

C. Typhoid fever

D. Measles

Answer:

1. Diarrhea

B. Clostridium difficile infection

2. Rash

D. Measles

3. Fever

C. Typhoid fever

4. Headache

A. Malaria

Exercise 9: True or False

Indicate whether the following statement is true or false:

Antibiotic resistance occurs when bacteria evolve and become resistant to the drugs used to treat them.

Answer:

True

Exercise 10: Fill in the blanks

Transcribe the following sentence:

The patient's __________ test result was negative, ruling out a common sexually transmitted infection.

Answer:

The patient's Chlamydia trachomatis test result was negative, ruling out a common sexually transmitted infection.

23. PEDIATRIC

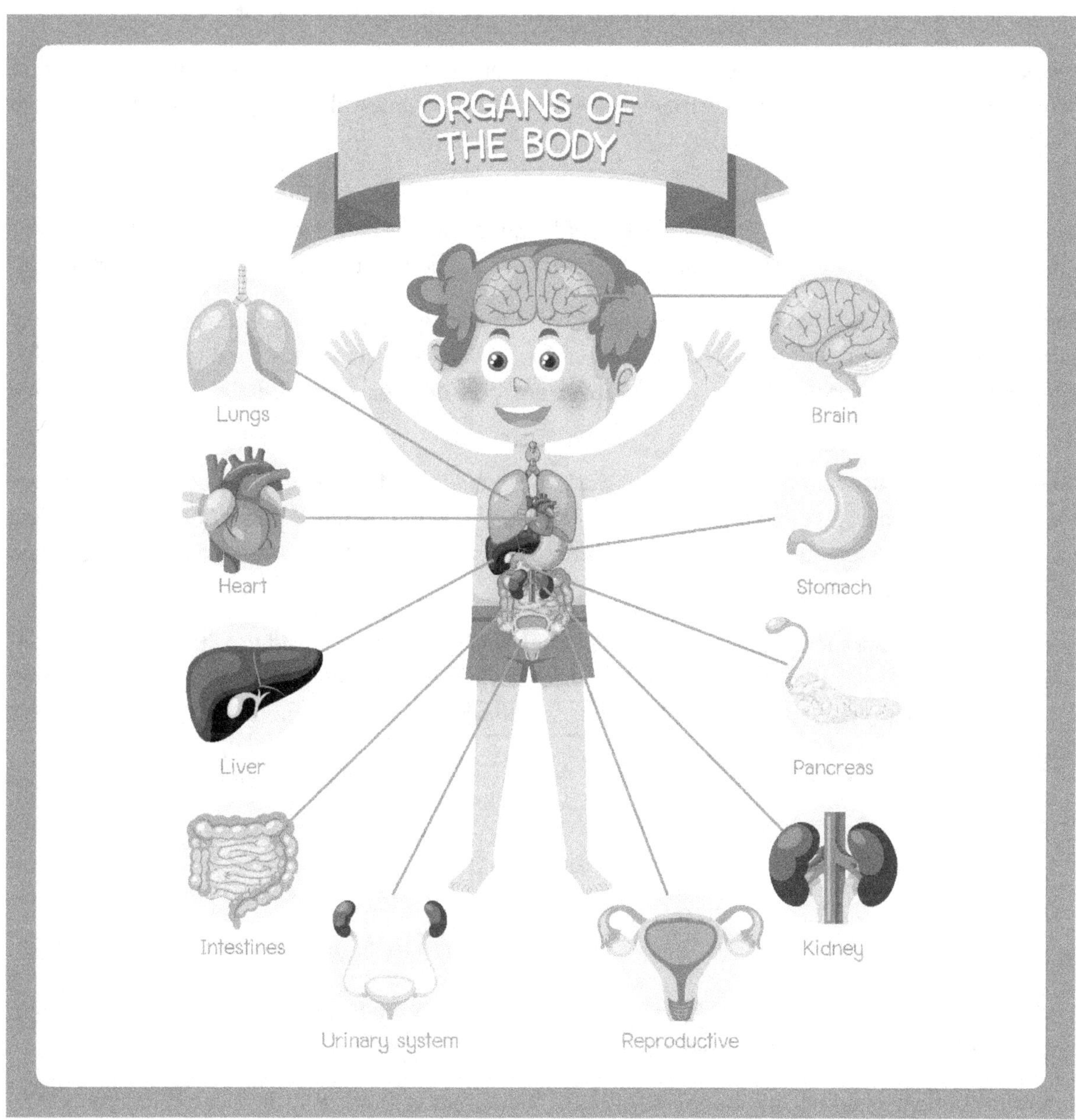

Understanding pediatrics and its specialized vocabulary

Pediatrics is a branch of medicine that involves the medical care of infants, children, and adolescents. The American Academy of Pediatrics recommends people be under pediatric care up to the age of 21. Pediatricians are medical doctors who manage the physical, behavioral, and mental health of children from birth until adulthood.

Here are some key points to understand as a beginner in this field:

1. Child-Centered Care: Pediatricians are trained to consider the well-being of the whole child, taking into account the unique developmental needs and growth patterns at each stage of childhood.

2. Preventive Care: A large part of pediatrics involves preventive health care, including routine check-ups, immunizations, and screenings. Pediatricians advise on nutrition, physical activity, and safety to prevent problems later.

3. Common Conditions: Pediatricians diagnose and treat a wide range of childhood illnesses, from minor health issues to serious diseases. This can include infections, injuries, genetic and congenital conditions, malignancies, and diseases affecting organs or systems such as the heart, lungs, or endocrine system.

4. Developmental and Behavioral Issues: Pediatricians monitor the growth, development, and behavior of children to detect any issues as early as possible. They are trained to manage conditions like attention deficit hyperactivity disorder (ADHD), autism spectrum disorder, learning disabilities, and behavioral problems.

5. Specialization: After general pediatrics, there are several subspecialties including neonatology (newborn infants), pediatric cardiology (heart and circulatory system), pediatric endocrinology (glands and hormones), pediatric hematology/oncology (blood and cancer), pediatric infectious diseases, and pediatric nephrology (kidneys), among others.

6. Family-Centered Approach: Pediatricians work closely with the family, considering the family's values, culture, and social context, and advocating for their patients in school and community settings. They often coordinate care with other specialists, educators, social workers, and therapists to comprehensively support a child's health and well-being.

Pediatric conditions, growth and development milestones, and treatments

I. Pediatric Conditions:

1. Asthma: A chronic condition characterized by inflammation and narrowing of the airways, leading to difficulty breathing, wheezing, and coughing.

2. Attention-Deficit/Hyperactivity Disorder (ADHD): A neurodevelopmental disorder characterized by inattention, hyperactivity, and impulsivity that often affects children's academic and social functioning.

3. Autism Spectrum Disorder (ASD): A developmental disorder characterized by challenges in social interaction, communication, and repetitive behaviors.

4. Cerebral Palsy: A group of neurological disorders that affect movement, muscle coordination, and posture, typically caused by brain damage before or during birth.

5. Down Syndrome: A genetic disorder caused by the presence of an extra copy of chromosome 21, resulting in developmental delays, intellectual disability, and distinct physical features.

6. Juvenile Diabetes (Type 1 Diabetes): A chronic condition in which the pancreas does not produce enough insulin, leading to high blood sugar levels and requiring lifelong insulin management.

7. Ear Infections (Otitis Media): Inflammation and infection of the middle ear, often causing ear pain, fever, and sometimes temporary hearing loss.

8. Allergies: Hypersensitivity reactions to certain substances, such as pollen, dust mites, or certain foods, leading to symptoms like sneezing, itching, and wheezing.

9. Gastroesophageal Reflux Disease (GERD): A condition in which stomach acid flows back into the esophagus, causing heartburn, regurgitation, and other digestive symptoms.

10. Congenital Heart Defects: Structural abnormalities of the heart present at birth, ranging from mild to severe conditions that may require medical intervention or surgery.

11. Cystic Fibrosis: A genetic disorder that primarily affects the lungs, pancreas, and digestive system, leading to mucus buildup, respiratory problems, and digestive difficulties.

12. Childhood Obesity: Excessive body weight in children, often resulting from a combination of genetic, behavioral, and environmental factors, with potential long-term health implications.

13. Pediatric Asthma: A chronic respiratory condition characterized by recurrent episodes of wheezing, coughing, and difficulty breathing in children.

14. Autism: A developmental disorder that affects communication, social interaction, and behavior, typically diagnosed in early childhood.

15. Pediatric Epilepsy: A neurological disorder characterized by recurrent seizures, caused by abnormal brain activity and affecting children of different ages.

16. Pediatric Migraines: Recurrent headaches characterized by moderate to severe pain, often accompanied by other symptoms such as nausea, sensitivity to light or sound, and visual disturbances.

17. Intellectual Disability: A developmental condition characterized by limitations in intellectual functioning and adaptive skills, affecting a child's overall cognitive abilities.

18. Developmental Delays: Delays in reaching developmental milestones in areas such as motor skills, language, cognition, or social-emotional development.

19. Pediatric Cancer: The development of cancer in children, including various types such as leukemia, brain tumors, and solid tumors.

20. Pediatric Sleep Disorders: Sleep-related conditions in children, including insomnia, sleep apnea, or restless leg syndrome, affecting sleep quality and daily functioning.

21. Pediatric Anxiety Disorders: Excessive and persistent worry or fear that significantly impacts a child's daily life, including generalized anxiety disorder, separation anxiety disorder, or specific phobias.

22. Pediatric Depression: Persistent feelings of sadness, hopelessness, or loss of interest in activities, impacting a child's emotional well-being and functioning.

23. Celiac Disease: An autoimmune disorder characterized by an inability to tolerate gluten, a protein found in wheat, barley, and rye, leading to digestive problems and nutrient deficiencies.

24. Pediatric Obesity: Excess body weight in children, often resulting from an imbalance between caloric intake and expenditure, with potential health complications.

25. Pediatric Allergies: Hypersensitivity reactions to specific allergens, such as food, pollen, or pet dander, leading to symptoms like itching, rash, nasal congestion, or difficulty breathing.

II. Growth and Development Milestones:

1. Lifting Head: Around 3-4 months, babies can lift their head while lying on their stomach, building neck and upper body strength.

2. Rolling Over: By 6 months, most babies can roll from their back to their tummy and vice versa, showcasing increased mobility.

3. Sitting Up: Around 6-8 months, babies can sit up with support and develop better head and trunk control.

4. Crawling: Typically occurring between 6-10 months, crawling involves moving on hands and knees, promoting gross motor skills and exploration.

5. Babbling: From around 6-9 months, babies start making repetitive sounds like "bababa" or "mamama," exploring vocal abilities and communication.

6. Pulling Up: Around 9-12 months, babies can pull themselves up to a standing position using furniture or support, preparing for walking.

7. First Steps: Between 9-15 months, babies take their first independent steps, marking a significant milestone in their gross motor development.

8. Using Utensils: By 12-18 months, toddlers start using spoons or forks to feed themselves, refining fine motor skills and self-feeding abilities.

9. Saying Words: Around 12-18 months, toddlers begin saying their first words, expanding their language and communication skills.

10. Parallel Play: Between 18-24 months, children engage in parallel play, playing alongside other children but not yet actively interacting or sharing.

11. Building Towers: From around 18-24 months, children can stack blocks or objects to create simple towers, enhancing hand-eye coordination and problem-solving skills.

12. Following Simple Instructions: By 2 years old, children can understand and follow simple instructions, demonstrating cognitive development and language comprehension.

13. Imaginative Play: Around 2-3 years old, children engage in imaginative play, using their creativity and social skills to pretend and role-play.

14. Riding a Tricycle: Typically around 3 years old, children can ride a tricycle, developing coordination, balance, and gross motor skills.

15. Counting and Recognizing Numbers: Between 3-4 years old, children start counting and recognizing numbers, beginning their mathematical understanding.

16. Dressing Themselves: Around 4-5 years old, children can dress themselves independently, refining fine motor skills and fostering self-help abilities.

17. Printing Letters: From around 4-6 years old, children can start printing letters and familiar words, laying the foundation for reading and writing.

18. Tying Shoelaces: Typically around 5-6 years old, children learn to tie their shoelaces, improving fine motor skills and independence.

19. Reading Simple Words: By 5-7 years old, children can read simple words and sentences, expanding their literacy and language skills.

20. Riding a Bicycle: Around 6-8 years old, children can ride a bicycle without training wheels, demonstrating balance, coordination, and motor skills.

21. Telling Time: Typically around 6-8 years old, children learn to tell time using analog clocks, developing time awareness and numerical understanding.

22. Independent Writing: From around 7-9 years old, children can write sentences and short stories independently, advancing their writing abilities.

23. Problem-Solving Skills: Throughout childhood, children develop problem-solving skills, learning to think critically, analyze situations, and find solutions.

24. Teamwork and Cooperation: As children grow, they learn the value of teamwork, collaboration, and cooperation, essential for social interactions and relationships.

25. Puberty: During adolescence, typically starting between 9-14 years old, children go through various physical and emotional changes, including the onset of puberty, marking the transition into adulthood.

III. Treatments:

1. Medication: The use of prescribed medications to manage symptoms, treat infections, or address specific conditions in children.

2. Physical Therapy: Therapeutic exercises, stretches, and activities to improve strength, mobility, and coordination in children with physical impairments or injuries.

3. Occupational Therapy: Interventions to help children develop or regain skills necessary for daily activities, such as self-care, fine motor tasks, and sensory processing.

4. Speech Therapy: Therapy sessions to improve speech and language skills, including articulation, comprehension, expressive language, and social communication.

5. Behavioral Therapy: Techniques and strategies to address behavioral issues, manage emotions, improve social skills, and promote positive behavior in children.

6. Play Therapy: Therapeutic approach using play to help children express themselves, process emotions, and resolve psychological or behavioral challenges.

7. Cognitive-Behavioral Therapy (CBT): A goal-oriented therapy that helps children identify and modify negative thoughts and behaviors, promoting healthier coping mechanisms.

8. Dietary Changes: Adjustments to a child's diet to manage allergies, sensitivities, or medical conditions such as diabetes, obesity, or gastrointestinal issues.

9. Assistive Devices: Provision of specialized equipment or devices to enhance mobility, communication, or independence in children with physical or sensory impairments.

10. Psychoeducation: Education and support for children and their families to better understand their condition, treatment options, and strategies for self-management.

11. Adaptive Skills Training: Teaching and developing skills necessary for daily living, such as self-care, personal hygiene, and household tasks, to promote independence.

12. Social Skills Training: Interventions to improve social interactions, communication, and relationship-building skills in children who struggle with socializing.

13. Parent-Child Interaction Therapy: A specialized therapy that focuses on improving the parent-child relationship, enhancing parenting skills, and addressing behavioral issues.

14. Sensory Integration Therapy: Aims to improve sensory processing and integration in children with sensory processing disorders, helping them better respond to sensory stimuli.

15. Breathing Exercises: Techniques and exercises to improve respiratory function, lung capacity, and breathing control in children with respiratory conditions or anxiety.

16. Biofeedback Therapy: Teaches children to control and regulate their physiological responses, such as heart rate or muscle tension, through relaxation techniques and feedback.

17. Surgical Interventions: Surgical procedures performed to address specific conditions or structural abnormalities in children, such as correcting congenital anomalies or removing tumors.

18. Behavior Modification: Strategies to reinforce positive behavior and discourage negative behavior through rewards, consequences, and consistent discipline techniques.

19. Family Therapy: Involving the entire family in therapy to address family dynamics, communication issues, and provide support during challenging times.

20. Respite Care: Temporary care provided to children with chronic illnesses or disabilities, offering relief for caregivers and ensuring the child's well-being.

21. Assistive Technology: Use of technology, such as communication devices, augmentative and alternative communication (AAC) systems, or computer adaptations, to facilitate communication and participation.

22. Emotional Support: Counseling, therapy, or support groups to address emotional difficulties, anxiety, depression, or trauma in children and provide coping strategies.

23. Special Education Services: Individualized education programs (IEPs), accommodations, or specialized instruction tailored to meet the unique learning needs of children with disabilities or learning difficulties.

24. Social-Emotional Learning Programs: Curriculum-based programs promoting emotional intelligence, self-awareness, empathy, and social skills in children.

25. Multidisciplinary Team Approach: Collaborative care involving healthcare professionals, therapists, educators, and support personnel working together to develop comprehensive treatment plans and support children's overall well-being.

Practice activities for transcribing pediatric reports effectively

Exercise 1: Fill in the blanks

Transcribe the following sentence:

The patient presented with a _________ fever, cough, and runny nose.

Answer:

The patient presented with a low-grade fever, cough, and runny nose.

Exercise 2: True or False

Indicate whether the following statement is true or false:

Rotavirus is a common cause of gastroenteritis in children.

Answer:

True

Exercise 3: Fill in the blanks

Transcribe the following sentence:

The patient's _________ percentile for height is below average for their age.

Answer:

The patient's 10th percentile for height is below average for their age.

Exercise 4: Matching

Match the childhood condition with its corresponding description:

1. Asthma

2. Attention-deficit/hyperactivity disorder (ADHD)

3. Autism spectrum disorder (ASD)

4. Croup

A. Chronic inflammation of the airways leading to wheezing and difficulty breathing

B. Developmental disorder characterized by inattention, hyperactivity, and impulsivity

C. Neurodevelopmental disorder affecting social interaction, communication, and behavior

D. Viral infection causing inflammation of the upper airway and barking cough

Answer:

1. Asthma

A. Chronic inflammation of the airways leading to wheezing and difficulty breathing

2. Attention-deficit/hyperactivity disorder (ADHD)

B. Developmental disorder characterized by inattention, hyperactivity, and impulsivity

3. Autism spectrum disorder (ASD)

C. Neurodevelopmental disorder affecting social interaction, communication, and behavior

4. Croup

D. Viral infection causing inflammation of the upper airway and barking cough

Exercise 5: Fill in the blanks

Transcribe the following sentence:

The patient's _________ examination revealed normal heart sounds and no murmurs.

Answer:

The patient's cardiac examination revealed normal heart sounds and no murmurs.

Exercise 6: True or False

Indicate whether the following statement is true or false:

The measles, mumps, and rubella (MMR) vaccine is routinely administered to children to prevent these infectious diseases.

Answer:

True

Exercise 7: Fill in the blanks

Transcribe the following sentence:

The patient's _________ development is within the expected range for their age.

Answer:

The patient's language development is within the expected range for their age.

Exercise 8: Matching

Match the pediatric procedure with its corresponding description:

1. Immunization

2. Well-child visit

3. Circumcision

4. Tonsillectomy

A. Administration of vaccines to protect against infectious diseases

B. Routine check-up to monitor growth, development, and general health

C. Surgical removal of the foreskin of the penis

D. Surgical removal of the tonsils

Answer:

1. Immunization

A. Administration of vaccines to protect against infectious diseases

2. Well-child visit

B. Routine check-up to monitor growth, development, and general health

3. Circumcision

C. Surgical removal of the foreskin of the penis

4. Tonsillectomy

D. Surgical removal of the tonsils

Exercise 9: True or False

Indicate whether the following statement is true or false:

Bronchiolitis is a common respiratory infection in infants and young children, usually caused by the respiratory syncytial virus (RSV).

Answer:

True

Exercise 10: Fill in the blanks

Transcribe the following sentence:

The patient's _________ results indicated a normal complete blood count and no signs of infection.

Answer:

The patient's laboratory results indicated a normal complete blood count and no signs of infection.

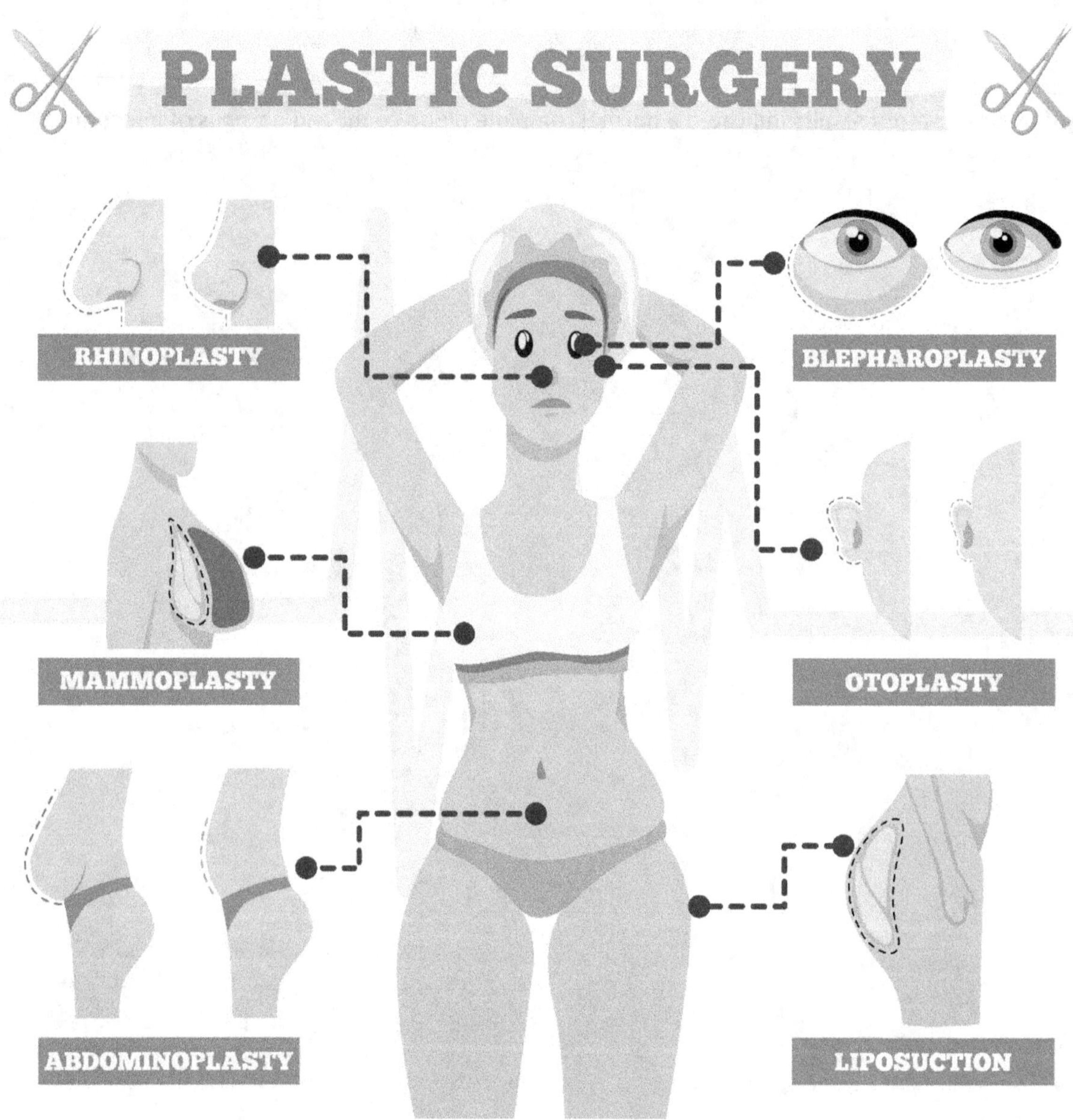

Overview of plastic surgery and its specific terminology

Plastic Surgery is a surgical specialty dedicated to the reconstruction of facial and body defects due to birth disorders, trauma, burns, and disease. It also involves aesthetic or 'cosmetic' surgery intended to improve appearance. The term 'plastic' in plastic surgery derives from the Greek word 'plastikos,' which means 'to mold' or 'to shape,' – it does not relate to synthetic plastic materials.

Here are some key points to understand as a beginner in this field:

1. Reconstructive and Cosmetic Surgery: Plastic surgery includes both reconstructive procedures (which restore function and normal appearance and correct deformities resulting from injury, disease, or birth disorders) and cosmetic or aesthetic procedures (which aim to improve appearance).

2. Common Procedures: Common reconstructive surgeries include tumor removal and reconstruction, laceration repair, scar revision, hand surgery, and breast reconstruction after mastectomy. Common cosmetic surgeries include breast augmentation, rhinoplasty (nose job), liposuction, tummy tucks, and facelifts.

3. Surgical Techniques: Plastic surgeons use a variety of techniques to carry out their procedures, including grafting (where tissue is moved from one site to another), implantation of devices, suturing of wounds and incisions, and various forms of 'flap' surgery where tissue is moved still attached to its blood supply.

4. Training: Plastic surgeons undergo rigorous training, including 4 years of medical school, a residency of at least 5 years, and often additional fellowship training, especially for subspecialties like hand surgery or craniofacial surgery.

5. Multidisciplinary Approach: Plastic surgery often involves a team approach with professionals from other medical specialties, particularly when dealing with complex reconstructive cases. For instance, a plastic surgeon might work with orthopedic surgeons in reconstructing a severely injured limb, or with oncologists in the reconstruction of a woman's breast after surgery for breast cancer.

6. Patient Safety and Expectations: In both reconstructive and cosmetic plastic surgery, a critical role for the surgeon is managing patient expectations and ensuring patient safety. This includes a comprehensive consultation to discuss the patient's goals, the potential risks and benefits of surgery, and to outline the course of recovery.

Cosmetic procedures, reconstructive surgeries, and aesthetic treatments

I. Cosmetic Procedures:

1. Botox Injections: Botulinum toxin injections used to reduce the appearance of wrinkles and fine lines by temporarily relaxing the muscles.

2. Dermal Fillers: Injectable substances used to restore volume and smooth out wrinkles and lines on the face.

3. Chemical Peel: A chemical solution applied to the skin to exfoliate the outer layer, improving texture and reducing fine lines, age spots, and acne scars.

4. Microdermabrasion: A non-invasive procedure that exfoliates the skin using tiny crystals or a diamond-tipped wand to improve skin tone and texture.

5. Laser Hair Removal: Laser technology used to remove unwanted hair by targeting and damaging hair follicles.

6. Lip Augmentation: Enhancing the size and shape of the lips through injectable fillers or surgical procedures.

7. Breast Augmentation: Surgical procedure to increase the size or alter the shape of the breasts using implants or fat transfer.

8. Rhinoplasty: Nose reshaping surgery to improve the appearance or function of the nose.

9. Facelift: Surgical procedure to tighten and lift sagging facial skin, reducing wrinkles and improving facial contours.

10. Liposuction: Surgical procedure to remove excess fat deposits and sculpt the body contours.

11. Tummy Tuck: Surgical procedure to remove excess abdominal skin and fat and tighten the underlying muscles.

12. Eyelid Surgery (Blepharoplasty): Surgical procedure to improve the appearance of droopy or sagging eyelids by removing excess skin and fat.

13. Breast Lift: Surgical procedure to raise and reshape sagging breasts, restoring a more youthful appearance.

14. Brow Lift: Surgical procedure to lift and tighten the forehead and brow area, reducing wrinkles and restoring a more youthful appearance.

15. Hair Transplantation: Surgical procedure to transplant hair follicles from a donor site to areas of hair loss or thinning.

16. Fat Grafting: Procedure that involves removing fat from one area of the body and transferring it to another area to enhance volume or shape.

17. Liposculpture: Minimally invasive procedure that uses laser or ultrasound technology to selectively remove fat and contour the body.

18. Cellulite Treatment: Non-surgical procedures, such as laser therapy or radiofrequency treatments, to reduce the appearance of cellulite.

19. Varicose Vein Treatment: Procedures, such as sclerotherapy or laser therapy, to reduce or eliminate the appearance of varicose veins.

20. Body Contouring: Surgical or non-surgical procedures to reshape and contour specific areas of the body, such as the abdomen, buttocks, or thighs.

21. Tattoo Removal: Laser treatments used to fade or remove unwanted tattoos.

22. Non-Surgical Facelift: Procedures such as thread lifting, ultrasound therapy, or radiofrequency treatments to lift and tighten the skin without surgery.

23. Injectable Fat Reduction: Non-surgical treatments that use injectable compounds to dissolve and reduce localized fat deposits.

24. Laser Skin Resurfacing: Laser technology used to improve skin texture, reduce wrinkles, and address skin concerns such as scars, sun damage, or age spots.

25. Scar Revision: Surgical or non-surgical procedures to improve the appearance of scars by minimizing their size, changing their shape, or improving their texture.

II. Reconstructive Surgeries:

1. Breast Reconstruction: Surgical procedure to rebuild the breast mound following mastectomy or breast-conserving surgery for breast cancer.

2. Cleft Lip and Palate Repair: Surgical procedure to correct birth defects in the lip and palate that can affect speech and facial appearance.

3. Burn Scar Reconstruction: Surgical procedures to improve the appearance and function of scars resulting from burn injuries.

4. Mohs Surgery: A specialized surgical technique used to remove skin cancer, layer by layer, preserving as much healthy tissue as possible.

5. Hand Surgery: Reconstructive procedures to restore function and appearance in individuals with hand injuries, deformities, or conditions such as carpal tunnel syndrome.

6. Facial Fracture Repair: Surgical procedures to realign and stabilize facial bones following fractures, restoring facial function and aesthetics.

7. Limb Reconstruction: Surgical procedures to reconstruct and restore function in limbs affected by trauma, tumors, or congenital conditions.

8. Microvascular Surgery: Complex surgical procedures that involve reconnecting blood vessels to restore blood flow in areas such as reattached amputated limbs or tissue reconstruction.

9. Scar Revision: Surgical procedures to minimize the appearance of scars and improve their texture, blending them with the surrounding skin.

10. Nasal Reconstruction: Surgical procedures to rebuild and reshape the nose after trauma, cancer removal, or congenital abnormalities.

11. Abdominal Wall Reconstruction: Surgical procedures to repair and restore the integrity of the abdominal wall, often necessary after extensive surgeries or trauma.

12. Tracheal Reconstruction: Surgical procedures to repair or reconstruct the trachea (windpipe), often needed due to trauma, tumors, or congenital abnormalities.

13. Lower Extremity Reconstruction: Surgical procedures to restore function and aesthetics in the lower limbs affected by trauma, tumors, or congenital conditions.

14. Orbital Reconstruction: Surgical procedures to reconstruct and restore the function and appearance of the eye socket following trauma or tumor removal.

15. Vaginal Reconstruction: Surgical procedures to repair and reconstruct the vaginal canal, often required due to congenital abnormalities or following cancer treatment.

16. Craniofacial Reconstruction: Complex surgical procedures to rebuild and reshape the skull and facial structures, often performed in individuals with congenital abnormalities or trauma.

17. Nipple and Areola Reconstruction: Surgical procedures to recreate the nipple and areola complex following mastectomy or breast reconstruction.

18. Joint Reconstruction: Surgical procedures to repair or replace damaged joints, such as the knee, hip, or shoulder, to restore function and alleviate pain.

19. Penile Reconstruction: Surgical procedures to reconstruct the penis in individuals with congenital abnormalities or following trauma or cancer treatment.

20. Vascular Reconstruction: Surgical procedures to repair or bypass damaged blood vessels to restore blood flow and prevent complications.

21. Craniosynostosis Repair: Surgical procedures to correct the premature fusion of skull sutures in infants, allowing for proper brain and skull growth.

22. Maxillofacial Reconstruction: Surgical procedures to reconstruct and restore function in the upper jaw, lower jaw, and facial structures affected by trauma or cancer removal.

23. Auricular Reconstruction: Surgical procedures to reconstruct the external ear in individuals with congenital abnormalities or following trauma or cancer removal.

24. Nerve Repair and Reconstruction: Surgical procedures to repair or graft damaged nerves to restore function and sensation in affected areas.

25. Pelvic Floor Reconstruction: Surgical procedures to repair and strengthen the pelvic floor muscles and tissues, often necessary in cases of pelvic organ prolapse or urinary incontinence.

III. Aesthetic Treatments:

1. Botox Injections: Injecting botulinum toxin to temporarily smooth out wrinkles and fine lines on the face.

2. Dermal Fillers: Injecting hyaluronic acid or other substances to restore volume and improve facial contours.

3. Chemical Peels: Applying a chemical solution to the skin to exfoliate and improve texture, reduce fine lines, and even out skin tone.

4. Laser Hair Removal: Using laser technology to remove unwanted hair permanently by targeting hair follicles.

5. Microdermabrasion: Exfoliating the skin with a special device to improve its texture and reduce the appearance of scars, age spots, and fine lines.

6. Platelet-Rich Plasma (PRP) Therapy: Using a patient's own plasma, enriched with platelets, to stimulate collagen production and rejuvenate the skin.

7. Lip Augmentation: Enhancing the volume and shape of the lips using dermal fillers or fat grafting.

8. Eyelid Surgery (Blepharoplasty): Removing excess skin and fat from the eyelids to rejuvenate the appearance and reduce puffiness.

9. Laser Skin Resurfacing: Using laser technology to improve skin texture, reduce wrinkles, and address pigmentation issues.

10. Rhinoplasty: Surgical procedure to reshape and enhance the appearance of the nose.

11. Liposuction: Removing excess fat deposits from specific areas of the body to improve contours.

12. Breast Augmentation: Surgical procedure to enhance the size and shape of the breasts using implants.

13. Tummy Tuck (Abdominoplasty): Removing excess skin and fat from the abdomen and tightening the underlying muscles to create a more toned appearance.

14. Facelift (Rhytidectomy): Surgical procedure to lift and tighten facial skin, reducing sagging and wrinkles.

15. Hair Transplantation: Transplanting hair follicles from one area of the body to areas with thinning or balding hair.

16. Non-Surgical Skin Tightening: Using ultrasound or radiofrequency technology to tighten and firm the skin without surgery.

17. Laser Tattoo Removal: Using laser technology to break down tattoo pigments and remove unwanted tattoos.

18. Body Contouring: Using a combination of surgical and non-surgical procedures to reshape and sculpt the body after significant weight loss.

19. Scar Revision: Surgical or non-surgical techniques to improve the appearance of scars, making them less noticeable.

20. Injectable Wrinkle Relaxers: Injecting substances like Dysport or Xeomin to temporarily relax facial muscles and reduce the appearance of wrinkles.

21. Cellulite Treatments: Using various techniques like radiofrequency, ultrasound, or massage to reduce the appearance of cellulite on the skin.

22. Skin Rejuvenation: Using a combination of treatments like lasers, chemical peels, and skin care products to improve overall skin quality and appearance.

23. Liposculpture: A more precise form of liposuction that focuses on sculpting and contouring specific areas of the body.

24. Thread Lift: Inserting dissolvable threads under the skin to lift and tighten sagging facial or neck tissues.

25. Intense Pulsed Light (IPL) Therapy: Using light-based technology to target skin imperfections like sunspots, freckles, and vascular lesions.

Exercises for transcribing plastic surgery reports accurately

Exercise 1: Fill in the blanks

Transcribe the following sentence:

The patient underwent a _________ to enhance the size and shape of her breasts.

Answer:

The patient underwent a breast augmentation to enhance the size and shape of her breasts.

Exercise 2: True or False

Indicate whether the following statement is true or false:

Rhinoplasty is a surgical procedure performed to reshape the nose.

Answer:

True

Exercise 3: Fill in the blanks

Transcribe the following sentence:

The patient received a _________ injection to reduce the appearance of wrinkles.

Answer:

The patient received a Botox injection to reduce the appearance of wrinkles.

Exercise 4: Matching

Match the plastic surgery procedure with its corresponding description:

1. Liposuction

2. Abdominoplasty

3. Facelift

4. Blepharoplasty

A. Surgical removal of excess fat deposits from specific areas of the body

B. Surgical procedure to reshape the nose

C. Surgical procedure to remove excess skin and tighten the abdominal muscles

D. Surgical procedure to rejuvenate the appearance of the face and neck

Answer:

1. Liposuction

A. Surgical removal of excess fat deposits from specific areas of the body

2. Abdominoplasty

C. Surgical procedure to remove excess skin and tighten the abdominal muscles

3. Facelift

D. Surgical procedure to rejuvenate the appearance of the face and neck

4. Blepharoplasty

B. Surgical procedure to reshape the nose

Exercise 5: Fill in the blanks

Transcribe the following sentence:

The patient's _________ implants were removed due to complications.

Answer:

The patient's breast implants were removed due to complications.

Exercise 6: True or False

Indicate whether the following statement is true or false:

A facelift is a surgical procedure performed to lift and tighten the facial skin, reducing sagging and wrinkles.

Answer:

True

Exercise 7: Fill in the blanks

Transcribe the following sentence:

The patient underwent a _________ procedure to remove excess skin and fat from her upper arms.

Answer:

The patient underwent a brachioplasty procedure to remove excess skin and fat from her upper arms.

Exercise 8: Matching

Match the plastic surgery term with its corresponding description:

1. Augmentation

2. Mastopexy

3. Rhinoplasty

4. Genioplasty

A. Surgical procedure to reshape the chin and jawline

B. Surgical procedure to lift and reshape sagging breasts

C. Surgical procedure to enhance the size and shape of the breasts

D. Surgical procedure to reshape the nose

Answer:

1. Augmentation

C. Surgical procedure to enhance the size and shape of the breasts

2. Mastopexy

B. Surgical procedure to lift and reshape sagging breasts

3. Rhinoplasty

D. Surgical procedure to reshape the nose

4. Genioplasty

A. Surgical procedure to reshape the chin and jawline

Exercise 9: True or False

Indicate whether the following statement is true or false:

Liposuction is a non-surgical procedure that uses ultrasound technology to remove excess fat.

Answer:

False

Exercise 10: Fill in the blanks

Transcribe the following sentence:

The patient underwent a _________ procedure to restore volume and fullness to her cheeks.

Answer:

The patient underwent a cheek augmentation procedure to restore volume and fullness to her cheeks.

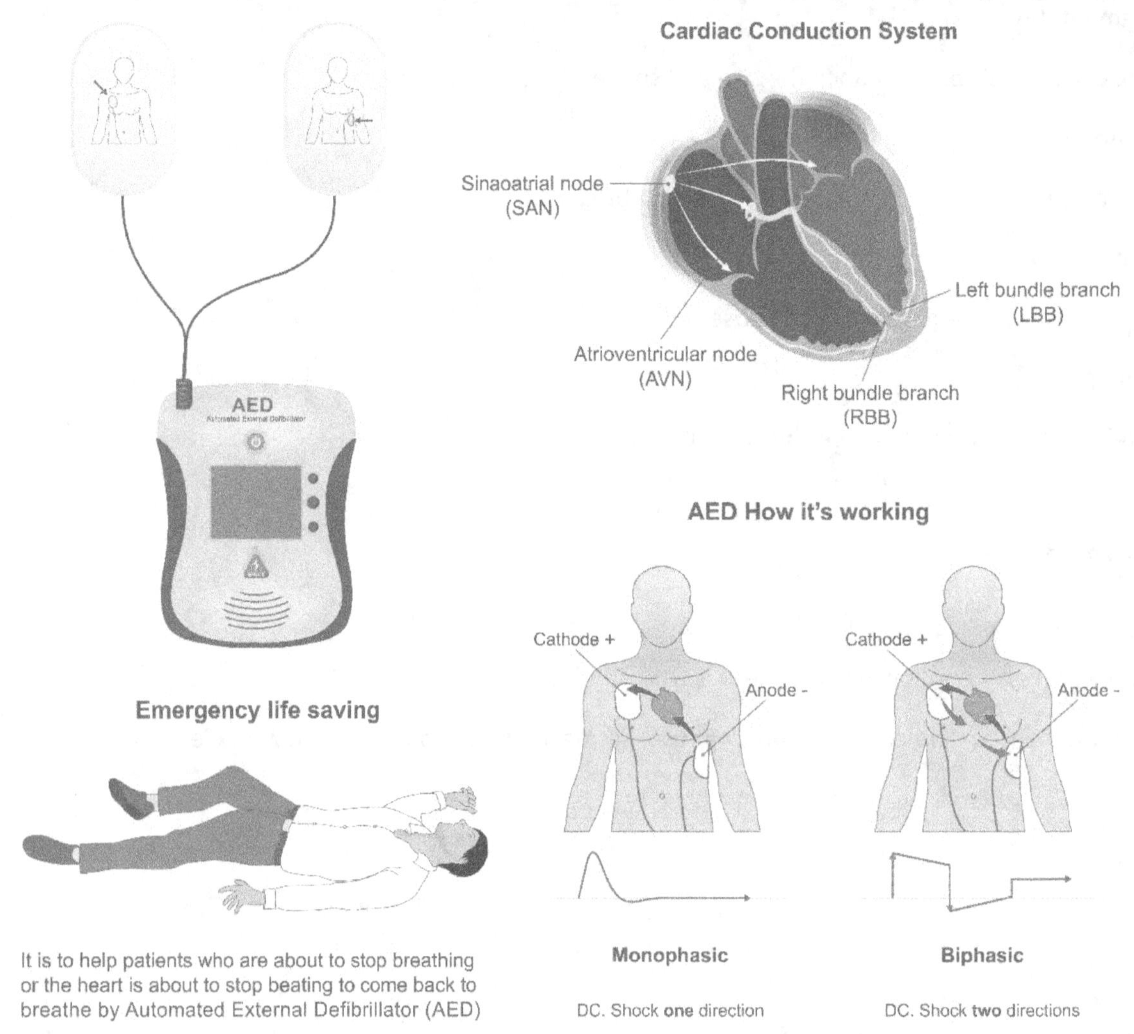

It is to help patients who are about to stop breathing or the heart is about to stop beating to come back to breathe by Automated External Defibrillator (AED)

Introduction to emergency medicine and its specialized terminology

Emergency Medicine is a medical specialty that focuses on the immediate evaluation, management, and treatment of patients with acute illnesses or injuries. Emergency physicians are trained to handle a wide range of medical conditions and emergencies in diverse settings such as emergency departments, ambulances, and pre-hospital care. Here are some key points to understand about emergency medicine as a beginner in this field:

1. Scope of Practice: Emergency physicians provide initial assessments, stabilize critically ill or injured patients, perform necessary procedures, coordinate care, and make disposition decisions (admission, discharge, or transfer) based on the patient's condition.

2. Time Sensitivity: Emergency medicine emphasizes rapid assessment and treatment of time-sensitive conditions where delay can result in adverse outcomes or complications.

3. Multidisciplinary Approach: Emergency physicians work closely with other healthcare professionals, including nurses, paramedics, radiologists, and specialists, to provide comprehensive and coordinated care to patients in emergency situations.

4. Triage: The process of triage, categorizing patients based on the severity of their condition, is a critical component of emergency medicine to ensure that the most critically ill or injured patients receive prompt care.

5. Emergency Medical Services (EMS): Emergency physicians often collaborate with EMS personnel to provide immediate medical care at the scene of an emergency and during transport to the hospital.

Common emergency medical conditions, procedures, and interventions

I. Common Emergency Medical Conditions:

1. Chest Pain: Evaluation and management of patients presenting with chest pain, including assessment for myocardial infarction (heart attack), pulmonary embolism, and other life-threatening conditions.

2. Stroke: Rapid assessment and initiation of appropriate interventions for patients with symptoms of stroke, including administration of clot-dissolving medication or thrombectomy.

3. Trauma: Evaluation and management of patients with traumatic injuries, including fractures, head injuries, burns, and severe bleeding.

4. Respiratory Distress: Assessment and treatment of patients experiencing difficulty breathing, such as acute asthma exacerbation, pneumothorax, or severe respiratory infections.

5. Sepsis: Early recognition and initiation of appropriate interventions for patients with sepsis, a life-threatening systemic infection.

6. Allergic Reactions: Evaluation and management of patients with severe allergic reactions (anaphylaxis), including administration of epinephrine and other supportive therapies.

7. Gastrointestinal Emergencies: Diagnosis and treatment of acute abdominal pain, gastrointestinal bleeding, pancreatitis, bowel obstructions, and other urgent conditions.

8. Mental Health Emergencies: Assessment and stabilization of patients with acute psychiatric emergencies, such as suicidal ideation, psychosis, or severe anxiety.

9. Poisoning and Overdose: Management of patients with toxic exposures or drug overdoses, including administration of antidotes and supportive care.

10. Pediatric Emergencies: Evaluation and treatment of acute illnesses and injuries in children, including fever, respiratory distress, seizures, and trauma.

11. Cardiac Arrest: Immediate initiation of cardiopulmonary resuscitation (CPR) and advanced cardiac life support (ACLS) measures for patients experiencing cardiac arrest.

12. Altered Mental Status: Evaluation and management of patients with altered mental status, including delirium, intoxication, or neurological conditions.

13. Acute Abdominal Pain: Assessment and diagnosis of patients presenting with severe abdominal pain, including conditions like appendicitis, bowel perforation, or gallbladder disease.

14. Acute Kidney Injury: Identification and management of patients with sudden impairment of kidney function, including addressing underlying causes and initiating appropriate therapies.

15. Ankle Sprains and Fractures: Evaluation and treatment of ankle injuries, including sprains, fractures, and ligament tears, to promote healing and restore function.

16. Diabetic Emergencies: Assessment and management of acute complications related to diabetes, such as diabetic ketoacidosis or hypoglycemia.

17. Psychiatric Crisis Intervention: Immediate evaluation and intervention for patients experiencing acute psychiatric crises, providing supportive care and appropriate referrals.

18. Heatstroke and Heat Exhaustion: Recognition and management of heat-related emergencies, including rapid cooling measures and fluid resuscitation.

19. Eye Emergencies: Diagnosis and treatment of urgent eye conditions, such as corneal abrasions, foreign body removal, or acute glaucoma.

20. Sports Injuries: Evaluation and management of acute sports-related injuries, including fractures, dislocations, and concussions.

21. Drowning and Near-Drowning: Assessment and resuscitation of patients who have experienced submersion in water, ensuring adequate oxygenation and preventing complications.

22. Psychogenic Non-Epileptic Seizures: Differentiation and management of seizures with non-epileptic causes, including psychological factors and stress.

23. Opioid Overdose: Immediate administration of naloxone and provision of supportive care for patients experiencing opioid overdose.

24. Electrical Injuries: Evaluation and management of patients with electrical injuries, including cardiac monitoring, wound care, and assessment for internal organ damage.

25. Acute Psychosis: Assessment and stabilization of patients presenting with acute psychosis, implementing appropriate interventions and ensuring patient safety.

II. Common Emergency Medical Procedures and Interventions:

1. Advanced Cardiac Life Support (ACLS): Resuscitation and management of cardiac arrest, including CPR, defibrillation, and medication administration.

2. Airway Management: Establishment and maintenance of a patent airway through techniques like intubation, supraglottic airway placement, or cricothyroidotomy.

3. Central Venous Access: Insertion of a catheter into a central vein for medication administration, fluid resuscitation, or hemodynamic monitoring.

4. Rapid Sequence Intubation (RSI): Rapid airway management technique involving the administration of induction agents and neuromuscular blockers for intubation.

5. Chest Tube Insertion: Placement of a tube in the pleural space to drain air, fluid, or blood in cases of pneumothorax, hemothorax, or pleural effusion.

6. Cardioversion: Conversion of abnormal heart rhythms back to normal sinus rhythm using electrical or pharmacological methods.

7. Procedural Sedation: Administration of sedatives to facilitate uncomfortable procedures while ensuring patient comfort and safety.

8. Fracture and Dislocation Reduction: Manipulation or realignment of fractured bones or dislocated joints to restore proper alignment and relieve pain.

9. Wound Management: Evaluation and treatment of various wounds, including cleaning, suturing, and dressing.

10. Lumbar Puncture: Insertion of a needle into the spinal canal to obtain cerebrospinal fluid for diagnostic purposes or therapeutic relief.

11. Point-of-Care Ultrasound: Utilization of bedside ultrasound for rapid assessment and diagnosis of conditions such as trauma, abdominal pain, or cardiac abnormalities.

12. Advanced Airway Management: Techniques beyond basic airway management, including video laryngoscopy, fiberoptic intubation, and surgical airway access.

13. Cardiovascular Procedures: Emergency cardiac catheterization, pericardiocentesis, and temporary pacing for cardiac rhythm disturbances.

14. Hemorrhage Control: Management of severe bleeding through direct pressure, tourniquets, hemostatic agents, or surgical interventions.

15. Orthopedic Procedures: Closed reduction and splinting of fractures and dislocations, joint aspirations, and compartment pressure measurements.

16. Intraosseous Access: Insertion of a needle into the bone marrow cavity for fluid and medication administration in patients with difficult vascular access or shock.

17. Rapid Diagnostic Testing: Utilization of point-of-care tests for rapid diagnosis of conditions such as influenza, streptococcal pharyngitis, or urinary tract infections.

18. Obstetric Emergencies: Evaluation and management of pregnant patients experiencing complications, including premature labor, eclampsia, or antepartum hemorrhage.

19. Thoracotomy: Emergency surgical procedure involving a chest incision to access and treat life-threatening injuries to the heart, lungs, or major blood vessels.

20. Transcutaneous Pacing: Non-invasive electrical stimulation of the chest to temporarily control or stabilize abnormal heart rhythms.

21. Rapid Blood Transfusion: Urgent administration of blood or blood products to replace significant blood loss in trauma or hemorrhagic emergencies.

22. Eye Irrigation: Flushing the eye with sterile fluids to remove foreign bodies, chemicals, or irritants.

23. Incision and Drainage: Surgical procedure to open and drain abscesses or infected fluid collections.

24. Pericardiocentesis: Insertion of a needle or catheter into the pericardial sac to remove excess fluid or blood in cases of cardiac tamponade.

25. Gastrointestinal Decompression: Insertion of a nasogastric tube to remove stomach contents, relieve gastric distention, or decompress the intestines

Exercises for transcribing emergency medicine reports accurately

Exercise 1: Fill in the blanks

Transcribe the following sentence:

The patient presented to the emergency department with complaints of severe _________ and shortness of breath.

Answer:

The patient presented to the emergency department with complaints of severe chest pain and shortness of breath.

Exercise 2: True or False

Indicate whether the following statement is true or false:

Emergency medicine focuses on the evaluation and management of non-urgent medical conditions.

Answer:

False

Exercise 3: Fill in the blanks

Transcribe the following sentence:

The patient was administered __________ for rapid sedation prior to a painful procedure.

Answer:

The patient was administered procedural sedation for rapid sedation prior to a painful procedure.

Exercise 4: Matching

Match the emergency medical procedure with its corresponding description:

1. Rapid Sequence Intubation (RSI)

2. Chest Tube Insertion

3. Cardioversion

4. Lumbar Puncture

A. Technique used to secure the airway rapidly by administering induction agents and neuromuscular blockers

B. Placement of a tube into the pleural space to drain air, fluid, or blood from the chest

C. Conversion of abnormal heart rhythms back to normal sinus rhythm using electrical or pharmacological methods

D. Insertion of a needle into the spinal canal to obtain cerebrospinal fluid for diagnostic or therapeutic purposes

Answer:

1. Rapid Sequence Intubation (RSI)

A. Technique used to secure the airway rapidly by administering induction agents and neuromuscular blockers

2. Chest Tube Insertion

B. Placement of a tube into the pleural space to drain air, fluid, or blood from the chest

3. Cardioversion

C. Conversion of abnormal heart rhythms back to normal sinus rhythm using electrical or pharmacological methods

4. Lumbar Puncture

D. Insertion of a needle into the spinal canal to obtain cerebrospinal fluid for diagnostic or therapeutic purposes

Exercise 5: Fill in the blanks

Transcribe the following sentence:

The patient underwent emergent _________ to control life-threatening bleeding.

Answer:

The patient underwent emergent surgery to control life-threatening bleeding.

Exercise 6: True or False

Indicate whether the following statement is true or false:

Point-of-care ultrasound is commonly used in emergency medicine to aid in the rapid assessment and diagnosis of various conditions.

Answer:

True

Exercise 7: Fill in the blanks

Transcribe the following sentence:

The patient's _________ revealed a displaced fracture of the left radius.

Answer:

The patient's X-ray revealed a displaced fracture of the left radius.

Exercise 8: Matching

Match the emergency medical condition with its corresponding description:

1. Stroke

2. Sepsis

3. Gastrointestinal Bleeding

4. Anaphylaxis

A. Acute condition characterized by inadequate blood flow to the brain, resulting in neurological deficits

B. Life-threatening allergic reaction characterized by airway compromise, hypotension, and other systemic symptoms

C. Loss of consciousness, cessation of breathing, and absence of pulse due to cardiac causes

D. Systemic inflammatory response to infection, leading to organ dysfunction and failure

Answer:

1. Stroke

A. Acute condition characterized by inadequate blood flow to the brain, resulting in neurological deficits

2. Sepsis

B. Life-threatening allergic reaction characterized by airway compromise, hypotension, and other systemic symptoms

3. Gastrointestinal Bleeding

C. Loss of consciousness, cessation of breathing, and absence of pulse due to cardiac causes

4. Anaphylaxis

D. Systemic inflammatory response to infection, leading to organ dysfunction and failure

Exercise 9: True or False

Indicate whether the following statement is true or false:

Emergency physicians collaborate with EMS personnel to provide immediate medical care at the scene of an emergency and during transport to the hospital.

Answer:

True

Exercise 10: Fill in the blanks

Transcribe the following sentence:

The patient's _________ revealed a dislocated shoulder that required immediate reduction.

Answer:

The patient's physical examination revealed a dislocated shoulder that required immediate reduction.

Circulatory System

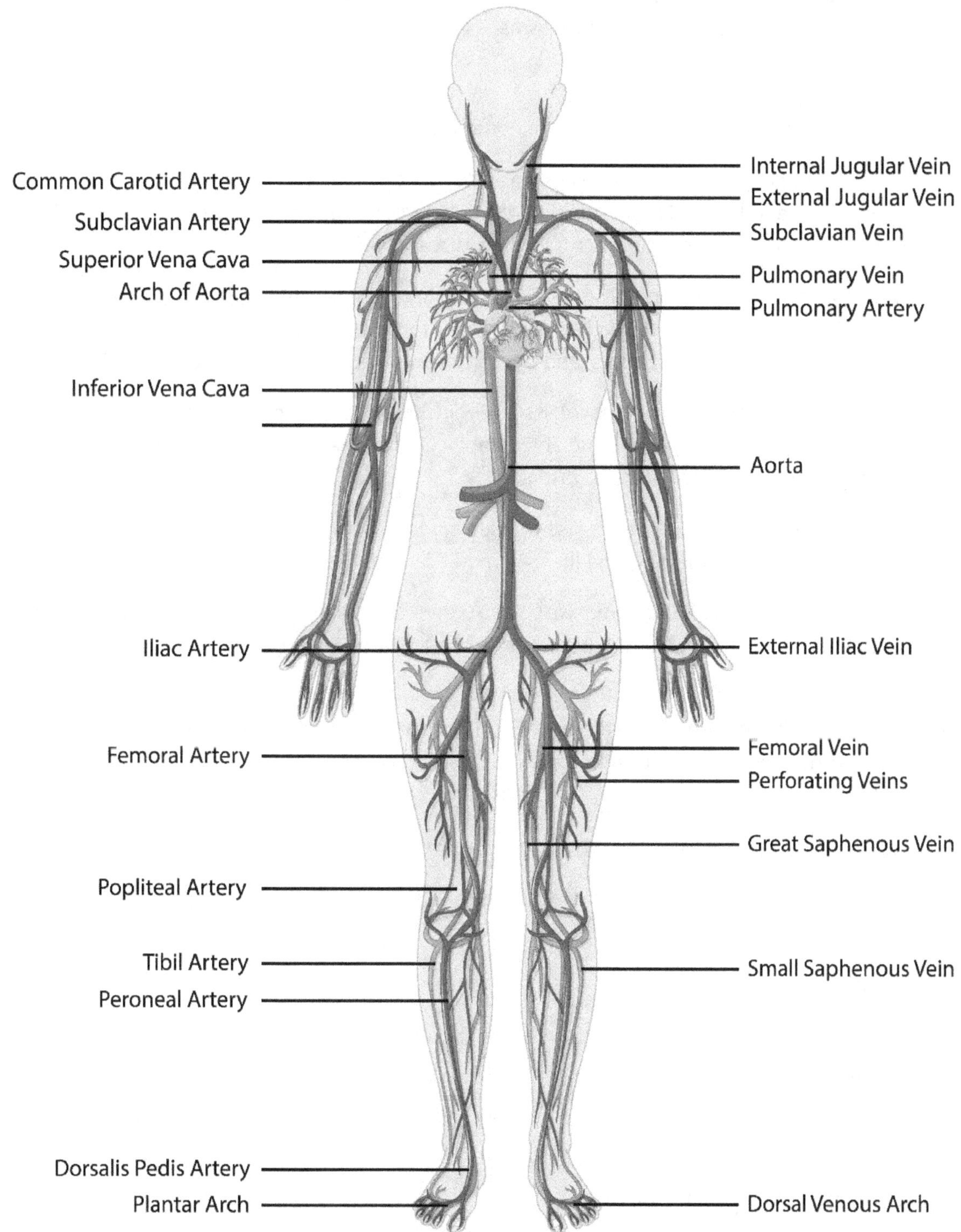

Vascular surgery is a surgical subspecialty that focuses on the treatment of diseases affecting the vascular system, which includes the arteries, veins, and lymphatic vessels. These diseases often involve blockages or weaknesses in these vessels, known as aneurysms.

Here are some key points to understand as a beginner in this field:

1. Disease Management: Vascular surgeons manage diseases in all parts of the vascular system except those within the heart and brain. Conditions they treat include peripheral artery disease, carotid artery disease, abdominal aortic aneurysm, deep vein thrombosis, and varicose veins.

2. Surgical Procedures: Vascular surgeons perform open surgeries and endovascular procedures, which involve inserting special instruments through small incisions to treat the inside of blood vessels. They also perform angioplasty, stenting, thrombolysis, and other procedures to repair or unblock vessels.

3. Diagnostic Tools: Diagnostic tools in vascular surgery include ultrasound, computed tomography (CT) scans, magnetic resonance imaging (MRI), and angiography. These imaging studies help vascular surgeons identify the location and severity of vascular diseases.

4. Comprehensive Care: Vascular surgeons also provide comprehensive vascular care, which may involve medical management, exercise therapy, and lifestyle modifications in addition to surgical interventions.

5. Specialization: Within the field, some vascular surgeons further specialize in particular types of conditions or procedures, such as treating diseases of the aorta or lower extremity peripheral vascular disease.

6. Interdisciplinary Collaboration: Given the systemic nature of vascular diseases, vascular surgeons often collaborate with other specialists, including cardiologists, interventional radiologists, neurologists, and others.

I. Vascular Conditions:

1.   Hypertension: A condition characterized by high blood pressure, which can lead to various cardiovascular complications.

2. Atherosclerosis: The buildup of plaque in the arteries, narrowing the blood vessels and restricting blood flow.

3. Coronary Artery Disease (CAD): The narrowing or blockage of the coronary arteries that supply blood to the heart muscle, often leading to chest pain or heart attacks.

4. Peripheral Artery Disease (PAD): The narrowing or blockage of the arteries outside the heart, typically affecting the lower extremities and causing leg pain and poor circulation.

5. Deep Vein Thrombosis (DVT): The formation of blood clots in the deep veins, usually in the legs, which can lead to complications if the clot breaks free and travels to other parts of the body.

6. Pulmonary Embolism (PE): A condition where a blood clot, often originating from the deep veins of the legs, blocks the blood vessels in the lungs.

7. Aneurysm: A bulging or weakened area in the blood vessel wall, which can potentially rupture and cause severe bleeding.

8. Stroke: A disruption of blood supply to the brain, typically caused by a blocked or ruptured blood vessel, leading to neurological impairment.

9. Varicose Veins: Enlarged, twisted veins that usually occur in the legs and can cause discomfort, pain, and cosmetic concerns.

10. Venous Insufficiency: A condition where the veins have difficulty returning blood from the legs to the heart, resulting in swelling, pain, and ulcers.

11. Thrombophlebitis: Inflammation of a vein, often accompanied by the formation of a blood clot, causing pain, redness, and swelling.

12. Raynaud's Disease: A condition characterized by the narrowing of blood vessels, usually in the fingers and toes, leading to coldness, color changes, and pain in response to cold or stress.

13. Aortic Aneurysm: A bulge or dilation in the wall of the aorta, the largest artery in the body, which can be life-threatening if it ruptures.

14. Carotid Artery Disease: The narrowing or blockage of the carotid arteries, which supply blood to the brain, increasing the risk of stroke.

15. Arteriovenous Malformation (AVM): An abnormal tangle of blood vessels connecting arteries and veins, which can cause symptoms or lead to complications.

16. Lymphedema: Swelling that occurs due to the accumulation of lymph fluid, often as a result of damage or obstruction in the lymphatic system.

17. Vasculitis: Inflammation of the blood vessels, which can affect various organs and tissues, leading to a range of symptoms depending on the affected area.

18. Varicocele: Enlarged veins within the scrotum, which can cause discomfort and affect fertility in males.

19. Arteriovenous Fistula: An abnormal connection between an artery and a vein, which can affect blood flow and circulation.

20. Kawasaki Disease: A rare childhood illness that involves inflammation of the blood vessels, primarily affecting young children and potentially leading to complications if not treated promptly.

21. Venous Thrombosis: The formation of blood clots in the veins, which can occur in different parts of the body, such as the legs, arms, or abdomen.

22. Hypotension: Low blood pressure, which can cause dizziness, fainting, and insufficient blood flow to vital organs.

23. Chronic Venous Insufficiency: A long-term condition characterized by poor blood flow from the leg veins back to the heart, often resulting in leg swelling, pain, and skin changes.

24. Lymphangitis: Infection and inflammation of the lymphatic vessels, usually caused by bacteria entering through a break in the skin, leading to red streaks and swollen lymph nodes.

25. Superficial Thrombophlebitis: Inflammation of the veins close to the skin's surface, often accompanied by the formation of a blood clot, causing pain, redness, and swelling.

II. Surgical Interventions:

1. Angioplasty: A procedure to open blocked or narrowed blood vessels using a balloon-like device, often combined with the placement of a stent to help keep the vessel open.

2. Endarterectomy: Surgical removal of plaque or fatty deposits from the inner lining of an artery, typically performed to improve blood flow in areas affected by atherosclerosis.

3. Bypass Surgery: A procedure in which a graft is used to create a new pathway for blood flow, bypassing a blocked or narrowed artery, commonly performed for coronary artery disease or peripheral artery disease.

4. Thrombectomy: Surgical removal of a blood clot from a blood vessel, usually performed in cases of deep vein thrombosis or arterial thrombosis.

5. Aneurysm Repair: Surgical treatment to repair or remove an aneurysm, which may involve open surgery or minimally invasive techniques such as endovascular stent grafting.

6. Carotid Endarterectomy: Surgical removal of plaque from the carotid arteries in the neck, reducing the risk of stroke in individuals with carotid artery disease.

7. Vascular Access Surgery: Creation of a vascular access point, such as an arteriovenous fistula or graft, for hemodialysis or other medical procedures requiring repeated access to the bloodstream.

8. Venous Stenting: Placement of a stent in a narrowed or obstructed vein to restore proper blood flow, often performed in cases of venous stenosis or thrombosis.

9. Varicose Vein Surgery: Surgical procedures, such as vein ligation and stripping or endovenous ablation, to remove or close off varicose veins, relieving symptoms and improving appearance.

10. Aortic Aneurysm Repair: Surgical repair of an aortic aneurysm, which may involve open surgery or endovascular stent grafting, depending on the location and characteristics of the aneurysm.

11. Deep Brain Stimulation: A surgical procedure involving the implantation of electrodes in specific areas of the brain to treat movement disorders like Parkinson's disease or essential tremor.

12. Limb Salvage Surgery: Surgical procedures aimed at preserving a limb affected by peripheral artery disease, using techniques such as angioplasty, bypass grafting, or endovascular therapy.

13. Atherectomy: A procedure to remove plaque buildup from arteries using specialized catheters or devices, improving blood flow and restoring vessel patency.

14. Embolectomy: Surgical removal of an embolus or blood clot from an artery, typically performed in cases of acute arterial occlusion.

15. Lymph Node Dissection: Surgical removal of lymph nodes in the affected area, often performed to stage and treat cancers that have spread to the lymphatic system.

16. Venous Ligation: Surgical tying off or sealing of a vein, usually performed to treat varicose veins or prevent further complications in cases of venous insufficiency.

17. Atrial Fibrillation Ablation: A procedure to correct abnormal electrical signals in the heart by creating scar tissue using heat or cold energy, restoring normal heart rhythm.

18. Port Placement: Surgical placement of a port-a-cath or similar device beneath the skin to provide long-term access for chemotherapy, blood transfusions, or intravenous medications.

19. Limb Revascularization: Surgical procedures to restore blood flow in a limb affected by peripheral artery disease, using techniques like angioplasty, bypass grafting, or endarterectomy.

20. Thoracic Outlet Decompression: Surgical release of structures in the thoracic outlet region, such as the scalene muscles or rib, to relieve compression of nerves or blood vessels.

21. Transjugular Intrahepatic Portosystemic Shunt (TIPS): Placement of a shunt between the portal vein and hepatic vein to redirect blood flow and reduce pressure in cases of portal hypertension.

22. Mesenteric Bypass: Surgical creation of a bypass graft to restore blood flow to the intestines and other abdominal organs in cases of mesenteric artery disease.

23. Dialysis Access Revision: Surgical revision or repair of a previously placed arteriovenous fistula or graft used for hemodialysis to ensure proper function and blood flow.

24. Vena Cava Filter Placement: Placement of a filter in the vena cava to prevent the migration of blood clots from the lower extremities or pelvis to the lungs.

25. Atrial Septal Defect Closure: Surgical repair or closure of a hole in the atrial septum, commonly performed using minimally invasive techniques or through open-heart surgery, depending on the size and location of the defect.

III. Endovascular Procedures:

1. Angioplasty: A minimally invasive procedure that uses a balloon-like device to open blocked or narrowed blood vessels, typically combined with the placement of a stent to help keep the vessel open.

2. Stent Placement: The insertion of a small metal or mesh tube (stent) into a narrowed or weakened blood vessel to provide structural support and restore proper blood flow.

3. Embolization: The injection of embolic agents, such as coils or particles, into abnormal blood vessels to block or reduce blood flow, often used to treat vascular malformations or control bleeding.

4. Thrombolysis: The administration of medication directly into a blood clot to dissolve it, restoring blood flow in cases of acute arterial or venous thrombosis.

5. Aneurysm Coiling: A minimally invasive procedure in which small platinum coils are inserted into an aneurysm to promote blood clotting and prevent rupture.

6. Atherectomy: The removal of plaque or fatty deposits from the inner lining of an artery using specialized devices or techniques, improving blood flow and vessel patency.

7. Endovascular Repair of Aortic Aneurysms: A minimally invasive procedure in which a stent graft is placed within the aorta to reinforce weakened areas and prevent aneurysm rupture.

8. Arterial Angiography: The injection of contrast dye into arteries to visualize blood flow and detect blockages or abnormalities using fluoroscopy or other imaging techniques.

9. Venous Angioplasty and Stenting: The use of balloons and stents to open and support narrowed or blocked veins, facilitating improved venous blood flow.

10. Transcatheter Valve Repair or Replacement: The repair or replacement of heart valves using catheter-based techniques, avoiding the need for open-heart surgery.

11. Endovascular Repair of Vascular Trauma: The use of endovascular techniques to repair injured blood vessels, often used in cases of traumatic arterial or venous injuries.

12. Inferior Vena Cava Filter Placement: The insertion of a filter into the inferior vena cava to prevent the migration of blood clots from the lower extremities to the lungs.

13. Intravascular Ultrasound (IVUS): The use of a specialized catheter with an ultrasound probe to visualize the inside of blood vessels and assess plaque buildup or vessel wall abnormalities.

14. Renal Artery Angioplasty and Stenting: The dilation of narrowed or blocked renal arteries using balloons and the placement of stents to restore proper blood flow to the kidneys.

15. Thrombectomy: The removal of a blood clot from a blood vessel using specialized devices or techniques, often performed in cases of acute arterial or venous thrombosis.

16. IVC Filter Retrieval: The removal of an inferior vena cava (IVC) filter using minimally invasive techniques once the risk of blood clots has subsided.

17. Arteriovenous Fistula Creation: The creation of a connection between an artery and vein, typically in the arm, to facilitate hemodialysis access in patients with end-stage renal disease.

18. Coil Embolization of Vascular Malformations: The placement of coils or other embolic agents within abnormal blood vessels to promote blood clotting and shrink the malformation.

19. Drug-Eluting Balloon Angioplasty: The use of a balloon coated with medication to treat narrowed or blocked blood vessels, preventing restenosis (re-narrowing) after angioplasty.

20. Transarterial Chemoembolization (TACE): The delivery of chemotherapy drugs directly to a tumor through an artery, combined with embolization to block blood supply to the tumor.

21. Transjugular Intrahepatic Portosystemic Shunt (TIPS): The creation of a shunt between the portal vein and hepatic vein to reduce pressure in the portal system in cases of portal hypertension.

22. Inferior Mesenteric Artery Embolization: The embolization of the inferior mesenteric artery to reduce blood flow and control bleeding in cases of gastrointestinal bleeding.

23. Uterine Artery Embolization (UAE): The blocking of the uterine arteries with embolic agents to treat symptomatic uterine fibroids or control heavy menstrual bleeding.

24. Percutaneous Transhepatic Biliary Drainage (PTBD): The placement of a tube through the liver to drain bile from the bile ducts in cases of biliary obstruction or strictures.

25. Radiofrequency Ablation (RFA): The use of radiofrequency energy to heat and destroy cancerous or abnormal tissues, often used in the treatment of liver or lung tumors.

Exercises for transcribing vascular surgery reports accurately

Exercise 1: Fill in the blanks

Transcribe the following sentence:

The patient underwent an _________ to remove a blood clot in the femoral artery.

Answer:

The patient underwent an embolectomy to remove a blood clot in the femoral artery.

Exercise 2: True or False

Indicate whether the following statement is true or false:

Endovascular repair is a minimally invasive procedure used to treat abdominal aortic aneurysms.

Answer:

True

Exercise 3: Fill in the blanks

Transcribe the following sentence:

The patient was diagnosed with __________ due to narrowing of the carotid arteries.

Answer:

The patient was diagnosed with carotid stenosis due to narrowing of the carotid arteries.

Exercise 4: Matching

Match the vascular surgery term with its corresponding description:

1. Arteriovenous fistula (AVF)

2. Aortic dissection

3. Peripheral arterial disease (PAD)

4. Varicose veins

A. Abnormal connection between an artery and a vein

B. Tear in the inner layer of the aorta, causing separation of the layers

C. Narrowing or blockage of the arteries that supply blood to the limbs

D. Enlarged and twisted veins, usually in the legs

Answer:

1. Arteriovenous fistula (AVF)

A. Abnormal connection between an artery and a vein

2. Aortic dissection

B. Tear in the inner layer of the aorta, causing separation of the layers

3. Peripheral arterial disease (PAD)

C. Narrowing or blockage of the arteries that supply blood to the limbs

4. Varicose veins

D. Enlarged and twisted veins, usually in the legs

Exercise 5: Fill in the blanks

Transcribe the following sentence:

The patient's _________ showed significant stenosis in the iliac arteries.

Answer:

The patient's angiogram showed significant stenosis in the iliac arteries.

Exercise 6: True or False

Indicate whether the following statement is true or false:

Aortic aneurysm repair can be performed using either open surgical techniques or endovascular stent grafts.

Answer:

True

Exercise 7: Fill in the blanks

Transcribe the following sentence:

The patient underwent _________ to improve blood flow in the lower extremities.

Answer:

The patient underwent bypass surgery to improve blood flow in the lower extremities.

Exercise 8: Matching

Match the vascular surgery intervention with its corresponding description:

1. Thrombectomy

2. Angioplasty

3. Stenting

4. Endarterectomy

A. Surgical removal of a blood clot

B. Minimally invasive procedure to open narrowed or blocked blood vessels

C. Placement of a small mesh tube to keep a narrowed or weakened artery open

D. Surgical removal of plaque buildup from inside an artery

Answer:

1. Thrombectomy

A. Surgical removal of a blood clot

2. Angioplasty

B. Minimally invasive procedure to open narrowed or blocked blood vessels

3. Stenting

C. Placement of a small mesh tube to keep a narrowed or weakened artery open

4. Endarterectomy

D. Surgical removal of plaque buildup from inside an artery

Exercise 9: True or False

Indicate whether the following statement is true or false:

Varicose vein stripping is a surgical procedure performed to remove large varicose veins.

Answer:

True

Exercise 10: Fill in the blanks

Transcribe the following sentence:

The patient's _________ revealed an abdominal aortic aneurysm measuring 5 centimeters in diameter.

Answer:

The patient's computed tomography (CT) scan revealed an abdominal aortic aneurysm measuring 5 centimeters in diameter.

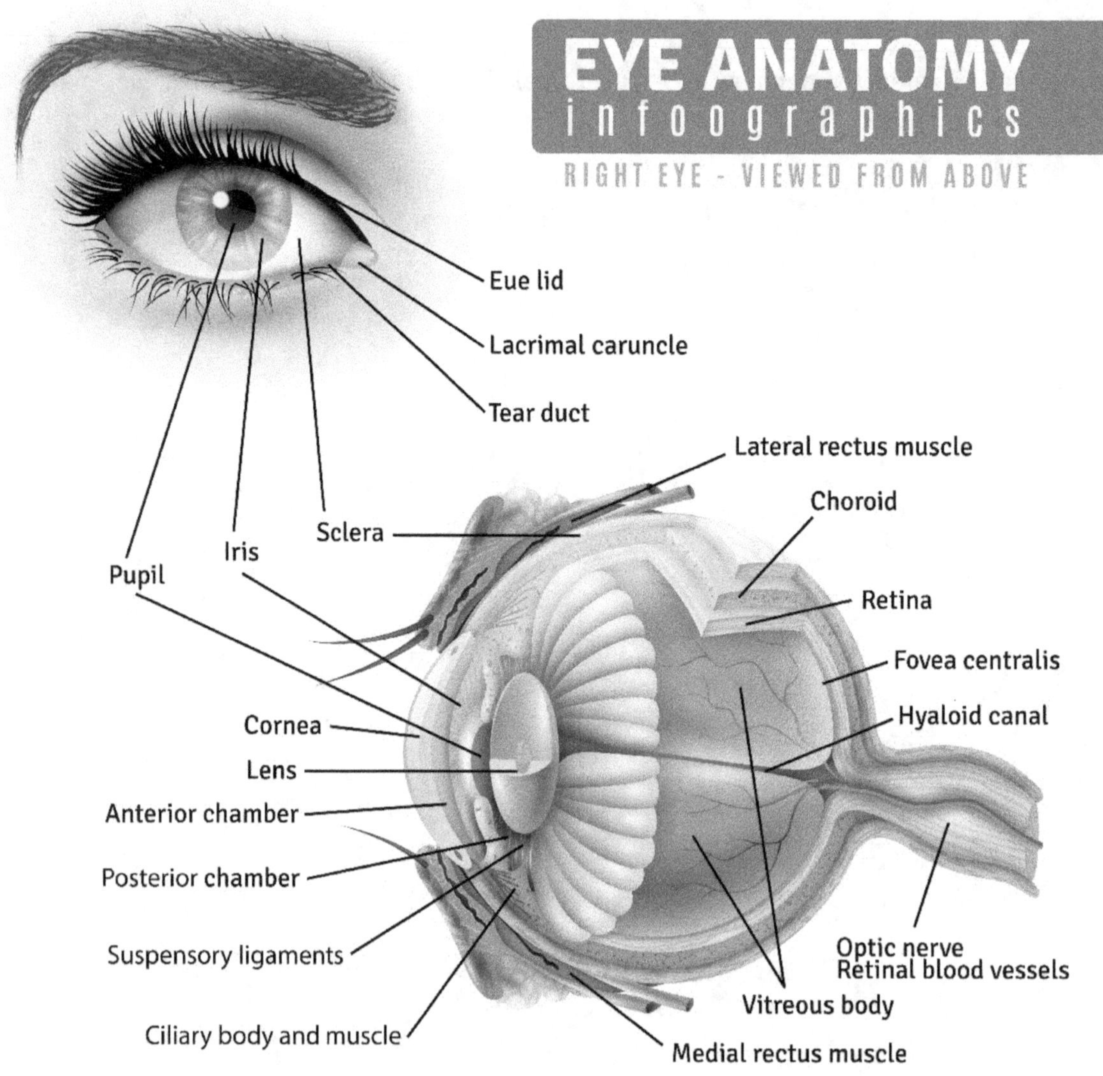

Overview of ophthalmology and its specific terminology

Ophthalmology is a branch of medicine that focuses on the diagnosis and treatment of diseases, disorders, and injuries of the eye. An ophthalmologist is a medical doctor who specializes in eye and vision care, performing eye exams, prescribing corrective lenses, diagnosing diseases, and carrying out surgical procedures.

Here are some key points to understand as a beginner in this field:

1. Eye Diseases and Conditions: Ophthalmologists treat a variety of conditions, including cataracts, glaucoma, macular degeneration, diabetic retinopathy, conjunctivitis, eye injuries, and vision issues such as nearsightedness, farsightedness, astigmatism, and presbyopia.

2. Diagnostic Tools: They use a variety of tools for diagnosis, such as slit lamps to examine the front of the eye, ophthalmoscopes to view the back of the eye, and tonometers to measure eye pressure. Specialized tests can also assess the field of vision, color perception, and the ability to focus.

3. Surgical Procedures: Ophthalmologists can perform surgeries including cataract removal, laser eye surgery (like LASIK), glaucoma surgeries, retinal detachment repair, and more. They can also perform plastic surgery procedures, such as those to repair droopy eyelids (blepharoplasty) or to smooth wrinkles around the eyes.

4. Corrective Lenses and Low Vision Aids: Ophthalmologists can prescribe glasses or contact lenses to correct vision problems. They can also provide low vision aids and vision therapy for conditions that cannot be completely corrected with glasses, contact lenses, medicine, or surgery.

5. Specialization: Some ophthalmologists choose to specialize in a particular aspect of eye health. Subspecialties can include cornea and external disease, glaucoma, neuro-ophthalmology, ophthalmic plastic surgery, pediatric ophthalmology, and vitreoretinal diseases.

6. Preventive Care: Ophthalmologists play a key role in preventive eye care, providing routine eye examinations to detect and treat eye diseases early, and educating patients about eye health and safety.

Eye conditions, vision tests, and ophthalmic surgeries

I. Eye Conditions:

1. Myopia (Nearsightedness): A condition where individuals have difficulty seeing objects at a distance but can see nearby objects clearly. It occurs when the eyeball is too long or the cornea is too curved.

2. Hyperopia (Farsightedness): A condition where individuals have difficulty seeing nearby objects clearly but can see distant objects more easily. It occurs when the eyeball is too short or the cornea is too flat.

3. Astigmatism: A condition where the cornea is irregularly shaped, causing blurred or distorted vision at both near and far distances.

4. Presbyopia: An age-related condition where individuals have difficulty focusing on near objects due to a loss of flexibility in the lens of the eye.

5. Cataracts: Clouding of the lens of the eye, resulting in blurry vision, sensitivity to light, and reduced color perception.

6. Glaucoma: A group of eye conditions characterized by increased pressure within the eye, leading to optic nerve damage and potential vision loss if left untreated.

7. Age-related Macular Degeneration (AMD): A progressive condition that affects the macula, leading to central vision loss and difficulty with activities like reading and recognizing faces.

8. Diabetic Retinopathy: A complication of diabetes that affects the blood vessels in the retina, potentially leading to vision loss if not properly managed.

9. Retinal Detachment: A condition where the retina separates from the underlying tissue, causing sudden vision loss or the appearance of flashing lights and floaters.

10. Dry Eye Syndrome: A condition characterized by insufficient tear production or poor tear quality, leading to eye discomfort, redness, and blurred vision.

11. Blepharitis: Inflammation of the eyelid margins, resulting in redness, itching, and crusting of the eyelashes.

12. Conjunctivitis (Pink Eye): Inflammation of the conjunctiva, the clear tissue covering the white part of the eye, often causing redness, itching, and discharge.

13. Keratoconus: A progressive condition where the cornea becomes thin and bulges outward, resulting in distorted vision and increased sensitivity to light.

14. Retinal Vascular Occlusion: Blockage of the blood vessels supplying the retina, leading to sudden vision loss or a sudden decrease in vision.

15. Uveitis: Inflammation of the uvea, the middle layer of the eye, causing eye redness, pain, and light sensitivity.

16. Macular Hole: A small break or defect in the macula, resulting in central vision loss or distortion.

17. Strabismus: A misalignment of the eyes, causing one or both eyes to turn inward, outward, upward, or downward.

18. Amblyopia (Lazy Eye): Reduced vision in one eye due to a lack of proper development during childhood, often requiring early intervention to prevent permanent vision loss.

19. Floaters: Small specks or cobweb-like shapes that float across the field of vision, usually caused by age-related changes in the jelly-like substance inside the eye.

20. Pinguecula: A yellowish bump or deposit on the conjunctiva, usually caused by long-term exposure to sunlight or environmental irritants.

21. Pterygium: A growth of fleshy tissue on the conjunctiva that may extend onto the cornea, often associated with prolonged sun exposure.

22. Ocular Hypertension: Elevated intraocular pressure without signs of optic nerve damage or vision loss, requiring close monitoring to prevent the development of glaucoma.

23. Corneal Abrasion: A scratch or injury to the cornea, often causing eye pain, redness, and blurred vision.

24. Refractive Errors: Conditions that cause blurred vision due to irregularities in the shape of the eye or its focusing ability, including myopia, hyperopia, and astigmatism.

25. Ptosis: Drooping of the upper eyelid, which can obstruct vision and affect the appearance of the eyes.

II. Vision Tests:

1. Visual Acuity Test: Measures the clarity and sharpness of your vision, usually conducted using an eye chart.

2. Refraction Test: Determines your exact eyeglass prescription by assessing how light bends as it enters your eyes.

3. Slit Lamp Examination: Uses a special microscope and bright light to examine the structures at the front of your eye, such as the cornea, iris, and lens.

4. Tonometry: Measures the pressure inside your eyes to check for glaucoma.

5. Color Vision Test: Evaluates your ability to perceive and differentiate colors, typically using color plates or specialized tests.

6. Cover Test: Checks for misalignment or imbalance in your eye muscles, which can indicate strabismus or other vision disorders.

7. Visual Field Test: Assesses your peripheral vision to detect any abnormalities or visual field loss.

8. Ocular Motility Test: Evaluates the range and coordination of eye movements in different directions.

9. Retinal Imaging: Captures detailed images of the retina to assess its health and detect any abnormalities or diseases.

10. Contrast Sensitivity Test: Measures your ability to distinguish between various shades of gray, which can be important for tasks like driving at night.

11. Stereopsis Test: Evaluates your depth perception by assessing your ability to perceive three-dimensional images.

12. Pupil Examination: Examines the size, shape, and response of your pupils to light, which can provide information about the function of your eye muscles and nerves.

13. Visual Field Testing: Maps your entire field of vision to detect any blind spots or areas of reduced vision.

14. Visual Evoked Potential (VEP) Test: Measures the electrical activity in your visual pathway to assess the function of your optic nerves and brain.

15. Autorefraction: Uses an automated device to measure the refractive error of your eyes quickly and accurately.

16. Retinoscopy: Involves shining a light into your eyes and observing the reflection to determine your eyeglass prescription.

17. Amsler Grid Test: Helps detect central vision abnormalities by evaluating your ability to see and interpret a grid pattern.

18. Cover-Uncover Test: Assesses eye alignment and detects any strabismus or tropia by observing how the eyes move when one eye is covered and then uncovered.

19. Keratometry: Measures the curvature of your cornea, which is crucial for determining the correct fit of contact lenses or the potential need for corneal surgery.

20. Visual Electrodiagnostic Test: Evaluates the electrical activity of the retina and optic nerves to diagnose certain eye conditions and assess overall visual function.

21. Refractive Error Assessment: Determines the type and severity of refractive errors, such as nearsightedness, farsightedness, or astigmatism.

22. Near Point of Convergence Test: Assesses how well your eyes coordinate when focusing on close objects.

23. Ophthalmoscopy: Allows the eye doctor to examine the internal structures of the eye, including the retina, optic nerve, and blood vessels.

24. Fundus Photography: Captures detailed images of the back of the eye, including the retina, macula, and optic disc, for diagnostic and monitoring purposes.

25. Digital Retinal Imaging: Uses advanced imaging technology to capture high-resolution images of the retina, providing detailed information for diagnosis and management of eye conditions.

III. Ophthalmic Surgeries:

1. Cataract Surgery: Removes the cloudy lens of the eye and replaces it with an artificial intraocular lens (IOL) to restore clear vision.

2. LASIK Surgery: Uses a laser to reshape the cornea, correcting refractive errors such as nearsightedness, farsightedness, and astigmatism.

3. Corneal Transplantation: Replaces a damaged or diseased cornea with a healthy donor cornea to improve vision and alleviate corneal conditions.

4. Glaucoma Surgery: Various surgical procedures, such as trabeculectomy or tube shunt implantation, are performed to reduce intraocular pressure and manage glaucoma.

5. Retinal Detachment Repair: Involves reattaching the detached retina to the back of the eye using techniques like scleral buckling, pneumatic retinopexy, or vitrectomy.

6. Vitrectomy: Removes the gel-like substance (vitreous) from the eye and may involve repairing retinal detachments, removing scar tissue, or treating macular holes.

7. Strabismus Surgery: Corrects misalignment of the eyes (strabismus) by adjusting the eye muscles to improve eye alignment and coordination.

8. Pterygium Excision: Removes a noncancerous growth called a pterygium that can affect the cornea and cause visual disturbances.

9. Ectropion Repair: Corrects the outward turning of the eyelid (ectropion) by tightening the eyelid muscles and tissues.

10. Entropion Repair: Corrects the inward turning of the eyelid (entropion) by repositioning the eyelid or tightening the eyelid muscles.

11. Eyelid Surgery (Blepharoplasty): Removes excess skin, fat, or muscle from the eyelids to improve their appearance or address functional concerns.

12. Ptosis Repair: Corrects drooping of the upper eyelid (ptosis) by tightening or reattaching the eyelid muscles.

13. Dacryocystorhinostomy (DCR): Creates a new drainage channel between the tear sac and the nose to treat a blocked tear duct.

14. Enucleation: Surgical removal of the eye, usually performed in cases of severe eye trauma, tumors, or unmanageable pain.

15. Orbital Decompression: Relieves pressure within the eye socket by removing or reshaping bone to treat conditions such as thyroid eye disease or orbital tumors.

16. Retinal Laser Photocoagulation: Uses a laser to seal leaking blood vessels or to create scars on the retina to treat conditions like diabetic retinopathy or retinal tears.

17. YAG Laser Capsulotomy: Uses a laser to create an opening in the cloudy posterior capsule that develops after cataract surgery, improving vision.

18. Trabeculotomy: Creates a tiny opening in the trabecular meshwork of the eye to improve drainage and reduce intraocular pressure in glaucoma.

19. Lamellar Keratoplasty: Partial-thickness corneal transplantation, typically performed to treat corneal conditions like keratoconus or corneal scarring.

20. Intacs Implantation: Inserts small plastic rings into the cornea to reshape it and improve vision in patients with keratoconus.

21. Refractive Lens Exchange: Removes the natural lens of the eye and replaces it with an artificial intraocular lens (IOL) to correct refractive errors.

22. LASEK/PRK Surgery: Uses laser technology to reshape the cornea's surface to correct refractive errors, similar to LASIK but without creating a corneal flap.

23. Punctal Plugs: Small silicone or collagen plugs inserted into the tear ducts to help retain tears and alleviate dry eye symptoms.

24. Lid Margin Repair: Repairs abnormalities or defects in the eyelid margin, such as eyelid notches or trichiasis, to improve eyelid function and comfort.

25. Neuro-Ophthalmic Surgery: Addresses conditions affecting the optic nerves, brain, or related structures, often involving procedures like optic nerve sheath fenestration or decompression surgeries.

Exercise 1: Fill in the blanks

Transcribe the following sentence:

The patient presented with complaints of blurred _________ and difficulty reading.

Answer:

The patient presented with complaints of blurred vision and difficulty reading.

Exercise 2: True or False

Indicate whether the following statement is true or false:

Cataract surgery is a common procedure performed to remove clouded lenses and restore vision.

Answer:

True

Exercise 3: Fill in the blanks

Transcribe the following sentence:

The ophthalmologist diagnosed the patient with _________ and prescribed eye drops for treatment.

Answer:

The ophthalmologist diagnosed the patient with glaucoma and prescribed eye drops for treatment.

Exercise 4: Matching

Match the ophthalmology term with its corresponding description:

1. Retinal detachment

2. Macular degeneration

3. Strabismus

4. Conjunctivitis

A. Separation of the retina from the underlying tissue

B. Progressive deterioration of the central portion of the retina

C. Misalignment of the eyes, causing them to point in different directions

D. Inflammation of the conjunctiva, resulting in redness and irritation

Answer:

1. Retinal detachment

A. Separation of the retina from the underlying tissue

2. Macular degeneration

B. Progressive deterioration of the central portion of the retina

3. Strabismus

C. Misalignment of the eyes, causing them to point in different directions

4. Conjunctivitis

D. Inflammation of the conjunctiva, resulting in redness and irritation

Exercise 5: Fill in the blanks

Transcribe the following sentence:

The patient's __________ revealed signs of diabetic retinopathy.

Answer:

The patient's fundus examination revealed signs of diabetic retinopathy.

Exercise 6: True or False

Indicate whether the following statement is true or false:

LASIK is a surgical procedure used to correct vision problems by reshaping the cornea.

Answer:

True

Exercise 7: Fill in the blanks

Transcribe the following sentence:

The ophthalmologist performed __________ to assess the optic nerve and diagnose glaucoma.

Answer:

The ophthalmologist performed visual field testing to assess the optic nerve and diagnose glaucoma.

Exercise 8: Matching

Match the ophthalmology intervention with its corresponding description:

1. Refractive surgery

2. Corneal transplantation

3. Retinal laser photocoagulation

4. Ptosis repair

A. Surgical procedures to correct refractive errors and reduce the need for glasses or contact lenses

B. Surgical replacement of damaged or diseased cornea with a healthy donor cornea

C. Use of laser energy to seal or cauterize leaking blood vessels in the retina

D. Surgical correction of drooping eyelids

Answer:

1. Refractive surgery

A. Surgical procedures to correct refractive errors and reduce the need for glasses or contact lenses

2. Corneal transplantation

B. Surgical replacement of damaged or diseased cornea with a healthy donor cornea

3. Retinal laser photocoagulation

C. Use of laser energy to seal or cauterize leaking blood vessels in the retina

4. Ptosis repair

D. Surgical correction of drooping eyelids

Exercise 9: True or False

Indicate whether the following statement is true or false:

Blepharoplasty is a surgical procedure performed to remove excess skin and fat from the eyelids.

Answer:

True

Exercise 10: Fill in the blanks

Transcribe the following sentence:

The patient underwent _________ to remove a cataract and implant an intraocular lens.

Answer:

The patient underwent cataract surgery to remove a cataract and implant an intraocular lens.

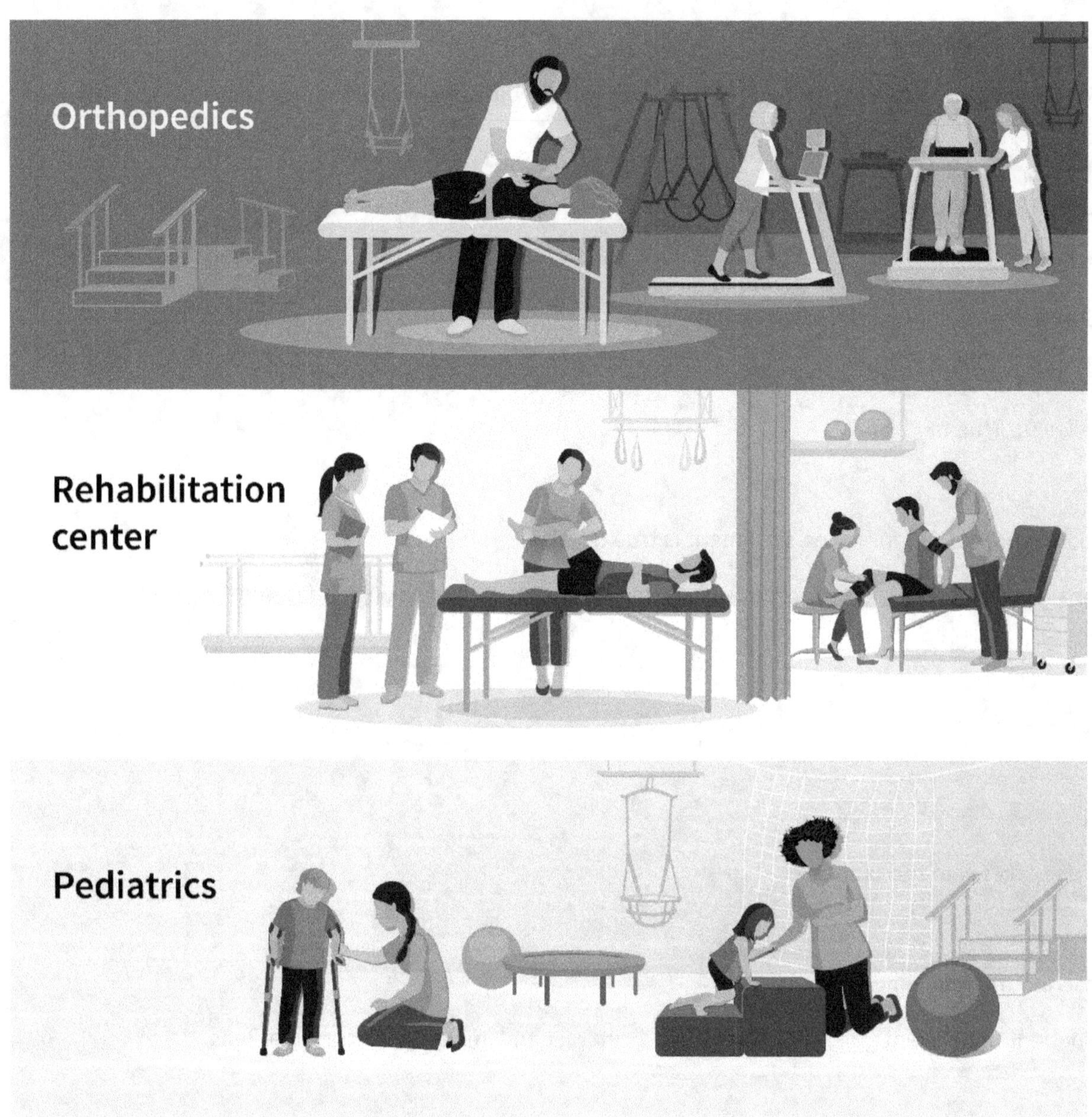

Principles and Techniques of Physiotherapy and Rehabilitation

Physiotherapy and rehabilitation are disciplines that aim to restore, maintain, and improve physical function and mobility, as well as alleviate pain and promote overall well-being. These practices involve a variety of principles and techniques designed to enhance the body's ability to recover from injury, surgery, or disease. Here are some key points to understand about physiotherapy and rehabilitation:

1. Holistic Approach: Physiotherapy and rehabilitation focus on the whole person, considering their physical, emotional, and social well-being. Treatment plans are tailored to each individual's specific needs and goals.

2. Assessment and Evaluation: A thorough assessment is conducted to evaluate the patient's condition, identify impairments, and determine the appropriate treatment approach. This may include physical examinations, functional tests, and the use of specialized tools and technologies.

3. Therapeutic Exercises: Therapeutic exercises play a crucial role in physiotherapy and rehabilitation. These exercises are designed to strengthen muscles, improve flexibility, enhance balance and coordination, and restore normal movement patterns. They can range from simple range-of-motion exercises to complex functional activities.

4. Manual Therapy: Manual therapy techniques involve hands-on interventions by the physiotherapist. These techniques may include joint mobilization, soft tissue mobilization, manual stretching, and manipulation to improve joint mobility, reduce pain, and enhance tissue healing.

5. Electrotherapy and Modalities: Electrotherapy modalities, such as electrical stimulation, ultrasound, and laser therapy, are commonly used in physiotherapy and rehabilitation. These modalities help manage pain, reduce inflammation, promote tissue healing, and improve muscle function.

6. Assistive Devices and Equipment: Physiotherapy may involve the use of assistive devices and equipment, such as crutches, walkers, canes, braces, and wheelchairs, to support mobility and facilitate rehabilitation.

7. Patient Education and Self-Management: Education is a vital component of physiotherapy and rehabilitation. Patients are empowered with knowledge about their condition, proper body mechanics, ergonomics, and techniques for self-management and injury prevention.

8. Progress Monitoring and Goal Setting: Regular monitoring of progress is essential in physiotherapy and rehabilitation. Functional assessments and outcome measures are used to track improvements and adjust treatment plans accordingly. Collaborative goal setting between the patient and the physiotherapist ensures that treatment targets are relevant and achievable.

Common Rehabilitation Exercises and Modalities

I. Rehabilitation Exercises:

1. Range of Motion (ROM) Exercises: These exercises aim to restore joint mobility and flexibility by moving the affected body part through its full range of motion.

2. Strengthening Exercises: These exercises target specific muscle groups to improve strength and endurance. They can involve the use of resistance bands, weights, or bodyweight exercises.

3. Balance and Coordination Exercises: These exercises focus on improving balance, stability, and coordination to enhance functional abilities and reduce the risk of falls.

4. Proprioception Exercises: Proprioception exercises help improve body awareness, joint position sense, and control, which are crucial for maintaining stability and preventing injuries.

5. Cardiovascular Conditioning: Aerobic exercises, such as walking, cycling, or swimming, are utilized to improve cardiovascular fitness, endurance, and overall physical conditioning.

6. Neuromuscular Re-education: These exercises focus on retraining movement patterns, motor control, and coordination, particularly in cases of neurological conditions or muscle imbalances.

7. Functional Training: Functional exercises simulate activities of daily living to improve the patient's ability to perform tasks and regain independence.

8. Core Stabilization Exercises: Core exercises target the muscles of the abdomen, back, and pelvis to improve stability, posture, and overall body mechanics.

9. Gait Training: Gait training involves specific exercises and techniques to restore normal walking patterns and improve mobility.

10. Endurance Training: Endurance exercises are designed to improve stamina and tolerance to physical activity, helping patients maintain performance over an extended period.

11. Flexibility Exercises: Flexibility exercises aim to improve the range of motion of muscles and joints, enhancing mobility and preventing stiffness.

12. Postural Correction Exercises: These exercises focus on correcting postural imbalances, improving alignment, and reducing the risk of musculoskeletal problems.

13. Resistance Training: Resistance training involves the use of external resistance, such as weights or resistance bands, to strengthen muscles and improve overall functional capacity.

14. Stretching Exercises: Stretching exercises help lengthen muscles and improve flexibility, reducing the risk of muscle strains and promoting optimal muscle function.

15. Isometric Exercises: Isometric exercises involve muscle contractions without joint movement, targeting specific muscle groups and improving muscle strength and stability.

16. Plyometric Exercises: Plyometric exercises involve quick and explosive movements to improve power, agility, and neuromuscular control.

17. Aquatic Therapy: Aquatic therapy utilizes water's buoyancy and resistance to facilitate exercises and improve strength, flexibility, and mobility with reduced impact on joints.

18. Manual Therapy Techniques: Manual therapy techniques, such as joint mobilization or soft tissue mobilization, are performed by therapists to improve joint mobility and reduce pain.

19. Respiratory Exercises: Respiratory exercises aim to improve lung function, breathing patterns, and overall respiratory capacity through techniques like deep breathing and coughing.

20. Functional Electrical Stimulation (FES): FES involves using electrical currents to stimulate muscles and assist with muscle activation and movement in individuals with neurological conditions.

21. Assistive Device Training: Assistive device training involves teaching patients how to properly use mobility aids, such as crutches, walkers, or wheelchairs, to improve mobility and independence.

22. Pain Management Techniques: Pain management techniques, including heat or cold therapy, transcutaneous electrical nerve stimulation (TENS), or ultrasound therapy, are used to alleviate pain and promote healing.

23. Task-Specific Training: Task-specific training involves practicing specific tasks or activities to improve functional abilities and promote independence in performing daily activities.

24. Cognitive Rehabilitation: Cognitive rehabilitation exercises aim to improve cognitive functions, such as memory, attention, problem-solving, and executive functioning, in individuals with cognitive impairments.

25. Virtual Reality Rehabilitation: Virtual reality rehabilitation utilizes virtual environments and interactive technology to simulate real-life scenarios and engage patients in therapeutic exercises, improving motor skills and functional outcomes.

II. Rehabilitation Modalities:

1. Electrical Stimulation: Electrical stimulation involves the use of electrical currents to stimulate muscles, promote muscle contraction or relaxation, and manage pain.

2. Ultrasound Therapy: Ultrasound utilizes high-frequency sound waves to generate deep heat within tissues, promoting tissue healing and reducing pain and inflammation.

3. Heat Therapy: Heat therapy, such as hot packs or warm baths, is applied to muscles and joints to increase blood flow, relax muscles, and alleviate pain and stiffness.

4. Cold Therapy: Cold therapy, such as ice packs or cold baths, is used to reduce inflammation, swelling, and pain by constricting blood vessels and numbing the area.

5. Traction: Traction is a technique that involves the application of a pulling force to the spine or extremities to relieve pressure, reduce pain, and improve mobility.

6. Massage Therapy: Massage techniques, including effleurage, kneading, and friction, are used to relax muscles, improve circulation, reduce pain, and enhance overall well-being.

7. Hydrotherapy: Hydrotherapy involves exercises and treatments performed in water, utilizing the buoyancy and resistance properties to support and challenge the body during rehabilitation.

8. Cryotherapy: Cryotherapy uses extremely cold temperatures, often through the use of ice or cryo-chambers, to reduce pain, inflammation, and swelling.

9. Laser Therapy: Low-level laser therapy applies low-intensity lasers or light-emitting diodes to stimulate tissue healing, reduce pain, and improve mobility.

10. Transcutaneous Electrical Nerve Stimulation (TENS): TENS units deliver low-level electrical currents to the skin to alleviate pain and promote relaxation.

11. Iontophoresis: Iontophoresis involves the use of a low-level electrical current to deliver medications through the skin, such as anti-inflammatory drugs, to reduce pain and inflammation.

12. Paraffin Wax Therapy: Paraffin wax therapy involves immersing body parts in warm paraffin wax to alleviate pain, increase blood flow, and promote joint mobility.

13. Therapeutic Ultrasound: Therapeutic ultrasound uses high-frequency sound waves to penetrate deep into tissues, promoting tissue healing, reducing inflammation, and improving range of motion.

14. Infrared Therapy: Infrared therapy uses infrared light to generate heat within tissues, promoting circulation, relieving muscle tension, and reducing pain and inflammation.

15. Taping Techniques: Taping techniques, such as kinesiology taping, are used to provide support, stabilize joints, improve muscle function, and reduce pain during movement.

16. Joint Mobilization: Joint mobilization techniques involve the skilled movement of joints by a therapist to improve joint range of motion, reduce stiffness, and restore function.

17. Therapeutic Exercise: Therapeutic exercises are customized exercises designed to restore strength, flexibility, endurance, and functional abilities specific to an individual's needs and condition.

18. Balance and Coordination Training: Balance and coordination training involves exercises and activities to improve balance, proprioception, and coordination for enhanced stability and functional movement.

19. Gait Training: Gait training focuses on improving an individual's walking pattern and efficiency through exercises, assistive devices, and gait re-education techniques.

20. Functional Training: Functional training mimics real-life movements and activities to improve an individual's ability to perform everyday tasks and activities with ease.

21. Neuromuscular Reeducation: Neuromuscular reeducation techniques are used to retrain and restore proper movement patterns, muscle control, and coordination following injury or neurological conditions.

22. Strength Training: Strength training involves exercises aimed at increasing muscle strength, power, and endurance to improve overall functional performance.

23. Range of Motion Exercises: Range of motion exercises aim to improve joint mobility, flexibility, and prevent contractures by moving the joints through their full range of motion.

24. Cardiovascular Conditioning: Cardiovascular conditioning exercises, such as cycling or swimming, are performed to improve cardiovascular fitness, endurance, and overall health.

25. Manual Therapy: Manual therapy techniques, including joint mobilization, soft tissue mobilization, and manual stretching, are used by therapists to improve joint and tissue mobility, reduce pain, and enhance function.

Exercises for Transcribing Physiotherapy and Rehabilitation Reports Accurately

Exercise 1: Fill in the blanks

Transcribe the following sentence:

The patient demonstrated good __________ and balance during the walking assessment.

Answer:

The patient demonstrated good gait and balance during the walking assessment.

Exercise 2: True or False

Indicate whether the following statement is true or false:

Ultrasound therapy is commonly used in physiotherapy to reduce pain and inflammation.

Answer:

True

Exercise 3: Fill in the blanks

Transcribe the following sentence:

The physiotherapist instructed the patient to perform __________ exercises to improve range of motion.

Answer:

The physiotherapist instructed the patient to perform range of motion exercises to improve range of motion.

Exercise 4: Matching

Match the physiotherapy and rehabilitation term with its corresponding description:

1. Core stabilization exercises

2. Transcutaneous Electrical Nerve Stimulation (TENS)

3. Neuromuscular re-education

4. Hydrotherapy

A. Exercises targeting muscles of the abdomen, back, and pelvis to improve stability and posture.

B. Delivery of medication through the skin using a low-level electrical current.

C. Exercises focusing on retraining movement patterns, motor control, and coordination.

D. Use of water for exercises and treatments, taking advantage of buoyancy and resistance.

5. Massage therapy

E. Manual techniques to relax muscles, improve circulation, and reduce pain.

Answer:

1. Core stabilization exercises

A. Exercises targeting muscles of the abdomen, back, and pelvis to improve stability and posture.

2. Transcutaneous Electrical Nerve Stimulation (TENS)

B. Delivery of medication through the skin using a low-level electrical current.

3. Neuromuscular re-education

C. Exercises focusing on retraining movement patterns, motor control, and coordination.

4. Hydrotherapy

D. Use of water for exercises and treatments, taking advantage of buoyancy and resistance.

5. Massage therapy

E. Manual techniques to relax muscles, improve circulation, and reduce pain.

Exercise 5: Fill in the blanks

Transcribe the following sentence:

The patient underwent _________ to reduce muscle tension and promote relaxation.

Answer:

The patient underwent massage therapy to reduce muscle tension and promote relaxation.

Exercise 6: True or False

Indicate whether the following statement is true or false:

Heat therapy is commonly used to increase blood flow and relax muscles in physiotherapy.

Answer:

True

Exercise 7: Fill in the blanks

Transcribe the following sentence:

The physiotherapist applied __________ to the patient's shoulder to reduce swelling and pain.

Answer:

The physiotherapist applied cold therapy to the patient's shoulder to reduce swelling and pain.

Exercise 8: Matching

Match the physiotherapy and rehabilitation intervention with its corresponding description:

1. Gait training

2. Traction

3. Ultrasound therapy

4. Cryotherapy

A. Specific exercises and techniques to restore normal walking patterns.

B. Application of a pulling force to relieve pressure on the spine or extremities.

C. Use of high-frequency sound waves to promote tissue healing and reduce pain.

D. Application of extremely cold temperatures to reduce pain and inflammation.

Answer:

1. Gait training

A. Specific exercises and techniques to restore normal walking patterns.

2. Traction

B. Application of a pulling force to relieve pressure on the spine or extremities.

3. Ultrasound therapy

C. Use of high-frequency sound waves to promote tissue healing and reduce pain.

4. Cryotherapy

D. Application of extremely cold temperatures to reduce pain and inflammation.

Exercise 9: True or False

Indicate whether the following statement is true or false:

Hydrotherapy utilizes water's buoyancy and resistance properties for exercises and treatments.

Answer:

True

Exercise 10: Fill in the blanks

Transcribe the following sentence:

The patient was prescribed _________ exercises to improve balance and stability.

Answer:

The patient was prescribed balance and stability exercises to improve balance and stability.

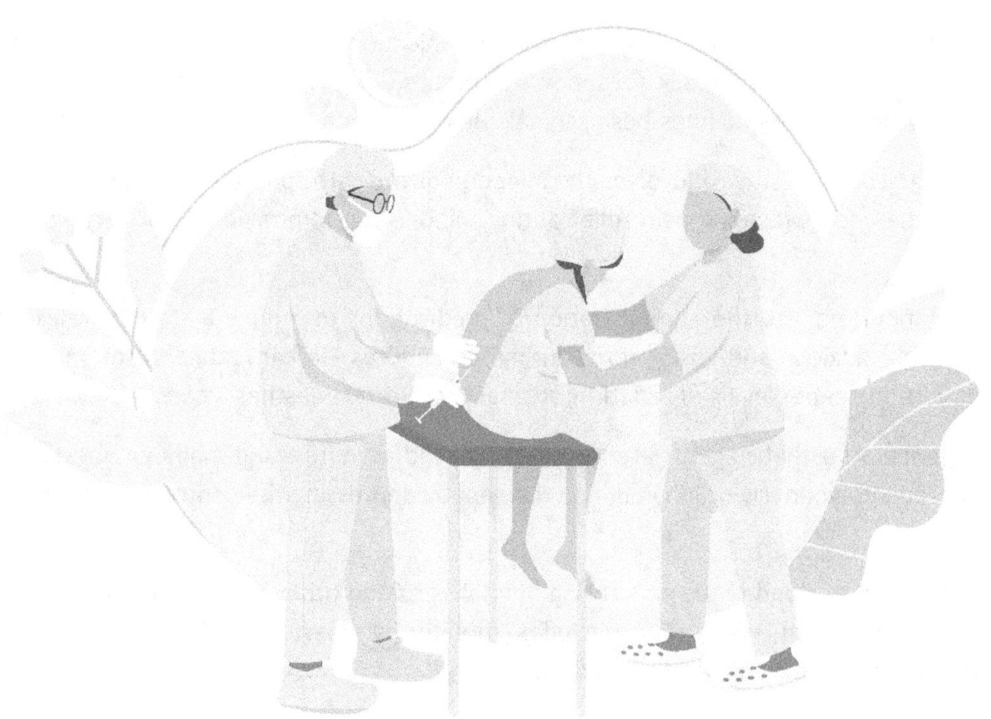

Introduction to Anesthesiology and Its Specialized Terminology

Anesthesiology is a medical specialty that focuses on providing anesthesia and perioperative care to patients undergoing surgical procedures. An anesthesiologist is a medical doctor who specializes in administering anesthesia, managing pain, monitoring vital signs, and ensuring patient safety and comfort throughout the surgical process.

Here are some key points to understand as a beginner in this field:

1. Anesthesia: Anesthesia is the use of medications to induce a reversible loss of sensation and consciousness, allowing for pain-free medical procedures. There are different types of anesthesia, including general anesthesia, regional anesthesia, and local anesthesia.

2. General Anesthesia: General anesthesia is a state of controlled unconsciousness induced through the administration of intravenous drugs and inhaled anesthetics. It involves complete loss of consciousness and pain sensation, allowing for major surgical procedures to be performed.

3. Regional Anesthesia: Regional anesthesia involves the injection of local anesthetic medication near specific nerves or nerve groups to block sensation in a specific region of the body. Common types of regional anesthesia include epidural anesthesia, spinal anesthesia, and peripheral nerve blocks.

4. Local Anesthesia: Local anesthesia involves the injection or topical application of anesthetics to numb a specific area of the body, providing pain relief during minor surgical procedures or certain diagnostic procedures.

5. Sedation: Sedation refers to the administration of medications to induce a state of relaxation and drowsiness, reducing anxiety and discomfort during procedures. It can range from mild sedation (conscious sedation) to deeper levels of sedation, such as monitored anesthesia care (MAC).

6. Anesthetic Agents: Anesthetic agents are medications used to induce and maintain anesthesia. They can be administered intravenously or inhaled, and they act by depressing the central nervous system and blocking pain signals.

7. Anesthesia Monitoring: Continuous monitoring of vital signs and other parameters is essential during anesthesia to ensure patient safety. This includes monitoring heart rate, blood pressure, oxygen saturation, end-tidal carbon dioxide levels, and temperature.

8. Perioperative Care: Perioperative care involves the management of patients before, during, and after surgery. It includes preoperative assessment and optimization, intraoperative monitoring and anesthesia administration, and postoperative pain management and recovery.

Anesthesia Techniques, Monitoring, and Perioperative Care

I. Anesthesia Techniques:

1. General Anesthesia: General anesthesia involves the administration of intravenous medications and inhaled anesthetics to induce unconsciousness and ensure pain control during surgery. It requires airway management and mechanical ventilation.

2. Regional Anesthesia: Regional anesthesia blocks nerve transmission in specific regions of the body, allowing for surgery or pain relief in the targeted area. Common techniques include epidural anesthesia, spinal anesthesia, and peripheral nerve blocks.

3. Local Anesthesia: Local anesthesia involves the injection or topical application of anesthetics to numb a specific area of the body. It is commonly used for minor surgical procedures or diagnostic procedures.

4. Monitored Anesthesia Care (MAC): MAC refers to the administration of sedation and analgesia to keep the patient comfortable during procedures while allowing them to maintain consciousness and protective reflexes.

5. Sedation: Sedation involves the administration of medications to induce a state of relaxation and reduce anxiety or discomfort during medical procedures, without necessarily causing complete loss of consciousness.

6. Epidural Anesthesia: Epidural anesthesia is a regional anesthesia technique in which an anesthetic agent is injected into the epidural space, providing pain relief and anesthesia for procedures such as childbirth or surgery in the lower body.

7. Spinal Anesthesia: Spinal anesthesia involves the injection of anesthetic medication into the cerebrospinal fluid in the spinal canal, numbing the lower body for surgery or pain relief.

8. Local Infiltration: Local infiltration is a technique in which anesthetic medication is directly injected into the surgical or treatment site to provide localized pain control.

9. Intravenous Regional Anesthesia (Bier Block): Intravenous regional anesthesia, also known as a Bier Block, involves the use of a tourniquet to isolate blood flow to a limb while injecting local anesthetics into the isolated area.

10. Topical Anesthesia: Topical anesthesia involves applying anesthetic agents in the form of creams, gels, or sprays directly to the skin or mucous membranes to provide localized numbness and pain relief.

II. Anesthesia Monitoring:

1. ECG Monitoring: Electrocardiogram (ECG) monitoring provides continuous monitoring of the electrical activity of the heart, allowing for the detection of any abnormalities or arrhythmias during anesthesia.

2. Blood Pressure Monitoring: Non-invasive blood pressure monitoring or invasive arterial blood pressure monitoring is used to monitor blood pressure throughout the surgical procedure, ensuring adequate perfusion to vital organs.

3. Pulse Oximetry: Pulse oximetry measures oxygen saturation in the blood, providing continuous monitoring of oxygen levels during anesthesia.

4. End-Tidal Carbon Dioxide Monitoring: End-tidal carbon dioxide monitoring measures the concentration of carbon dioxide at the end of expiration, helping assess the effectiveness of ventilation and detect any potential issues, such as airway obstruction or hypoventilation.

5. Temperature Monitoring: Temperature monitoring is crucial during anesthesia to prevent hypothermia or hyperthermia, as anesthesia can affect the body's ability to regulate temperature.

6. Anesthetic Gas Monitoring: Anesthetic gas monitoring measures the concentration of inhaled anesthetic agents in the patient's respiratory gases, ensuring appropriate levels are maintained for anesthesia induction and maintenance.

7. Depth of Anesthesia Monitoring: Depth of anesthesia monitoring helps assess the patient's level of consciousness and anesthesia depth, ensuring adequate anesthesia and minimizing the risk of awareness during surgery.

8. Neuromuscular Monitoring: Neuromuscular monitoring assesses the patient's neuromuscular function to determine the level of muscle relaxation, which is important for surgical procedures and preventing complications related to inadequate paralysis or prolonged muscle relaxation.

9. Capnography: Capnography is a monitoring technique that measures the concentration of carbon dioxide in exhaled breath, providing valuable information about the patient's respiratory status and the effectiveness of ventilation.

10. Hemodynamic Monitoring: Hemodynamic monitoring involves assessing parameters such as heart rate, blood pressure, cardiac output, and fluid status to ensure adequate perfusion and oxygen delivery to the body's organs during anesthesia.

III. Perioperative Care:

1. Preoperative Assessment: Preoperative assessment involves evaluating the patient's medical history, conducting physical examinations, and ordering relevant tests to ensure optimal preparation for surgery. This includes assessing the patient's anesthesia risks, allergies, medications, and overall health status.

2. Intraoperative Care: Intraoperative care involves the administration and management of anesthesia, ensuring patient safety, and providing adequate pain control during surgery. The anesthesiologist monitors vital signs, adjusts anesthesia levels, manages airway, and administers fluids and medications as needed.

3. Postoperative Pain Management: Postoperative pain management focuses on controlling pain after surgery to enhance patient comfort and facilitate recovery. This may involve the use of medications, regional anesthesia techniques, or other pain management modalities.

4. Post-Anesthesia Care Unit (PACU) Care: PACU care involves monitoring patients in the recovery phase after surgery, ensuring stable vital signs, managing pain and nausea, and ensuring a smooth transition to the next phase of care.

5. Airway Management: Ensuring the patient's airway is open and maintained during surgery, which may involve intubation, use of airway devices, or specialized techniques.

6. Fluid and Electrolyte Management: Monitoring and regulating the patient's fluid and electrolyte balance during surgery to maintain stable physiological function.

7. Anesthetic Drug Administration: Administering and titrating anesthetic drugs to achieve and maintain the desired level of anesthesia throughout the surgical procedure.

8. Hemodynamic Monitoring: Continuously monitoring the patient's cardiovascular function, including blood pressure, heart rate, and oxygenation, to ensure stability and detect any abnormalities.

9. Infection Control: Implementing measures to prevent and control infections in the surgical environment, including sterile techniques, proper disinfection, and adherence to infection control protocols.

10. Emergency Preparedness: Being prepared to respond to emergencies during surgery, including managing complications, providing resuscitation, and ensuring patient safety.

Practice Activities for Transcribing Anesthesiology Reports Effectively

Exercise 1: Fill in the blanks

Transcribe the following sentence:

The patient received _________ anesthesia for a knee arthroscopy.

Answer:

The patient received regional anesthesia for a knee arthroscopy.

Exercise 2: True or False

Indicate whether the following statement is true or false:

An anesthesiologist monitors the patient's vital signs during surgery to ensure their safety and well-being.

Answer:

True

Exercise 3: Fill in the blanks

Transcribe the following sentence:

The anesthesiologist administered _________ to induce and maintain general anesthesia.

Answer:

The anesthesiologist administered intravenous medications and inhaled anesthetics to induce and maintain general anesthesia.

Exercise 4: Matching

Match the anesthesia technique with its corresponding description:

1. Regional anesthesia

2. Monitored Anesthesia Care (MAC)

3. Local anesthesia

4. General anesthesia

A. Blocks nerve transmission in a specific region of the body.

B. Administration of sedation and analgesia to keep the patient comfortable during procedures.

C. Numbs a specific area of the body for minor surgical procedures or diagnostic procedures.

D. Induces unconsciousness and pain control through intravenous medications and inhaled anesthetics.

Answer:

1. Regional anesthesia

A. Blocks nerve transmission in a specific region of the body.

2. Monitored Anesthesia Care (MAC)

B. Administration of sedation and analgesia to keep the patient comfortable during procedures.

3. Local anesthesia

C. Numbs a specific area of the body for minor surgical procedures or diagnostic procedures.

4. General anesthesia

D. Induces unconsciousness and pain control through intravenous medications and inhaled anesthetics.

Exercise 5: Fill in the blanks

Transcribe the following sentence:

During surgery, the anesthesiologist monitored the patient's _________ to ensure adequate ventilation.

Answer:

During surgery, the anesthesiologist monitored the patient's end-tidal carbon dioxide levels to ensure adequate ventilation.

Exercise 6: True or False

Indicate whether the following statement is true or false:

Perioperative care involves managing patients before, during, and after surgery, including preoperative assessment, intraoperative monitoring, and postoperative pain management.

Answer:

True

Exercise 7: Fill in the blanks

Transcribe the following sentence:

The patient received _________ for postoperative pain management.

Answer:

The patient received medications and regional anesthesia techniques for postoperative pain management.

Exercise 8: Matching

Match the anesthesia monitoring technique with its corresponding description:

1. ECG monitoring

2. Blood pressure monitoring

3. Pulse oximetry

4. End-tidal carbon dioxide monitoring

A. Continuous monitoring of the electrical activity of the heart during anesthesia.

B. Measurement of blood pressure throughout the surgical procedure.

C. Continuous monitoring of oxygen saturation in the blood during anesthesia.

D. Measurement of carbon dioxide concentration at the end of expiration to assess ventilation.

Answer:

1. ECG monitoring

A. Continuous monitoring of the electrical activity of the heart during anesthesia.

2. Blood pressure monitoring

B. Measurement of blood pressure throughout the surgical procedure.

3. Pulse oximetry

C. Continuous monitoring of oxygen saturation in the blood during anesthesia.

4. End-tidal carbon dioxide monitoring

D. Measurement of carbon dioxide concentration at the end of expiration to assess ventilation.

Exercise 9: True or False

Indicate whether the following statement is true or false:

The post-anesthesia care unit (PACU) is where patients recover immediately after surgery under the care of specialized nurses.

Answer:

True

Exercise 10: Fill in the blanks

Transcribe the following sentence:

The anesthesiologist closely monitored the patient's _________ and adjusted anesthesia levels accordingly.

Answer:

The anesthesiologist closely monitored the patient's vital signs, including blood pressure, heart rate, and oxygen saturation, and adjusted anesthesia levels accordingly.

MODULE III. WEEKLY TRANSCRIPTION MASTERCLASS: CONFORMING TO TRANSCRIPTION GUIDELINES FOR ACCURACY

1. INTRODUCTION TO TRANSCRIPTION GUIDELINES

In the field of medical transcription, adhering to transcription guidelines is essential for ensuring accuracy and consistency in medical reports. Following these guidelines helps maintain quality and facilitates effective communication among healthcare professionals. Common industry-standard guidelines and style manuals include those provided by the Association for Healthcare Documentation Integrity (AHDI) and the American Medical Association (AMA).

Example:

Case Study: A medical transcriptionist receives a dictation from a healthcare provider and transcribes the report following the established transcription guidelines. By adhering to the guidelines, the transcriptionist ensures that the report is accurately documented, with proper formatting, abbreviations, and terminology usage.

Usual Values:

- AHDI Guidelines for Healthcare Documentation: The AHDI provides comprehensive guidelines on grammar, punctuation, medical terms, abbreviations, and formatting.

- AMA Manual of Style: The AMA manual offers guidelines specific to medical terminology, citation, reference formatting, and writing style for medical reports and publications.

By familiarizing themselves with these guidelines, medical transcriptionists can produce accurate and consistent medical reports that meet industry standards.

2. ABBREVIATIONS AND ACRONYMS

Abbreviations and acronyms play a significant role in medical reports. It is essential to follow guidelines for their proper usage and expansion to ensure clarity and accuracy.

Guidelines:

- Use standard and approved abbreviations according to industry guidelines and style manuals.

- Expand abbreviations upon their first use, followed by the abbreviation in parentheses.

- Avoid excessive use of abbreviations to maintain readability and understanding.

- Ensure consistency in the usage and formatting of abbreviations throughout the report.

Commonly Used Medical Abbreviations and Proper Usage:

- BP: Blood pressure

- HR: Heart rate

- EKG: Electrocardiogram

- C-section: Cesarean section

- UTI: Urinary tract infection

- CAD: Coronary artery disease

Exercises:

1. Identify the expanded form of the following abbreviations:

   a) NPO

   b) SOB

   c) MRI

   d) ICU

2. Expand the following abbreviations correctly:

   a) qd

   b) stat

c) BM

d) ADL

By adhering to the guidelines for using and expanding abbreviations and acronyms, accurate and consistent documentation can be achieved in medical reports. Regular practice and familiarization with commonly used medical abbreviations are key to mastering their usage in transcription.

3. HANDLING AGES IN TRANSCRIPTION

Handling ages in transcription requires following specific rules and conventions to accurately document age-related information in medical reports.

Rules and Conventions:

- Use numerical values to express ages, unless instructed otherwise.

- Specify the unit of measurement, such as years (y), months (mo), or days (d), after the numerical value.

- Use the appropriate abbreviation for the unit of measurement based on the context and style guidelines.

- Use hyphens when expressing age ranges, such as "2-3 years old."

- Be consistent in the format and style used for ages throughout the report.

Examples:

- 45 years

- 6 months (6 mo)

- 10 days (10 d)

- Age range: 2-5 years old

Practice Activities:

1. Transcribe the following age-related information:

   a) The patient is a 65-year-old male.

   b) The child is 9 months old.

   c) The patient's age is 40 years.

   d) The age range for the study participants is 18-25 years old.

2. Correctly format the following age expressions:

   a) 5 yrs

   b) 7 mo

   c) 15 days

d) Age range: 10-15 yrs

4. PROPER USAGE OF AMPERSAND (&)

The ampersand symbol (&) is commonly used in various contexts, including medical reports. However, its usage must adhere to specific guidelines to maintain professionalism and clarity.

Guidelines for Using the Ampersand Symbol:

1. Use the ampersand symbol in place of "and" only in specific situations, such as:

   - Official names of organizations or institutions (e.g., NIH & CDC).

   - Commonly recognized abbreviations or logos (e.g., AT&T).

   - Title of a study, research project, or publication (e.g., Smith et al.).

   - Commonly used phrases or expressions (e.g., R&D, Q&A).

2. In general, use "and" instead of the ampersand symbol in formal writing, especially in medical reports.

Exercises:

1. Determine whether the ampersand or "and" should be used in the following sentences:

   a) The patient presented with hypertension & diabetes.

   b) Please consult with Dr. Johnson and Dr. Smith.

   c) The study was conducted by Dr. Brown & Dr. White.

   d) The patient is scheduled for a CT scan and an MRI.

2. Rewrite the following sentences, replacing the ampersand with "and" where appropriate:

   a) The patient requires a consultation with Dr. Johnson & Dr. Smith.

   b) The laboratory results show an increase in RBC count & WBC count.

   c) The patient is currently taking medication for hypertension & diabetes.

5. TRANSCRIBING APGAR SCORES

The Apgar scoring system is a standardized method used to assess the physical condition of newborns immediately after birth. It evaluates five criteria: appearance (skin color), pulse (heart rate), grimace (reflex irritability), activity (muscle tone), and respiration (breathing effort). Each criterion is assigned a score of 0, 1, or 2, with a total score ranging from 0 to 10.

Guidelines for Transcribing Apgar Scores in Medical Reports:

1. Document the Apgar scores in the format "Apgar score at 1 minute: __/10" and "Apgar score at 5 minutes: __/10" to indicate the scores obtained at different time points.

2. Use the appropriate abbreviations (e.g., min for minute, HR for heart rate) to maintain brevity and clarity.

3. Ensure accuracy in transcribing the Apgar scores, as they play a crucial role in assessing the newborn's condition and may influence subsequent medical decisions.

Practice Exercises:

1. Transcribe the Apgar scores based on the given information:

   a) Apgar score at 1 minute: 7/10

   b) Apgar score at 5 minutes: 9/10

2. Identify any errors or inaccuracies in the following transcriptions of Apgar scores and correct them:

   a) Apgar score at 1 min: 6/10

   b) Apgar score at 5 minutes: 8 out of 10

Transcribing blood count values accurately is essential in medical reports as it provides crucial information about a patient's hematological status. The blood count typically includes measurements of red blood cells (RBCs), white blood cells (WBCs), and platelets.

Proper Transcription of Blood Count Values:

1. Document the blood count values in the appropriate format, such as "RBC count: __ (units of measurement)" for red blood cells, "WBC count: __ (units of measurement)" for white blood cells, and "Platelet count: __ (units of measurement)" for platelets.

2. Use the correct units of measurement for each blood component. Common units include cells per microliter (cells/μL) for RBCs and WBCs, and platelets per microliter (platelets/μL) for platelet counts.

3. Pay attention to any specified reference ranges or normal values to ensure accurate transcription.

Understanding Units of Measurement in Blood Counts:

1. Red Blood Cells (RBCs): The RBC count represents the number of red blood cells in a given volume of blood. The usual unit of measurement is cells per microliter (cells/μL).

2. White Blood Cells (WBCs): The WBC count indicates the number of white blood cells in a specified blood volume. The units of measurement are typically cells per microliter (cells/μL).

3. Platelets: Platelet count measures the number of platelets present in a given blood volume. It is expressed as platelets per microliter (platelets/μL).

Exercises for Transcribing Blood Count Values Accurately:

1. Transcribe the blood count values based on the given information:

  a) RBC count: 4.5 million cells/μL

  b) WBC count: 8,000 cells/μL

  c) Platelet count: 250,000 platelets/μL

2. Fill in the blanks with the appropriate units of measurement for each blood count:

  a) RBC count: 5.2 _________

  b) WBC count: 10,500 _________

  c) Platelet count: 180,000 _________

7. TRANSCRIBING BLOOD PRESSURE READINGS

Transcribing blood pressure readings accurately is crucial in medical reports as it provides valuable information about a patient's cardiovascular health. Blood pressure is typically measured using two values: systolic and diastolic.

Guidelines for Transcribing Blood Pressure Readings:

1. Document the blood pressure measurements in the appropriate format, such as "Blood pressure: __ / __ mmHg" for systolic and diastolic values.

2. Use the proper formatting for representing systolic and diastolic values with a forward slash (/) separating the two values.

3. Include the unit of measurement, which is millimeters of mercury (mmHg), after each value.

4. Follow the standard order of systolic value first, followed by diastolic value.

Proper Formatting and Placement of Blood Pressure Readings:

1. Place the blood pressure reading in the appropriate section of the medical report, such as vital signs or relevant examination findings.

2. Use the correct formatting to distinguish systolic and diastolic values, ensuring clear separation between the two measurements.

3. Avoid unnecessary punctuation or symbols that may cause confusion or misinterpretation.

Practice Activities for Transcribing Blood Pressure Accurately:

1. Transcribe the blood pressure readings based on the given information:

   a) Blood pressure: 120/80 mmHg

   b) Blood pressure: 140/90 mmHg

   c) Blood pressure: 110/70 mmHg

2. Fill in the blanks with the appropriate systolic and diastolic values for each blood pressure reading:

   a) Blood pressure: ___ / ___ mmHg

   b) Blood pressure: ___ / ___ mmHg

   c) Blood pressure: ___ / ___ mmHg

8. TRANSCRIBING BUILDING, STRUCTURE, AND ROOM NAMES

Transcribing building, structure, and room names accurately is important in medical reports to ensure clear communication and proper identification of locations within healthcare facilities. Here are some guidelines for transcribing building, structure, and room names:

Proper Transcription of Building and Structure Names:

1. Use the correct spelling and punctuation when transcribing the names of hospitals, clinics, and medical facilities.

2. Follow any specific formatting guidelines provided by the facility or transcription style manual.

3. If an abbreviation or acronym is commonly used for a building or structure name, expand it when first mentioned and use the expanded form consistently throughout the report.

Guidelines for Transcribing Room Names and Numbers:

1. Transcribe room names and numbers exactly as they appear, paying attention to any capitalization or punctuation.

2. Include the appropriate designation for room types, such as "Room," "Suite," or "Unit," if specified.

3. Use numerals for room numbers unless otherwise instructed or if there is a specific style guideline to use spelled-out numbers.

Examples of Transcribing Building and Room Names:

1. Medical Center: St. Mary's Hospital

   - Proper transcription: St. Mary's Hospital

2. Clinic: Johnson Family Clinic, Suite 205

   - Proper transcription: Johnson Family Clinic, Suite 205

3. Outpatient Surgery Center: City Medical Center, Operating Room 3

   - Proper transcription: City Medical Center, Operating Room 3

Exercises for Accurately Transcribing Building and Room Names:

1. Transcribe the following building names accurately:

   a) Children's Hospital of Philadelphia

   b) Memorial Sloan Kettering Cancer Center

   c) Mayo Clinic

2. Fill in the blanks with the appropriate room names and numbers:

   a) Main __________, Room 302

   b) ________ Medical Center, Suite 101

   c) ___________ Hospital, Emergency Department

9. CANCER CLASSIFICATION TERMINOLOGY

Understanding cancer classification terminology is crucial for accurately transcribing cancer-related information in medical reports. Here are the key points to consider:

Classification and Staging of Cancer:

1. Learn the basic principles of cancer classification, including the primary site of the tumor and the histological type.

2. Familiarize yourself with the different cancer types, such as carcinoma, sarcoma, lymphoma, and leukemia.

3. Understand the grading and staging systems used to determine the extent and severity of the cancer.

Transcribing Cancer Types, Grades, and Stages:

1. Use the appropriate medical terminology when transcribing the type of cancer. For example, "adenocarcinoma," "squamous cell carcinoma," or "melanoma."

2. Follow the guidelines for capitalization and punctuation specific to cancer classification terms.

3. Clearly document the grade of the cancer, which indicates how abnormal the cells appear under a microscope.

4. Accurately transcribe the cancer stage, which describes the size of the tumor and its spread to nearby lymph nodes or other organs.

Practice Exercises for Transcribing Cancer Classification Terms:

1. Match the following cancer types with their corresponding definitions:

  a) Carcinoma

  b) Sarcoma

  c) Lymphoma

  d) Leukemia

  i. A cancer that arises from connective tissues, such as bones or muscles.

  ii. A cancer of the blood or bone marrow.

  iii. A cancer that starts in epithelial cells, which are the cells that line the organs and tissues.

iv. A cancer that begins in the cells of the immune system.

2. Fill in the blanks with the correct cancer classification terms:

a) The patient was diagnosed with _______________, a type of cancer that affects the lymphocytes.

b) The biopsy results confirmed the presence of _______________, a malignant tumor originating from glandular cells.

c) The pathologist identified the tumor as _______________, which arises from the soft tissues.

10. CAPITALIZATION RULES IN TRANSCRIPTION

Understanding capitalization rules is essential for accurate transcription in medical reports. Here's an overview of capitalization guidelines in transcription:

Guidelines for Capitalizing Medical Terms, Headings, and Proper Nouns:

1. Capitalize proper nouns, including names of individuals, places, organizations, and specific medical terms (e.g., Parkinson's disease).

2. Capitalize the first word of a sentence, headings, and subheadings in medical reports.

3. Capitalize acronyms and abbreviations if they represent proper nouns or the first letter of each abbreviated word (e.g., MRI, AIDS).

Rules for Capitalizing Specific Words and Phrases in Medical Reports:

1. Capitalize anatomical terms that are derived from proper nouns (e.g., Achilles tendon).

2. Capitalize trade names of medications, medical devices, and equipment (e.g., Advil, MRI scanner).

3. Capitalize names of medical specialties, departments, and units (e.g., Cardiology Department, Neonatal Intensive Care Unit).

4. Capitalize specific diagnostic tests, procedures, or surgical techniques (e.g., Electrocardiogram, Magnetic Resonance Imaging, Laparoscopic Cholecystectomy).

Exercises for Practicing Correct Capitalization in Transcription:

1. Correct the capitalization errors in the following sentence:

   "The patient presented with chest pain and was admitted to the cardiology Department for further evaluation."

2. Identify the correct capitalization in the following medical term:

   "intravenous fluids"

3. Rewrite the following sentence with correct capitalization:

   "the patient underwent a CT scan of the brain to rule out any abnormalities."

11. HANDLING COMPOUND MODIFIERS

Properly handling compound modifiers is crucial for accurate transcription in medical reports. Here's a breakdown of the guidelines for transcribing compound modifiers:

Rules for Transcribing Compound Modifiers and Hyphenated Terms:

1. Use a hyphen to connect two or more words that act together as a single modifying unit before a noun (e.g., well-known surgeon).

2. Hyphenate compound modifiers when they come before a noun but not after a verb (e.g., high-risk pregnancy).

3. Avoid using hyphens with adverbs ending in "-ly" (e.g., widely used drug).

4. If the compound modifier follows the noun, no hyphen is needed (e.g., the surgeon is well known).

Understanding the Proper Placement of Hyphens in Compound Modifiers:

1. Hyphens are used to prevent confusion or ambiguity in meaning.

2. They help convey a specific relationship between words in a compound modifier.

Practice Activities for Transcribing Compound Modifiers Accurately:

1. Identify the correct placement of the hyphen in the following phrase:

   "The patient has a long-term history of diabetes."

2. Rewrite the following sentence with the appropriate hyphenation:

   "The patient has a history of smoking related lung disease."

3. Determine whether the following phrase needs hyphenation or not:

   "The patient has an age related condition."

12. TRANSCRIBING COMPOUND WORDS

Transcribing compound words accurately is important for maintaining clarity and consistency in medical reports. Here are the guidelines for transcribing compound words:

Guidelines for Transcribing Compound Words in Medical Reports:

1. Determine if the compound word is written as one word, hyphenated, or separate words.

2. Consult reputable medical dictionaries and style guides for guidance on specific compound words.

3. Follow established hyphenation rules when required, especially for clarity and avoiding ambiguity.

4. Pay attention to any changes in meaning or pronunciation when a compound word is hyphenated or written as separate words.

5. Use proper spacing and formatting to ensure readability and adherence to transcription guidelines.

Proper Spacing and Hyphenation Rules for Compound Words:

1. Closed Form: Some compound words are written as one word without any spaces or hyphens (e.g., bloodstream, healthcare).

2. Hyphenated Form: Some compound words are hyphenated to clarify meaning or aid in pronunciation (e.g., well-being, self-care).

3. Open Form: Some compound words are written as separate words (e.g., medical transcription, patient care).

Examples and Exercises for Transcribing Compound Words Correctly:

1. Identify the correct form of the compound word in the following phrase:

   "The patient is undergoing a longterm treatment plan."

2. Determine whether the compound word should be hyphenated or written as separate words:

   "The patient has a well defined condition."

3. Rewrite the following sentence with the appropriate compound word format:

   "The patient is receiving outpatient care services."

13. TRANSCRIBING DATES

When transcribing dates in medical reports, it is crucial to follow specific rules and conventions to ensure accuracy and clarity. Here are the guidelines for transcribing dates:

Rules for Transcribing Dates in Medical Reports:

1. Format: Follow the standard format of day, month, and year (e.g., 15th May 2023).

2. Punctuation: Use a comma after the day and a comma after the year (e.g., May 15, 2023).

3. Abbreviations: Use the appropriate abbreviations for months (e.g., Jan for January, Feb for February).

4. Spelling: Spell out the month if it appears at the beginning of a sentence or in narrative sections.

5. Leading Zeros: Include a leading zero for single-digit days (e.g., 05th May 2023).

6. Context: Consider the context of the report and use the most appropriate format (e.g., numerical vs. written-out dates).

Proper Use of Punctuation and Abbreviations in Date Transcription:

1. Example 1: 15th May 2023

2. Example 2: May 15, 2023

3. Example 3: 05/15/23 (numeric format, commonly used in some regions or systems)

4. Example 4: January 3rd, 2024 (spelled out month with ordinal indicator)

Practice Exercises for Accurately Transcribing Dates:

1. Transcribe the following date: March 10, 2022.

2. Rewrite the following date using the numeric format: 21st June 2023.

3. Correctly transcribe the date in the following sentence: The patient's appointment is scheduled for 5th December 2023.

When transcribing decimal numbers in medical reports, it is important to follow specific guidelines to ensure accuracy and precision. Here are the guidelines for transcribing decimals:

Guidelines for Transcribing Decimals in Medical Reports:

1. Decimal Point Placement: Place the decimal point according to the correct position in the number.

2. Leading Zeroes: Include leading zeroes for values between 0 and 1 (e.g., 0.5).

3. Precision: Transcribe the decimal number with the appropriate level of precision indicated in the original report.

4. Units of Measurement: Ensure that the decimal is correctly associated with the corresponding unit of measurement.

Understanding Decimal Point Placement and Precision:

1. Decimal point placement: The decimal point separates the whole number from the fractional part of the number.

2. Precision: Pay attention to the precision indicated in the original report. It may vary depending on the context and the significance of the measurement.

Exercises for Transcribing Decimals Accurately:

1. Transcribe the decimal value: 2.75.

2. Rewrite the following decimal number with the appropriate precision: 0.0035.

3. Correctly transcribe the decimal in the following sentence: The patient's body temperature is 37.5°C.

15. DIABETES MELLITUS TERMINOLOGY

When transcribing diabetes mellitus terminology in medical reports, it is important to have a clear understanding of the different types, treatment options, and complications associated with this condition. Here are the key points for transcribing diabetes-related information:

Transcribing Diabetes Mellitus Terminology:

1. Types of Diabetes: Familiarize yourself with the different types of diabetes, such as Type 1, Type 2, gestational diabetes, and other less common types.

2. Treatment Modalities: Understand the various treatment modalities used in managing diabetes, including insulin therapy, oral medications, lifestyle modifications, and dietary interventions.

3. Complications: Be aware of the potential complications associated with diabetes, such as diabetic neuropathy, retinopathy, nephropathy, and cardiovascular complications.

Guidelines for Documenting Diabetes-Related Information:

1. Accurate Representation: Ensure that you transcribe the correct type of diabetes, treatment modalities, and any associated complications based on the information provided in the medical report.

2. Consistency: Use consistent terminology and abbreviations when documenting diabetes-related terms to maintain clarity and avoid confusion.

3. Contextual Understanding: Consider the context of the patient's condition, treatment plan, and any comorbidities when transcribing diabetes-related information.

Practice Activities for Transcribing Diabetes-Related Terms:

1. Transcribe the following diabetes-related terms accurately: insulin, hyperglycemia, hypoglycemia, diabetic ketoacidosis, diabetic retinopathy.

2. Given a medical report describing a patient with Type 2 diabetes, transcribe the treatment plan and any complications mentioned.

3. Practice transcribing diabetes-related terms in various scenarios, such as outpatient clinic notes, hospital discharge summaries, or endocrinology consultations.

16. DRUG TERMINOLOGY IN TRANSCRIPTION

When transcribing drug-related information in medical reports, it is crucial to have a solid understanding of drug names, dosages, frequencies, and routes of administration. Here are the key points for transcribing drug terminology accurately:

Understanding Drug Terminology:

1. Drug Names: Familiarize yourself with the generic and brand names of commonly prescribed medications.

2. Dosages: Understand the different units of measurement used for dosages, such as milligrams (mg), micrograms (mcg), or international units (IU).

3. Frequencies: Learn the abbreviations and terms used to indicate the frequency of medication administration, such as "daily," "twice daily," "as needed," or specific time intervals.

4. Routes of Administration: Be aware of the various routes through which medications can be administered, such as oral (PO), intravenous (IV), intramuscular (IM), or topical.

Guidelines for Transcribing Drug-Related Information:

1. Accurate Representation: Ensure that you transcribe the correct drug name, dosage, frequency, and route of administration based on the information provided in the medical report.

2. Clarity and Consistency: Use clear and consistent terminology and abbreviations when documenting drug-related information to avoid confusion and ensure accurate interpretation.

3. Contextual Understanding: Consider the patient's medical condition, other medications they are taking, and any specific instructions provided by the healthcare provider when transcribing drug-related information.

Examples of Drug Terminology:

1. Drug Name: Transcribe "Ibuprofen" for a generic name or "Advil" for a brand name.

2. Dosage: Transcribe "10 mg" for a dosage of 10 milligrams.

3. Frequency: Transcribe "Twice daily" or "BID" for a medication to be taken two times a day.

4. Route of Administration: Transcribe "PO" for oral administration or "IV" for intravenous administration.

Practice Activities for Transcribing Drug Terminology:

1. Transcribe a prescription for a common medication, including the drug name, dosage, frequency, and route of administration.

2. Given a medical report describing a patient's medication regimen, accurately transcribe the names, dosages, frequencies, and routes of administration of the prescribed drugs.

3. Practice transcribing drug-related information in different scenarios, such as hospital medication orders, outpatient medication lists, or medication reconciliation forms.

17. TRANSCRIBING EPONYMS

When transcribing medical reports, you may encounter eponyms, which are medical terms derived from people's names. Here are the key points to consider when transcribing eponyms accurately:

Guidelines for Transcribing Eponyms:

1. Familiarize Yourself: Learn the commonly used eponyms in the medical field, such as Parkinson's disease, Alzheimer's disease, or Crohn's disease.

2. Proper Capitalization: Eponyms derived from people's names are usually capitalized, such as Hodgkin's lymphoma or Addison's disease.

3. Avoid Possessive Forms: Do not include an apostrophe or "s" after the name when transcribing eponyms, as it is not required. For example, it is Hodgkin's lymphoma, not Hodgkin's's lymphoma.

4. Consistency: Maintain consistency in the capitalization and formatting of eponyms throughout the medical report.

Understanding the Proper Capitalization and Formatting of Eponyms:

1. Capitalize the Eponym: Capitalize the eponym as it is derived from a person's name. For example, transcribe "Parkinson's disease," not "parkinson's disease."

2. Maintain Consistency: Ensure that the eponym is capitalized consistently each time it appears in the medical report.

3. Consider Sentence Structure: Apply proper capitalization rules for eponyms within sentences, such as capitalizing the eponym when it begins a sentence.

Practice Exercises for Transcribing Eponyms Accurately:

1. Given a list of eponyms, transcribe them accurately, ensuring proper capitalization and formatting.

2. Review medical reports containing eponyms and practice transcribing them accurately, following the guidelines for capitalization and formatting.

3. Create a list of sentences or paragraphs containing eponyms, and transcribe them, focusing on consistent capitalization and formatting.

When transcribing medical reports, you may encounter genetic terminology related to genes, mutations, and genetic disorders. Here are the key points to consider when transcribing genetic terminology accurately:

Transcribing Genetic Terms:

1. Familiarize Yourself: Learn the commonly used genetic terms in medical transcription, such as DNA, RNA, gene mutations, genetic disorders, etc.

2. Accurate Spelling: Ensure the correct spelling of genetic terms as they are crucial for conveying accurate information.

3. Proper Formatting: Follow the formatting conventions for genetic terms, such as capitalization and italicization, as specified by the transcription guidelines or style manual.

Guidelines for Documenting Genetic Information:

1. Use Standard Nomenclature: Utilize the accepted standard nomenclature for genes, genetic variants, and genetic disorders, such as HGVS (Human Genome Variation Society) nomenclature.

2. Consistency: Maintain consistency in the use of abbreviations and acronyms for genetic terms throughout the report.

3. Understand Context: Understand the context in which the genetic information is being documented to accurately transcribe the relevant details.

Exercises for Transcribing Genetic Terminology Correctly:

1. Practice Transcription: Transcribe genetic reports, including the names of genes, genetic variants, and genetic disorders, paying close attention to accurate spelling and formatting.

2. Review Genetic Reports: Analyze real-world genetic reports and identify the genetic terms used. Practice transcribing those terms accurately based on the established guidelines.

3. Create Transcription Scenarios: Create scenarios involving genetic information and transcribe them, focusing on using the appropriate genetic terminology in the given context.

19. TRANSCRIBING GENUS AND SPECIES NAMES

When transcribing genus and species names in medical reports, it is important to ensure accuracy and follow specific guidelines. Here are the key points to consider:

Proper Transcription of Genus and Species Names:

1. Familiarize Yourself: Learn the correct spelling and pronunciation of commonly encountered genus and species names in medical reports.

2. Understand Binomial Nomenclature: Genus and species names follow the binomial nomenclature system, where the genus name is capitalized and the species name is lowercase, both in italics (or underlined).

3. Use Correct Formatting: Follow the appropriate formatting conventions for genus and species names as specified by the transcription guidelines or style manual.

Guidelines for Formatting and Capitalizing Genus and Species Names:

1. Capitalization: Capitalize the first letter of the genus name, and ensure that the species name is entirely lowercase.

2. Italics or Underlining: Italicize or underline both the genus and species names to distinguish them from the surrounding text.

3. Abbreviations: Use standard abbreviations for genus and species names when instructed by the guidelines or style manual.

Practice Activities for Accurately Transcribing Genus and Species Names:

1. Review Medical Reports: Analyze real-world medical reports that include genus and species names. Practice transcribing those names accurately while adhering to the proper formatting and capitalization guidelines.

2. Create Transcription Scenarios: Create scenarios involving genus and species names and transcribe them, focusing on applying the correct formatting and capitalization rules.

3. Self-Assessment: Test your skills by comparing your transcriptions of genus and species names with authoritative sources or reference materials to ensure accuracy.

20. TRANSCRIBING GEOGRAPHIC NAMES

When transcribing geographic names in medical reports, it is important to follow specific guidelines to ensure accuracy and consistency. Here are the key points to consider:

Guidelines for Transcribing Geographic Names:

1. Familiarize Yourself: Be familiar with the correct spelling and capitalization of commonly encountered geographic names, including cities, states, countries, and regions.

2. Use Official Sources: Consult reliable sources, such as official geographical databases, maps, or reputable references, to verify the correct spelling and capitalization of specific geographic names.

3. Follow Capitalization Rules: Capitalize the proper nouns in geographic names, such as the names of cities, states, countries, and specific regions.

4. Spelling Accuracy: Ensure that the geographic names are spelled accurately, paying attention to any diacritical marks or special characters.

5. Use Standard Conventions: Follow standard conventions for abbreviating or shortening geographic names, as specified by the transcription guidelines or style manual.

Practice Activities for Transcribing Geographic Names:

1. Review Medical Reports: Analyze medical reports that include geographic names and practice transcribing them accurately, focusing on proper capitalization and spelling.

2. Create Transcription Scenarios: Create scenarios involving various geographic names and transcribe them, paying attention to capitalization and spelling rules.

3. Self-Assessment: Compare your transcriptions of geographic names with reliable sources or reference materials to assess their accuracy.

21. TRANSCRIBING GLOBULINS

When transcribing globulins in medical reports, it is essential to have a good understanding of the different types of globulins and follow specific guidelines for accurate transcription. Here's what you need to know:

Understanding the Different Types of Globulins:

1. Alpha-Globulins: These are a group of proteins that include alpha-1 globulins and alpha-2 globulins. They play various roles in the body, including transport and immune function.

2. Beta-Globulins: Beta-globulins are a group of proteins involved in transport and immune response. They include beta-1 globulins and beta-2 globulins.

3. Gamma-Globulins: Gamma-globulins are a class of proteins that consist of antibodies (immunoglobulins) and play a crucial role in the immune system.

Guidelines for Transcribing Globulin Values:

1. Use Proper Notation: When transcribing globulin values, use the appropriate units of measurement, such as grams per deciliter (g/dL) or grams per liter (g/L).

2. Accuracy and Precision: Ensure that the values are transcribed accurately and with the correct number of decimal places, according to the specific laboratory or reference ranges.

3. Context and Format: Transcribe the globulin values in the context of the complete blood test results and follow the formatting guidelines specified by the transcription guidelines or style manual.

Practice Exercises for Transcribing Globulins:

1. Review Blood Test Results: Analyze blood test reports that include globulin values and practice transcribing them accurately, focusing on proper notation, units of measurement, and precision.

2. Create Transcription Scenarios: Create scenarios involving different globulin values and transcribe them, adhering to the guidelines for notation and format.

3. Self-Assessment: Compare your transcriptions of globulin values with the original reports or reference materials to assess their accuracy.

22. TRANSCRIBING LABORATORY DATA AND VALUES

When transcribing laboratory data and values in medical reports, it is crucial to adhere to specific guidelines to ensure accuracy and consistency. Here are the key points to consider:

Proper Transcription of Laboratory Data and Values:

1. Understand Test Results: Familiarize yourself with different laboratory tests and their corresponding values, including reference ranges and units of measurement.

2. Use Standard Notation: Transcribe laboratory data using the standard notation or symbols commonly used for each specific test. This may include abbreviations, numerical values, or specific units of measurement.

3. Document Reference Ranges: Include the appropriate reference ranges for each laboratory test, indicating what is considered normal or abnormal.

4. Maintain Consistency: Ensure consistency in formatting laboratory data throughout the medical report, such as using the same units of measurement and notation style.

Guidelines for Formatting and Documenting Laboratory Data:

1. Proper Placement: Place laboratory data and values in the appropriate sections of the medical report, such as under the corresponding test or in a separate laboratory results section.

2. Clear Labeling: Clearly label each laboratory value with the corresponding test name and the units of measurement.

3. Use Standard Units: Transcribe laboratory values using the standard units of measurement, such as milligrams per deciliter (mg/dL), international units per liter (IU/L), or parts per million (ppm).

4. Avoid Ambiguity: Be mindful of potential ambiguities when transcribing laboratory data, such as different abbreviations or symbols that may have similar meanings but different units of measurement.

5. Follow Style Guidelines: Adhere to any specific style guidelines or requirements provided by the transcription guidelines or the facility where you are working.

Exercises for Accurately Transcribing Laboratory Data and Values:

1. Practice Transcribing Results: Review sample laboratory reports and practice transcribing the data and values accurately, including the appropriate units of measurement and reference ranges.

2. Test Interpretation Exercises: Engage in exercises where you interpret laboratory results and transcribe the relevant data, paying attention to the proper formatting and documentation.

3. Role-Play Scenarios: Simulate scenarios where you are transcribing laboratory data based on simulated patient cases, reinforcing your skills in accurately transcribing and documenting the results.

23. TRANSCRIBING NAMES IN MEDICAL REPORTS

When transcribing names in medical reports, it is essential to follow specific guidelines to ensure accuracy and maintain proper formatting. Here are the key points to consider:

Guidelines for Transcribing Names in Medical Reports:

1. Patient Names: Transcribe patient names as they are provided, paying close attention to spelling and any specific formatting requested by the facility or transcription guidelines.

2. Healthcare Professionals' Names: Transcribe healthcare professionals' names, including physicians, nurses, and specialists, using their full names or the preferred form they provide.

3. Proper Capitalization: Follow proper capitalization rules for names, including capitalizing the first letter of each name and any surnames or titles that are part of the name.

4. Maintain Consistency: Use the same spelling and formatting for names throughout the medical report, ensuring consistency.

5. Note Special Characters: Take note of any special characters or diacritical marks in names and include them accurately in the transcription.

6. Privacy and Confidentiality: Ensure that patient privacy and confidentiality are maintained when transcribing names by following the facility's policies and guidelines.

Proper Formatting and Capitalization of Names:

1. Patient Names: Format patient names in the standard order of given name(s) followed by the surname. Capitalize the first letter of each name.

2. Healthcare Professionals' Names: Format healthcare professionals' names with the appropriate title and surname, following the preferred form they provide or the facility's guidelines.

Practice Activities for Transcribing Names Accurately:

1. Name Transcription Exercises: Engage in exercises where you practice transcribing different names accurately, focusing on correct spelling and proper formatting.

2. Case Studies: Work on case studies that involve transcribing patient names and healthcare professionals' names, ensuring accurate transcription while maintaining patient privacy.

3. Review Real-World Examples: Review medical reports and documents that include names, and practice transcribing those names accurately, paying attention to specific formatting and capitalization rules.

24. TRANSCRIBING NUMBERS IN MEDICAL REPORTS

When transcribing numbers in medical reports, it is important to follow specific rules and guidelines to ensure accuracy and consistency. Here are the key points to consider:

Rules for Transcribing Numbers:

1. Whole Numbers: Transcribe whole numbers as they appear in the original document, without changing the value or format.

2. Fractions: Transcribe fractions using the appropriate notation, such as writing them in numerical form (e.g., 1/2) or in word form (e.g., one-half).

3. Percentages: Transcribe percentages using the percent symbol (%), following the numeric value. For example, 50% represents fifty percent.

4. Decimal Numbers: Transcribe decimal numbers by accurately placing the decimal point and retaining the specified precision. Use leading zeros before the decimal point if required (e.g., 0.5) and avoid trailing zeros after the decimal point if not necessary (e.g., 2.0).

Proper Formatting and Placement of Numbers:

1. Consistent Style: Maintain consistency in the formatting of numbers throughout the medical report. Follow any specific style guidelines provided by the transcription guidelines or the facility where you are working.

2. Appropriate Units: Ensure that numbers are accompanied by the correct units of measurement, if applicable, to provide accurate context. For example, transcribing a blood pressure reading as "120/80 mmHg" includes both the systolic and diastolic values as well as the unit of measurement (millimeters of mercury).

3. Placement within Text: Insert numbers in the appropriate positions within the text, ensuring they are placed correctly and make sense in the context of the sentence or paragraph.

Examples and Exercises for Transcribing Numbers Accurately:

1. Practice Transcribing Medical Measurements: Review sample medical reports containing measurements such as blood pressure, body temperature, heart rate, or laboratory values. Practice transcribing these numbers accurately, including the appropriate units of measurement.

2. Fill-in-the-Blanks Exercises: Engage in exercises where you are provided with sentences or paragraphs with missing numbers. Fill in the correct numbers based on the given context and units of measurement.

3. Role-Play Scenarios: Simulate scenarios where you transcribe numbers based on simulated patient cases, reinforcing your skills in accurately transcribing and formatting numerical values in medical reports.

25. OBSTETRICS TERMINOLOGY IN TRANSCRIPTION

Transcribing obstetrics terminology requires a thorough understanding of the specialized vocabulary related to pregnancy, childbirth, and postpartum care. Here are the key points to consider when transcribing obstetrics-related information:

Transcribing Terminology:

1. Pregnancy Terminology: Familiarize yourself with terms related to different stages of pregnancy, such as trimesters, gestational age, and fetal development.

2. Labor and Delivery Terminology: Learn terms associated with the stages of labor, including contractions, dilation, effacement, and station.

3. Postpartum Terminology: Understand terminology related to the immediate period after childbirth, such as lochia, episiotomy, breastfeeding, and postpartum care.

Guidelines for Accurate Documentation:

1. Spelling and Capitalization: Ensure proper spelling and capitalization of obstetrics-related terms, following the specific guidelines and style manuals used in medical transcription.

2. Contextual Understanding: Transcribe obstetrics terminology in the appropriate context, considering the patient's medical history, current condition, and relevant diagnostic findings.

3. Accuracy and Consistency: Maintain accuracy and consistency in documenting obstetrics-related information, ensuring that it aligns with the physician's dictation and the patient's medical record.

Practice Activities for Transcribing Obstetrics Terminology:

1. Transcription Exercises: Engage in transcription exercises that focus on obstetrics-related dictations, including prenatal visits, labor progress notes, delivery summaries, and postpartum assessments. Practice accurately transcribing the terminology used in these types of reports.

2. Case Studies: Analyze case studies involving obstetrics-related scenarios. Transcribe the relevant medical terminology used in each case, including diagnoses, procedures, and treatments.

3. Dictation Practice: Practice listening to obstetrics-related dictations and transcribing them accurately. Focus on understanding the context and properly documenting the relevant obstetrics terminology used in the dictation.

26. TRANSCRIBING PERCENTAGES

Transcribing percentages in medical reports requires attention to detail and adherence to specific guidelines. Here are the key considerations when transcribing percentages:

Guidelines for Transcribing Percentages:

1. Formatting: Percentages are typically represented by the percent symbol (%). Ensure that the percent symbol is placed immediately after the numeric value, without any spaces.

2. Numeric Representation: Percentages can be expressed as whole numbers or decimals. Follow the given format in the transcription and accurately transcribe the numeric representation.

3. Contextual Understanding: Consider the context in which the percentage is mentioned and ensure that it aligns with the information provided in the medical report.

Understanding the Proper Placement of the Percent Symbol:

1. Percent Symbol (%): The percent symbol (%) is always placed immediately after the numeric value without any spaces. For example, 25%.

2. Numerical Representation: The numerical value can be a whole number or a decimal, depending on the context. For example, 50% or 0.5%.

Practice Exercises for Accurately Transcribing Percentages:

1. Transcription Exercises: Engage in transcription exercises that involve percentages, such as documenting laboratory test results, medication dosages, or statistical data that includes percentages. Practice transcribing the percentages accurately and in the correct format.

2. Dictation Practice: Listen to dictations that mention percentages and practice transcribing them. Pay attention to the placement of the percent symbol and accurately represent the numeric value.

27. TRANSCRIBING PLURALS IN MEDICAL TERMS

When transcribing medical terms, it's essential to understand the rules for forming plurals and apply them accurately. Here are the key considerations for transcribing plurals in medical terms:

Rules for Forming Plurals of Medical Terms:

1. Regular Plurals: Most medical terms follow the regular pluralization patterns used in English. This involves adding an "s" to the end of the singular form. For example, "cells" is the plural form of "cell."

2. Pluralization of "s" Sounds: If a medical term ends with an "s" sound, such as "cystitis" (inflammation of the bladder), the plural form is created by adding "es" instead of just "s." The plural of "cystitis" is "cystitises."

3. Irregular Plurals: Some medical terms have irregular plural forms that do not follow the regular rules. For example, "bacterium" becomes "bacteria" in the plural form.

Understanding Different Pluralization Patterns in Medical Terminology:

1. Greek and Latin Roots: Many medical terms are derived from Greek and Latin roots. Understanding the pluralization patterns associated with these roots can help in transcribing the correct plural form. For example, the plural of "diagnosis" (singular) is "diagnoses" (plural).

2. Contextual Awareness: Consider the context in which the medical term is used and determine the appropriate pluralization based on the specific word and its root.

Examples and Exercises for Transcribing Plurals Correctly:

1. Transcription Exercises: Engage in transcription exercises that involve medical terms and practice transcribing their plural forms. This will help reinforce your understanding of pluralization patterns and improve your accuracy in transcribing plurals.

2. Word Recognition Practice: Familiarize yourself with common medical terms and their corresponding plural forms. Practice identifying and pronouncing the plural forms to strengthen your knowledge of plurals in medical terminology.

When transcribing medical reports, it is important to accurately indicate possession in medical terms and phrases. Here are some guidelines to follow when transcribing possession:

Guidelines for Indicating Possession in Medical Terms and Phrases:

1. Singular Possessive: To indicate possession for singular nouns, use an apostrophe followed by the letter "s." For example, "the patient's condition" indicates that the condition belongs to the patient.

2. Plural Possessive: To indicate possession for plural nouns, add an apostrophe after the "s" if the noun is already plural. For example, "the doctors' opinions" shows that the opinions belong to multiple doctors.

3. Plural Nouns Ending in "s": If the plural noun already ends in "s," add an apostrophe after the "s" without an additional "s." For example, "the patients' records" denotes that the records belong to multiple patients.

4. Possessive Pronouns: Possessive pronouns, such as "his," "her," "its," and "their," already indicate possession and do not require an apostrophe.

Proper Use of Apostrophes to Indicate Possession:

1. Place the apostrophe before the "s" to indicate possession for singular nouns and plural nouns that do not end in "s."

2. Place the apostrophe after the "s" for plural nouns that end in "s."

Practice Activities for Transcribing Possession Accurately:

1. Sentence Completion Exercises: Complete sentences by correctly indicating possession using apostrophes. For example, "The nurse's assessment" or "The surgeons' expertise."

2. Transcription Practice: Engage in transcription exercises that involve possessive medical terms and phrases. Practice transcribing them accurately, ensuring the correct placement of apostrophes.

When transcribing medical reports, you may encounter ratios that represent relationships between different values or measurements. Here are some guidelines for transcribing ratios accurately:

Rules for Transcribing Ratios in Medical Terms and Measurements:

1. Numerical Format: Write the ratio using numbers, with a colon (:) between the values. For example, a ratio of 2:1 represents a relationship where the first value is twice as much as the second value.

2. Proper Spacing: Place a space before and after the colon in the ratio. For example, 3:2, not 3:2.

3. No Plural Form: Ratios are not pluralized, so there is no need to add an "s" after the values.

Understanding the Formatting and Interpretation of Ratios:

1. Interpreting Ratios: Ratios can represent various types of relationships, such as proportions, concentrations, or risk factors. Understanding the context and purpose of the ratio will help in its interpretation.

2. Simplifying Ratios: In some cases, ratios can be simplified by dividing both values by their greatest common divisor. This simplification can make the ratio easier to read and understand.

Exercises for Transcribing Ratios Accurately:

1. Ratio Calculation: Given a set of values, calculate the ratio and write it in the proper format. For example, given 8 boys and 12 girls, the ratio of boys to girls is 8:12.

2. Transcription Practice: Engage in transcription exercises that involve ratios in medical terms and measurements. Practice transcribing them accurately, ensuring the correct numerical format and spacing.

30. TRANSCRIBING REFLEXES IN NEUROLOGICAL EXAMINATIONS

When transcribing neurological examinations, documenting reflex responses accurately is essential. Here are some guidelines for transcribing reflexes in neurological assessments:

Guidelines for Transcribing Reflexes in Neurological Assessments:

1. Use Standard Notation: Transcribe reflex responses using standardized notation, typically using abbreviations or symbols. Commonly used reflex abbreviations include:

- Biceps reflex: B

- Triceps reflex: T

- Patellar reflex: K

- Achilles reflex: A

2. Note the Response Level: Indicate the level of reflex response, such as "normal," "diminished," "hyperactive," or "absent." You can use abbreviations like "N," "D," "H," or "A" to represent these responses.

3. Specify Side and Body Part: Specify the side (right or left) and the body part where the reflex was tested. For example, "R Biceps reflex" indicates the biceps reflex on the right side.

4. Document the Grade or Scale: Some reflex assessments use a grading scale (e.g., 0 to 4) to indicate the strength or intensity of the reflex response. Transcribe the grade or scale used in the assessment.

Proper Notation and Interpretation of Reflex Responses:

1. Accurate Recording: Ensure accurate transcription of the reflex response, noting any abnormalities or significant findings. Use clear and concise language to describe the reflex response.

2. Interpretation: Understanding the significance of different reflex responses is crucial. Familiarize yourself with the expected responses for each reflex and how deviations from the norm may indicate neurological conditions or abnormalities.

Examples and Practice Activities for Transcribing Reflexes Correctly:

1. Transcription Examples: Provide examples of neurological examination findings that include reflex responses. Ask students to transcribe the reflex responses accurately, following the guidelines discussed.

2. Reflex Response Practice: Conduct practice activities where students are given reflex testing scenarios, and they must transcribe the reflex responses based on the standardized notation and guidelines provided.

31. TRANSCRIBING SERIES IN MEDICAL REPORTS

When transcribing series in medical reports, it is important to follow proper formatting and transcription guidelines to ensure clarity and accuracy. Here are some guidelines for transcribing series in medical reports:

Proper Formatting and Transcription of Series:

1. Use Bulleted or Numbered Lists: When presenting a series of items, use either bulleted or numbered lists to clearly separate each item. Bulleted lists are typically used when the order of the items is not significant, while numbered lists are used when the order is important.

2. Consistent Formatting: Maintain consistent formatting throughout the list, including indentation, spacing, and punctuation. Use a consistent style for bullet points (e.g., dashes, circles) or numbering (e.g., Arabic numerals, Roman numerals).

3. Clear Separation of Items: Ensure that each item in the series is clearly separated from the others. Use proper spacing and indentation to distinguish between items.

Guidelines for Using Appropriate Punctuation and Numbering in Series:

1. Use Commas: When listing items in a series within a sentence, use commas to separate the items. For example, "The patient presented with symptoms such as fever, cough, and fatigue."

2. Use Semicolons: If the items in the series themselves contain commas, use semicolons to separate the items. For example, "The laboratory tests included complete blood count, white blood cell differential; comprehensive metabolic panel; and urinalysis."

3. Use Colons: In some cases, a colon may be used to introduce a series. For example, "The following diagnostic tests were ordered: chest X-ray, electrocardiogram, and echocardiogram."

Practice Exercises for Transcribing Series Accurately:

1. Transcription Examples: Provide examples of medical reports that include series of items. Ask students to transcribe the series accurately, following the proper formatting and punctuation guidelines.

2. List Formation Practice: Conduct exercises where students are given a list of items, and they must transcribe the list using the appropriate formatting, punctuation, and numbering.

32. TRANSCRIBING SUTURE SIZES IN SURGICAL REPORTS

When transcribing suture sizes in surgical reports, it is essential to understand the different suture size measurements and their representation in medical reports. Here are some guidelines for accurately documenting suture sizes:

Understanding Suture Sizes:

1. Suture Size Measurement: Suture sizes are typically measured using a numerical scale. The higher the number, the smaller the suture size. For example, a size 2-0 suture is larger than a size 4-0 suture.

2. Number and Dash: Suture sizes are represented with a number followed by a dash and another number. The first number indicates the size, and the second number after the dash denotes the number of zeroes (0) associated with the size. For example, 2-0 represents a larger suture size compared to 4-0.

Guidelines for Documenting Suture Sizes:

1. Use Hyphens: When documenting suture sizes in medical reports, use hyphens to separate the two numbers. For example, "The incision was closed using a 4-0 suture."

2. Omit the Leading Zero: In some cases, the leading zero of the second number (number of zeroes) is omitted. For example, "The wound was sutured with a 3-0 suture."

3. Be Consistent: Maintain consistency in the representation of suture sizes throughout the medical report. Use the same format (number-dash-number or number-0) for all suture size mentions.

Exercises for Transcribing Suture Sizes Correctly:

1. Transcription Practice: Provide sample surgical reports that include mentions of suture sizes. Ask students to transcribe the suture sizes accurately using the proper format and representation.

2. Matching Exercise: Create a matching exercise where students are given a list of suture sizes and they have to match them with their corresponding numerical representation (e.g., 2-0, 4-0, 5-0).

33. TRANSCRIBING TELEPHONE NUMBERS IN MEDICAL REPORTS

When transcribing telephone numbers in medical reports, it is important to follow certain guidelines to ensure accuracy and consistency. Here are some guidelines for transcribing telephone numbers:

Guidelines for Transcribing Telephone Numbers:

1. Use Digits Only: Transcribe telephone numbers using digits only, without any special characters or punctuation marks.

2. Include Area Code: Include the area code, which is the three-digit code that identifies the specific geographic region or telephone service area.

3. Use Hyphens: Separate the telephone number into segments using hyphens for readability. Typically, telephone numbers are divided into three segments: area code, central office code, and line number.

4. Proper Formatting: Follow the standard formatting for telephone numbers based on the region or country. For example, in the United States, the format is usually (XXX) XXX-XXXX, where X represents a digit.

5. Leading Zeros: Do not include any leading zeros in the telephone number. Only include the actual digits.

Examples of Properly Transcribed Telephone Numbers:

1. (555) 123-4567

2. 123-456-7890

3. 9876543210

Practice Activities for Transcribing Telephone Numbers Accurately:

1. Transcription Exercise: Provide a list of contact information with telephone numbers and ask students to transcribe them accurately using the proper format and notation.

2. Formatting Practice: Provide incomplete telephone numbers and ask students to format them correctly by adding the missing digits and hyphens.

34. TRANSCRIBING TEMPERATURE AND TEMPERATURE SCALES

When transcribing temperature measurements in medical reports, it is essential to follow specific guidelines to ensure accurate and consistent representation. Here are some guidelines for transcribing temperatures:

Guidelines for Transcribing Temperature Measurements:

1. Use the Appropriate Scale: Determine the scale used for the temperature measurement, such as Celsius (°C) or Fahrenheit (°F), and transcribe the value accordingly.

2. Include the Degree Symbol: Use the degree symbol (°) to indicate temperature values. Place the degree symbol immediately after the numerical value without any spaces.

3. Use Numeric Values: Transcribe temperature values using numeric digits without any textual representation. For example, use "37.5°C" instead of "thirty-seven-point-five degrees Celsius."

4. Consistent Scale Conversion: If there is a need to convert temperatures between different scales, follow the appropriate conversion formula and ensure consistency in the transcribed values.

5. Decimal Point Placement: Be precise in transcribing decimal values for temperatures. Place the decimal point in the correct position to maintain accuracy.

Examples of Properly Transcribed Temperature Measurements:

1. 37.5°C

2. 98.6°F

3. -10°C (for below-zero temperatures)

Practice Exercises for Accurately Transcribing Temperature Values:

1. Transcription Exercise: Provide a list of temperature measurements in various scales and ask students to transcribe them accurately using the proper format and scale representation.

2. Conversion Practice: Provide temperature values in one scale and ask students to convert them to the other scale and transcribe the converted values accurately.

35. TRANSCRIBING TIME IN MEDICAL REPORTS

When transcribing time references in medical reports, it is important to follow specific rules to ensure consistency and accuracy. Here are some guidelines for transcribing time:

Rules for Transcribing Time References:

1. Use the 24-Hour Clock: In medical transcription, it is common to use the 24-hour clock format for indicating time. This format eliminates confusion between AM and PM designations.

2. Include Leading Zeroes: When transcribing time, include leading zeroes for single-digit hours and minutes. For example, 09:30 instead of 9:30.

3. Use a Colon (:) as the Separator: Use a colon (:) to separate hours and minutes. For example, 14:45.

4. Include Seconds, if Applicable: If the time reference includes seconds, transcribe them as well. For example, 10:15:30.

5. Use Numeric Digits: Transcribe time using numeric digits. Do not use textual representations or spell out the numbers.

Examples of Properly Transcribed Time References:

1. 09:00 (9:00 AM)

2. 14:30 (2:30 PM)

3. 23:45 (11:45 PM)

4. 08:15:30 (8 hours, 15 minutes, 30 seconds)

Exercises for Transcribing Time Accurately:

1. Transcription Exercise: Provide a list of time references in different formats and ask students to transcribe them accurately using the proper notation.

2. Time Calculation Practice: Provide time-related scenarios, such as calculating durations or adding/subtracting time intervals, and ask students to transcribe the results accurately.

36. TRANSCRIBING ACCORDING TO USPS GUIDELINES

When transcribing addresses in medical reports, it is important to follow the guidelines provided by the United States Postal Service (USPS) to ensure accurate and consistent formatting. Here are some key points to consider when transcribing addresses according to USPS guidelines:

Understanding USPS Guidelines for Addressing:

1. Correct Address Format: Use the correct format for the address, including the recipient's name, street address, city, state, and ZIP code.

2. Proper Spacing and Punctuation: Use proper spacing between address elements and include punctuation marks where necessary (e.g., commas, periods).

3. Capitalization: Follow the USPS guidelines for capitalization of address elements. Typically, all capital letters are used for the city name, and proper capitalization is used for other address elements.

4. Abbreviations: Use USPS-approved abbreviations for street types (e.g., St. for Street, Ave. for Avenue) and directional indicators (e.g., N for North, SW for Southwest).

5. ZIP Code: Include the correct ZIP code for the address. Verify the ZIP code to ensure accuracy.

Practice Activities for Transcribing Addresses:

1. Address Formatting Exercise: Provide a list of addresses in various formats and ask students to transcribe them correctly following USPS guidelines.

2. Abbreviation Usage Exercise: Give students a list of full street names and ask them to use USPS-approved abbreviations to transcribe the addresses.

37. TRANSCRIBING VIRGULE (SLASH) IN MEDICAL TERMS

When transcribing medical terms and abbreviations, the use of the virgule or slash symbol (/) may be required in certain cases. Here are some guidelines to consider when using the virgule in medical terms:

Guidelines for Using the Virgule in Medical Terms:

1. Separating Terms: The virgule can be used to separate two terms that are closely related or used interchangeably. For example, "hypertension/high blood pressure" or "acute/chronic pain."

2. Indicating Options: The virgule can indicate options or alternatives within a medical term. For example, "cardiovascular/cardiorespiratory" or "nasogastric/enteral tube."

3. Expressing Ranges: The virgule can be used to express a range of values or measurements. For example, "0.5/1.0 mg" or "20/40 vision."

Proper Placement and Interpretation of the Virgule:

1. Proper Spacing: Ensure there is proper spacing before and after the virgule. Avoid using spaces immediately before or after the symbol.

2. Contextual Understanding: Consider the context of the medical term and the intended meaning when interpreting the virgule. Understand whether it signifies a separation, options, or a range.

Examples and Exercises for Transcribing Virgule Accurately:

1. Matching Exercise: Provide a list of medical terms with virgules and ask students to match them with their corresponding meanings or options.

2. Transcription Exercise: Present medical terms with missing virgules, and students are required to transcribe them accurately, including the appropriate placement of the virgule.

In this appendix, we will provide you with a selection of practice transcription files. Due to the text-based nature of this book, we cannot provide audio files here, but you can find medical dictation practice files on various online platforms such as MTPractice (https://www.mtpractice.com/), StenoSpeed (http://stenospeed.com), and The Practice Zone (http://www.practicezone.com).

Below is an example of a short transcription:

A 59-year-old female presents with complaints of chest pain and shortness of breath. The patient has a past medical history significant for hypertension, diabetes mellitus, and hyperlipidemia. Her medications include lisinopril, metformin, and atorvastatin. Physical examination was unremarkable. An EKG showed no acute changes. Will schedule for stress test.

Here is an exhaustive list of the various types of medical reports commonly transcribed in the healthcare field:

1. History and Physical Examination Reports (H&P): These are detailed reports documenting a patient's medical history and the findings from a physical examination.

2. Consultation Reports: These reports document a specialist's opinion and advice about a patient's condition.

3. Operative Reports: These are detailed narratives of surgical procedures performed, including pre- and post-operative diagnoses, specific details of the procedure and the patient's condition after the surgery.

4. Discharge Summary: This is a comprehensive report providing an overview of a patient's hospitalization, including the reason for admission, major findings, procedures performed, treatment provided, and the patient's condition at discharge.

5. Progress Notes: These are regular updates documenting the course of treatment during a patient's stay in a hospital or long-term care facility.

6. Radiology Reports: These reports describe the findings and interpretations of imaging studies, such as X-rays, MRI scans, and ultrasounds.

7. Pathology Reports: These detail the findings of examinations performed on tissues and cells, including biopsy and surgical specimen analyses.

8. Emergency Room Reports: These document the care a patient received in the emergency department, including the reason for the visit, observations, treatment given, and the outcome.

9. Autopsy Reports: These reports detail the findings of a post-mortem examination.

10. SOAP Notes (Subjective, Objective, Assessment, and Plan): These are typically used in outpatient or ambulatory care settings, and detail a patient's visit with a healthcare provider.

11. Lab Reports: These document the results of laboratory tests, such as blood tests, cultures, and other analyses.

12. Death Summaries: These provide a summary of the events leading to a patient's death and can include post-mortem examination findings.

13. Referral Letters: These are written by doctors to refer a patient to a specialist or another doctor.

14. Psychiatric Evaluations: These reports detail a patient's mental health, including any diagnoses and treatment plans.

15. Rehabilitation Notes: These reports detail a patient's progress during rehabilitation from injury or illness.

16. Pre-Anesthesia Evaluations: These document a patient's fitness for anesthesia and surgery.

17. Anesthesia Reports: These detail the type of anesthesia administered, the procedure, and any complications or notable events.

18. Telehealth or Telemedicine Consultations: These are reports based on a remote consultation where the healthcare provider and patient are not physically present with each other. Using technology, physicians can assess, diagnose, intervene, confer, monitor, and provide education remotely.

Let's see more comprehensive examples:

1. History and Physical Examination Reports (H&P)

a. Patient: Mr. Smith

Age/Sex: 57-year-old male

Chief Complaint: Annual physical examination

Past Medical History: Hypertension, type 2 diabetes

Past Surgical History: None

Medications: Metformin, Lisinopril

Social History: Non-smoker, occasional alcohol use

Family History: Father with heart disease, mother with diabetes

Review of Systems: Negative for chest pain, shortness of breath, recent illness

Physical Exam: Vital signs are stable. Head, eyes, ears, nose, throat examination normal. Chest clear. Heart sounds normal. Abdomen soft, non-tender. Extremities without edema.

Assessment: Well-controlled hypertension and type 2 diabetes

Plan: Continue current medications. Encourage diet and exercise. Schedule follow-up in 6 months.

b. Patient: Ms. Johnson

Age/Sex: 34-year-old female

Chief Complaint: Confirmation of pregnancy and initial prenatal care

Past Medical History: None

Past Surgical History: Appendectomy 10 years ago

Medications: Prenatal vitamins

Social History: Non-smoker, no alcohol or drug use

Family History: Mother with gestational diabetes

Review of Systems: Positive for nausea, no vomiting. Negative for headache, vision changes, chest pain, shortness of breath, vaginal bleeding.

Physical Exam: Vital signs are stable. Abdominal exam reveals uterus consistent with approximately 10 weeks gestation. No abnormalities noted on the breast exam.

Assessment: Early pregnancy, approximately 10 weeks

Plan: Continue prenatal vitamins. Schedule ultrasound for dating and nuchal translucency. Discuss prenatal screening options.

2. Consultation Reports

a. Consultation Request: Dr. Johnson has requested a Cardiology consultation for Mr. Davis, a 62-year-old male with a recent history of chest pain.

History: Mr. Davis has been experiencing intermittent chest pain over the past month. It's pressure-like, located in the middle of his chest, and sometimes radiates to his left arm. It usually occurs with exertion and improves with rest.

Past Medical History: Hypertension, hyperlipidemia

Social History: Ex-smoker, quit 5 years ago

Family History: Father had a myocardial infarction at age 55

Physical Exam: Vital signs are stable. Heart sounds are normal with no murmurs. There are no jugular venous distension, peripheral edema, or chest wall tenderness.

Assessment: Stable angina

Plan: Initiate medical therapy with aspirin, statin, and beta-blocker. Order stress test to assess for ischemia.

b. Consultation Request: Dr. Anderson requests a Rheumatology consultation for Ms. Patel, a 27-year-old female with joint pain and morning stiffness.

History: Ms. Patel reports a 6-month history of pain and stiffness in her hands and knees. Symptoms are worse in the morning and improve with activity.

Past Medical History: None

Family History: Mother with rheumatoid arthritis

Physical Exam: There is synovial swelling in the metacarpophalangeal joints and knees. No erythema or warmth.

Assessment: Likely rheumatoid arthritis

Plan: Order rheumatoid factor and anti-CCP antibodies. Initiate NSAIDs for symptom relief. Discuss potential disease-modifying anti-rheumatic drugs (DMARDs) pending test results.

3. Operative Reports

a. Procedure: Left Total Hip Arthroplasty

Surgeon: Dr. William

Preoperative Diagnosis: Left hip osteoarthritis

Postoperative Diagnosis: Same

Procedure in Detail: Patient was given general anesthesia. The left hip was prepped and draped in the usual sterile fashion. A standard posterior approach to the hip was used. The hip was dislocated. The femoral head was removed. Acetabulum was reamed and a cup was press-fitted into place. A liner was placed inside the cup. Femoral canal was prepared. The femoral stem was placed inside the femoral canal. A femoral head was placed on the femoral stem and the hip was reduced. The wound was closed in layers. The patient tolerated the procedure well. There were no intraoperative complications.

b. Procedure: Appendectomy

Surgeon: Dr. Thompson

Preoperative Diagnosis: Acute appendicitis

Postoperative Diagnosis: Same

Procedure in Detail: The patient was given general anesthesia. The abdomen was prepped and draped in the usual sterile fashion. A laparoscopic approach was used with three trocar placements. The inflamed appendix was identified, mobilized, and divided using a surgical stapler. The specimen was retrieved in a bag and removed. The abdomen was inspected for hemostasis and irrigated. The trocars were removed and the incisions were closed. The patient tolerated the procedure well. There were no intraoperative complications.

4. Discharge Summary

a. Patient: Mr. Robinson

   Age: 65

   Admitting Diagnosis: Congestive heart failure

   Procedure: Cardiac catheterization

Hospital Course: The patient was admitted with shortness of breath. His echocardiogram showed decreased ejection fraction. He was treated with intravenous diuretics. His symptoms improved and he underwent a cardiac catheterization which showed non-obstructive coronary artery disease. He was started on medical therapy for heart failure.

   Discharge Medications: Furosemide, Lisinopril, Carvedilol, Aspirin, Atorvastatin

   Follow-Up: Cardiology clinic in one week

b. Patient: Mrs. Jones

   Age: 72

   Admitting Diagnosis: Hip fracture

   Procedure: Total hip arthroplasty

Hospital Course: The patient was admitted after a fall at home resulting in a left hip fracture. She underwent a total hip arthroplasty. Postoperatively, she had physical therapy and her pain was controlled with medications.

   Discharge Medications: Acetaminophen, Ibuprofen, Aspirin

   Follow-Up: Orthopedic clinic in two weeks, physical therapy

5. Progress Notes

a. Patient: Mr. Johnson

Date: 07/01/2023

Chief Complaint: Persistent headache and fever.

Medications: Tylenol 500mg, as needed for fever.

Physical Examination: Alert, oriented, appears uncomfortable. Temperature: 38.6 C, Pulse: 90 bpm, Respiratory rate: 16/min, BP: 130/85 mmHg.

Assessment: Patient is febrile with persistent headache, the cause of which is still unknown. No meningeal signs. Covid-19 test is negative.

Plan: Continue current medications. Perform additional diagnostic tests including complete blood count, CRP, and MRI brain.

b. Patient: Mrs. Martinez

Date: 07/15/2023

Chief Complaint: Difficulty breathing.

Medications: Albuterol inhaler as needed.

Physical Examination: Patient is anxious. Respiratory rate: 26/min, Pulse: 100 bpm, BP: 135/90 mmHg. Lung examination revealed wheezing.

Assessment: Acute exacerbation of asthma likely.

Plan: Increase dosage of Albuterol, administer steroids and provide supplemental oxygen. Monitor vitals closely. Consider hospitalization if there is no improvement.

6. Radiology Reports

a. Radiology Report

Exam: CT scan of the abdomen and pelvis

Referring Physician: Dr. John Murphy

Radiologist: Dr. David Evans

Indications: Recurrent abdominal pain and weight loss. Possible neoplasm.

Findings: There are several hypodense lesions in the liver, suggestive of metastatic disease. The largest lesion measures approximately 3 cm in diameter. The spleen, kidneys, and adrenal glands are unremarkable. No significant lymphadenopathy is present. There is a small amount of free fluid in the pelvis.

Impression: Findings are suggestive of metastatic disease in the liver. Recommend biopsy for further evaluation.

b. Radiology Report

Exam: Chest X-ray

Referring Physician: Dr. Amy Davis

Radiologist: Dr. Peter Clark

Indications: Persistent cough and shortness of breath.

Findings: There is a 2 cm mass in the right upper lobe. No pleural effusion or pneumothorax. Heart size is normal. No lymphadenopathy.

Impression: Mass in the right upper lobe suggestive of possible lung cancer. Recommend CT chest for further evaluation and characterisation of the mass.

7. Pathology Reports

a. Pathology Report

Specimen Type: Left breast biopsy

Clinical History: A 55-year-old female with a palpable mass in the left breast.

Gross Description: Received in formalin is a 1.5 cm portion of breast tissue with an associated mass.

Microscopic Description: Sections show infiltrating ductal carcinoma. The tumor is estrogen and progesterone receptor positive and HER2/neu negative. There is no lymphovascular invasion identified.

Diagnosis: Invasive ductal carcinoma, left breast.

b. Pathology Report

Specimen Type: Colon biopsy

Clinical History: A 66-year-old male with a history of rectal bleeding.

Gross Description: Received in formalin are two fragments of colonic tissue each measuring 0.5 cm in diameter.

Microscopic Description: Sections show fragments of colonic mucosa with a tubular adenoma. The adenoma shows high-grade dysplasia. There is no evidence of invasive carcinoma.

Diagnosis: Tubular adenoma with high-grade dysplasia, colon.

8. Emergency Room Reports

a. Emergency Room Report

Patient: John Doe

Gender: Male

Age: 45

Chief Complaint: Chest Pain

History of Present Illness: Patient reports chest pain onset while mowing the lawn, described as a heavy, squeezing sensation in the chest associated with shortness of breath. No history of similar episodes. Denies associated nausea or vomiting.

Past Medical History: Hypertension

Physical Exam: Patient in mild distress. Vital signs stable. Cardiac exam: Regular rhythm, no murmurs. Lungs clear to auscultation.

Assessment: Chest pain, possible angina.

Plan: Administer nitroglycerin. Order EKG and cardiac enzymes. Admit for observation and further workup.

b. Emergency Room Report

Patient: Jane Smith

Gender: Female

Age: 28

Chief Complaint: Abdominal Pain

History of Present Illness: Patient presents with severe right lower quadrant pain, onset this morning. Pain is sharp, non-radiating, and associated with nausea. No urinary symptoms.

Past Medical History: None

Physical Exam: Patient appears uncomfortable. Abdomen is tender in right lower quadrant with rebound tenderness.

Assessment: Suspected appendicitis.

Plan: Order complete blood count, urinalysis, and abdominal ultrasound. Consult general surgery for possible appendectomy.

9. Autopsy Reports

a. Autopsy Report

Deceased: George Brown

Age: 60

Date of Death: 21 May 2023

Cause of Death: Myocardial Infarction

Gross Description: Body is that of a well-nourished, adult male. There is severe atherosclerosis in the coronary arteries, with complete occlusion of the left anterior descending artery. The heart is enlarged with left ventricular hypertrophy. There are old infarcts present in the myocardium.

Microscopic Description: Examination of the heart tissue shows myocardial necrosis with contraction bands and neutrophilic infiltrates.

Summary: Findings are consistent with a recent myocardial infarction leading to death. The severe atherosclerosis and left ventricular hypertrophy suggest a history of ischemic heart disease.

b. Autopsy Report

Deceased: Mary Thompson

Age: 80

Date of Death: 23 May 2023

Cause of Death: Stroke

Gross Description: Brain is swollen with a large hemorrhagic area in the left hemisphere. Atherosclerotic plaques are noted in the cerebral arteries.

Microscopic Description: Histologic examination of the cerebral tissue shows extensive hemorrhage with necrosis and gliosis.

Summary: The findings are consistent with a hemorrhagic stroke. The presence of atherosclerosis in the cerebral arteries indicates a risk factor for cerebrovascular disease.

10. SOAP Notes (Subjective, Objective, Assessment, and Plan)

a. SOAP Note 1

Subjective: Patient is a 52-year-old male with a history of Type 2 Diabetes, presenting with complaints of increased urination and thirst over the last two weeks. The patient denies nausea, vomiting, or abdominal pain.

Objective: BP 130/85, HR 78, RR 20, BMI 28. Physical examination is unremarkable. Lab results show elevated blood glucose and HbA1c levels.

Assessment: Poorly controlled Type 2 Diabetes.

Plan: Increase Metformin dosage, initiate lifestyle counselling focusing on diet and exercise, schedule a follow-up visit in two weeks.

b. SOAP Note 2

Subjective: Patient is a 36-year-old female complaining of right lower quadrant pain for the past 24 hours. The pain is described as sharp and intermittent. The patient also reports nausea but no vomiting or fever.

Objective: BP 120/75, HR 88, RR 16, Temp 98.6°F. Physical exam reveals tenderness in the right lower quadrant.

Assessment: Suspected acute appendicitis.

Plan: Order abdominal ultrasound to confirm diagnosis, consult with general surgery for possible appendectomy if the ultrasound is positive.

11. Lab Reports

a. Lab Report 1

Patient: John Doe, 45-year-old male.

Test Ordered: Complete Blood Count (CBC).

Date Sampled: 1/15/2023

Results:

  - Hemoglobin: 16 g/dL (Normal range: 13-17 g/dL)

  - Hematocrit: 46% (Normal range: 38-50%)

  - White Blood Cell (WBC) count: 6,000 cells/mm3 (Normal range: 4,500-11,000 cells/mm3)

  - Platelet count: 250,000 cells/mm3 (Normal range: 150,000-450,000 cells/mm3)

Interpretation: All values within normal range.

b. Lab Report 2

Patient: Jane Doe, 50-year-old female.

Test Ordered: Lipid Panel.

Date Sampled: 1/20/2023

Results:

  - Total cholesterol: 250 mg/dL (Desirable: Less than 200 mg/dL)

  - HDL (good cholesterol): 45 mg/dL (Low: Less than 50 mg/dL in women)

  - LDL (bad cholesterol): 160 mg/dL (High: 160-189 mg/dL)

  - Triglycerides: 180 mg/dL (Borderline high: 150-199 mg/dL)

Interpretation: High total cholesterol, high LDL, low HDL, and borderline high triglycerides suggest a high risk of heart disease.

12. Death Summaries

a. Death Summary 1

Patient: Mr. John Smith, 85 years old male.

Admission Date: 04/10/2023

Death Date: 04/15/2023

Principal Diagnosis: Stage IV Lung Cancer with Metastasis

Brief Summary: Mr. Smith, a known case of stage IV lung cancer, was admitted with complaints of difficulty breathing and severe weakness. Despite supportive measures, his condition progressively worsened. He developed severe respiratory distress and was placed on end-of-life care as per family's wishes. Mr. Smith peacefully expired on the afternoon of April 15, 2023.

b. Death Summary 2

Patient: Mrs. Jane Doe, 73 years old female.

Admission Date: 05/05/2023

Death Date: 05/10/2023

Principal Diagnosis: Advanced Alzheimer's Disease

Brief Summary: Mrs. Doe was admitted to the hospital following a fall at home due to severe disorientation. In the hospital, her condition continued to deteriorate with increased confusion and agitation. Her existing health complications, including Alzheimer's disease, made recovery difficult. Despite the best efforts of the medical team, Mrs. Doe passed away peacefully in her sleep on the night of May 10, 2023.

13. Referral Letters

a. Referral Letter 1

Date: 20/05/2023

Referring Physician: Dr. James Peterson, Primary Care Physician

Patient: Mr. Michael Johnson, 52 years old male

Dear Dr. Stewart,

I am writing to refer my patient, Mr. Johnson, who has been complaining of persistent lower back pain for the last six months. He has tried physical therapy and over-the-counter pain relievers, but there has been no significant improvement. Recent imaging suggests possible disc herniation. Given your expertise in orthopedic conditions, I believe that he would benefit from your evaluation and treatment. His medical records are enclosed for your reference.

Thank you for considering this referral.

Sincerely,

Dr. James Peterson

b. Referral Letter 2

Date: 25/05/2023

Referring Physician: Dr. Laura Allen, Endocrinologist

Patient: Mrs. Lisa Davis, 46 years old female

Dear Dr. Simmons,

I am referring my patient, Mrs. Davis, who has recently been diagnosed with Type II Diabetes. Despite dietary changes and oral hypoglycemic agents, her blood glucose levels remain poorly controlled. Given your expertise in managing complex cases of diabetes, I believe your input would be beneficial. I am enclosing her latest lab reports and medical records.

I appreciate your assistance in this matter.

Regards,

Dr. Laura Allen

14. Psychiatric Evaluations

a. Psychiatric Evaluation 1

Patient: Mr. John Smith

Age: 32

Referring Physician: Dr. Lisa Walker

Chief Complaint: Anxiety and occasional panic attacks.

History of Present Illness: Mr. Smith has been suffering from anxiety for the last six months. The patient describes a constant feeling of dread and worry that he finds hard to control. The patient also reports experiencing sudden, intense episodes of fear that peak within a few minutes, which he identifies as panic attacks. These episodes are accompanied by shortness of breath, rapid heartbeat, and a strong desire to escape.

Past Psychiatric History: No previous psychiatric history.

Mental Status Examination: The patient appears his stated age and is cooperative and communicative. He displays signs of anxiety and appears mildly agitated. His thought process seems coherent and goal-oriented.

Diagnosis: Generalized Anxiety Disorder and Panic Disorder.

Plan: Initiate Cognitive Behavioral Therapy (CBT) and consider a short-term medication trial.

b. Psychiatric Evaluation 2

Patient: Ms. Jane Doe

Age: 45

Referring Physician: Dr. Michael Brown

Chief Complaint: Depression and thoughts of suicide.

History of Present Illness: Ms. Doe reports feeling sad and losing interest in activities she once enjoyed for the past year. She also reports significant weight loss, difficulty sleeping, decreased energy, and recurrent thoughts of death and suicide.

Past Psychiatric History: The patient has a history of recurrent major depressive episodes, first diagnosed in her early twenties. Previous treatments included psychotherapy and various antidepressant medications.

Mental Status Examination: The patient appears older than her stated age and looks fatigued. She exhibits signs of profound sadness and despair. Her speech is slow, and her responses are brief.

Diagnosis: Major Depressive Disorder, Recurrent, Severe.

Plan: Immediate safety assessment and hospitalization considering the patient's suicidal ideation. Treatment plan includes modification of current medication regimen and intensive psychotherapy.

15. Rehabilitation Notes

a. Rehabilitation Note 1

Patient: Mr. Thomas Hardy

Age: 67

Referring Physician: Dr. George Watson

Chief Complaint: Limited mobility post hip replacement surgery.

History of Present Illness: Mr. Hardy underwent left hip replacement surgery two weeks ago. He is having difficulty walking and is currently using a walker for support.

Current Medications: Paracetamol for pain as needed.

Physical Therapy Assessment: Patient displays reduced strength and range of motion in the left hip. Difficulty noted in weight bearing and balance activities.

Plan: Develop an individualized rehabilitation program focusing on strength, balance, and gait training. Patient will attend physical therapy sessions three times per week.

b. Rehabilitation Note 2

Patient: Ms. Emma Johnson

Age: 72

Referring Physician: Dr. Anna Martin

Chief Complaint: Difficulties with daily living activities post-stroke.

History of Present Illness: Ms. Johnson suffered a stroke one month ago, which resulted in right-sided weakness and difficulties with speech and swallowing.

Current Medications: Blood pressure medication and a daily aspirin.

Occupational Therapy Assessment: The patient has significant right-sided weakness affecting her ability to perform self-care activities. She also has mild difficulties with speech and swallowing.

Plan: Initiate an individualized rehabilitation program focusing on functional independence in self-care tasks, including dressing, grooming, and feeding. Speech therapy will be initiated to manage speech and swallowing difficulties.

16. Pre-Anesthesia Evaluations

a. Pre-Anesthesia Evaluation 1

Patient: Mrs. Rebecca Smith

Age: 59

Referring Physician: Dr. Amelia Turner

Procedure: Total knee replacement surgery

Past Medical History: Hypertension controlled with medication. No known allergies.

Current Medications: Amlodipine for hypertension.

Physical Examination: Vital signs stable. No obvious signs of infection. Airway appears patent.

Laboratory Results: Blood count and coagulation profile within normal limits. Electrocardiogram showed normal sinus rhythm.

Anesthesia Plan: The patient will undergo general anesthesia with an endotracheal tube. Postoperative pain will be managed with a combination of systemic opioids and local anesthesia delivered via a peripheral nerve block.

b. Pre-Anesthesia Evaluation 2

Patient: Mr. Robert Williams

Age: 68

Referring Physician: Dr. Edward Miller

Procedure: Coronary artery bypass graft surgery

Past Medical History: Coronary artery disease, previous heart attack, diabetes type 2.

Current Medications: Aspirin, Metformin, and Atorvastatin.

Physical Examination: Vital signs stable. No respiratory distress. Airway appears patent. Cardiac examination reveals a regular rhythm without murmurs.

Laboratory Results: Complete blood count, kidney and liver function tests, and coagulation profile within normal limits. Electrocardiogram showed no acute changes.

Anesthesia Plan: The patient will undergo general anesthesia with an endotracheal tube. Care will be taken to ensure hemodynamic stability given his past heart attack. Postoperative pain will be managed with systemic opioids.

17. Anesthesia Reports

a. Anesthesia Report 1

Patient: Mr. John Anderson

Age: 72

Procedure: Right hip replacement

Anesthetic Technique: General Anesthesia

Induction: Induction of anesthesia was achieved with Propofol, Fentanyl, and Rocuronium.

Maintenance: Maintenance was done with Sevoflurane in a mixture of air and oxygen. Bolus doses of Fentanyl and Vecuronium were used as needed for analgesia and muscle relaxation.

Intraoperative Period: Blood pressure, heart rate, oxygen saturation, and end-tidal CO_2 were monitored and maintained within normal limits throughout the procedure. The patient's temperature was monitored and a warming blanket was used.

Emergence: The patient was extubated upon meeting the extubation criteria.

Postoperative Pain Management: Patient received a single dose of IV Morphine for postoperative pain management.

Anesthesia Recovery: The patient was transferred to the post-anesthesia care unit (PACU) in a stable condition.

b. Anesthesia Report 2

Patient: Mrs. Margaret Taylor

Age: 49

Procedure: Abdominal hysterectomy

Anesthetic Technique: Combined General and Regional (Epidural) Anesthesia

Induction and Maintenance: Induction was achieved with Propofol and Fentanyl. A thoracic epidural was inserted for intraoperative and postoperative pain control. Maintenance of anesthesia was done with Sevoflurane and intermittent boluses of Fentanyl and Rocuronium.

Intraoperative Period: All monitored parameters remained stable throughout the surgery.

Emergence: The patient was extubated smoothly in the operating room.

Postoperative Pain Management: The epidural was utilized for postoperative pain control with a continuous infusion of Bupivacaine and Hydromorphone.

Anesthesia Recovery: The patient was transported to the PACU in stable condition. The functioning of the epidural was assessed and found to be satisfactory.

18. Telehealth Visit Reports

a. Telehealth Visit Report 1

Patient: Ms. Sarah Johnson

Date of Visit: March 10, 2023

Provider: Dr. Emily Roberts

Reason for Visit: Follow-up for hypertension management

Summary: During the telehealth visit, the patient's blood pressure readings were reviewed, and medication adjustments were made to optimize blood pressure control. Lifestyle modifications, such as dietary changes and increased physical activity, were discussed. The patient's questions and concerns regarding medication side effects and potential interactions were addressed. Follow-up visit scheduled in 3 months.

b. Telehealth Visit Report 2

Patient: Mr. David Martinez

Date of Visit: April 5, 2023

Provider: Dr. Jennifer Adams

Reason for Visit: Mental health counseling

Summary: The telehealth visit focused on assessing the patient's mental health symptoms, including anxiety and depression. The provider conducted a detailed interview to understand the patient's concerns and stressors. Coping strategies, relaxation techniques, and potential treatment options, including therapy and medication, were discussed. A follow-up appointment was scheduled in 2 weeks to monitor progress and adjust the treatment plan if necessary.

NOTE: Each of these reports serves a unique purpose in providing a comprehensive picture of a patient's health and the care they have received.   For more practice, you can use online resources that include medical dictation files and their transcriptions. Practice regularly to improve your listening skills, speed, and accuracy in transcription.

APPENDIX B: COMMON PITFALLS IN MEDICAL TRANSCRIPTION: HANDLING SOUND-ALIKES, PRONUNCIATION VARIATIONS, AND MORE

As a medical transcriptionist, it is not just essential to understand the medical jargon and language rules, but also to be aware of the common pitfalls that can lead to transcription errors. These include sound-alikes, pronunciation variations, and often misunderstood terms. Let's delve into these aspects and explore ways to handle them effectively.

Understanding Sound-alikes

One of the most common challenges in medical transcription is dealing with sound-alikes - words that sound similar but have different meanings. An example of sound-alikes are the words "illicit" (forbidden by law) and "elicit" (to draw out a response). While these two words sound very similar, their meanings are entirely different. Mixing them up in a medical transcription could lead to serious misunderstandings.

In order to handle sound-alikes effectively:

1. Context Is Key: Pay close attention to the context in which the word is being used. This can often provide clues to the correct word. For example, the sentence "The doctor asked the patient to _______ a response" is likely referring to "elicit", not "illicit".

2. Cross-check with Reliable Sources: If you're unsure about a particular term, cross-check it with reliable medical dictionaries or resources.

3. Continuous Learning: Continuously expand your medical vocabulary. The more familiar you are with medical terminology, the easier it will be to distinguish between sound-alikes.

Handling Different Pronunciations

Just as people across different regions speak English with varying accents, medical terms can also be pronounced differently. A common example is the word "often", which some people pronounce with a silent 't', while others do not. These variations in pronunciation can lead to transcription errors.

In order to effectively deal with different pronunciations:

1. Familiarize Yourself with Different Accents: Expose yourself to different accents by listening to varied audio sources. This could be audio books, podcasts, or medical dictation samples from different regions.

2. Use Phonetic Spellings: Phonetic spellings can be a helpful guide in deciphering the correct word, especially for medical terms. For example, the term "dyspnea" could be pronounced differently, but its phonetic spelling "[disp-nee-uh]" provides a clear guide.

3. Seek Clarification: If a particular pronunciation is unclear, don't hesitate to seek clarification. It's better to ask than to risk making a mistake.

Commonly Misunderstood Terms

Medical transcription also comes with its share of commonly misunderstood terms. These are typically medical terms that are complex or sound similar to other words. An example is the term "prostate" and "prostrate". While "prostate" is a male gland, "prostrate" means to lie face down. Misunderstanding these terms can lead to transcription errors.

In order to deal with misunderstood terms:

1. Expand Your Medical Vocabulary: As with sound-alikes, expanding your medical vocabulary is crucial. The more terms you're familiar with, the less likely you are to misunderstand them.

2. Double-check Unclear Terms: If you come across a term that you're unsure about, double-check it with reliable sources.

3. Practice, Practice, Practice: The more you practice medical transcription, the more familiar you'll become with the medical terminology.

In the following section, we will look at ways to prevent and correct these common errors:

1. accept/except: 'Accept' means to receive or agree to something (ex: The transcriptionist accepted the new assignment), while 'except' means apart from or excluding (ex: The transcriptionist completed all the files except one).

2. adopt/adept/adapt: 'Adopt' means to take up or start to use (ex: The transcriptionist adopted a new typing technique); 'adept' means very skilled (ex: The transcriptionist is adept at medical terminology); 'adapt' means to adjust to new conditions (ex: The transcriptionist had to adapt to the doctor's accent).

3. adverse/averse: 'Adverse' means harmful or unfavorable (ex: The transcriptionist faced adverse conditions due to poor sound quality); 'averse' means having a strong dislike or opposition to something (ex: The transcriptionist was averse to working late hours).

4. advice/advise: 'Advice' is a noun meaning guidance or recommendations (ex: The transcriptionist received advice on improving speed); 'advise' is a verb meaning to give advice (ex: The senior transcriptionist advised the trainee on handling difficult files).

5. affect/effect: 'Affect' is a verb that means to have an impact on (ex: The poor sound quality affected the transcriptionist's accuracy); 'effect' is a noun that means a result (ex: The effect of the training was evident in the transcriptionist's improved speed).

6. all right/alright: 'All right' is a formal way to say that everything is correct or satisfactory (ex: The transcriptionist checked that all the transcriptions were all right). 'Alright' is a more informal variant of the same, although in professional writing, 'all right' is preferred.

7. altar/alter: 'Altar' is a table used in religious services (not generally used in medical transcription); 'alter' means to change something (ex: The transcriptionist had to alter the file based on the doctor's additional notes).

8. alternate/alternative: 'Alternate' as a verb means to switch back and forth between two things; as an adjective, it means every other (ex: The transcriptionist decided to work on alternate files); 'alternative' means a second option (ex: The transcriptionist sought an alternative solution to the problem).

9. altogether/all together: 'Altogether' means completely or on the whole (ex: Altogether, the transcriptionist had to work on 100 files); 'all together' means everyone or everything in one place (ex: The transcriptionist put all the files together for final review).

10. ambiguous/ambivalent: 'Ambiguous' means unclear or open to more than one interpretation (ex: The doctor's dictation was ambiguous); 'ambivalent' means having mixed feelings (ex: The transcriptionist was ambivalent about working overtime).

11. amount/number: 'Amount' is used for uncountable nouns (ex: The transcriptionist was overwhelmed by the amount of work), while 'number' is used for countable nouns (ex: The number of medical reports that needed to be transcribed was increasing).

12. anecdote/antidote: 'Anecdote' means a short amusing or interesting story about a real incident or person (not often used in medical transcription), while 'antidote' is a medicine taken or given to counteract a particular poison (ex: The medical report mentioned an antidote administered to the patient).

13. appraise/apprise: 'Appraise' means to assess (ex: The transcriptionist's work was appraised for accuracy), while 'apprise' means to inform or tell (ex: The team leader apprised the transcriptionist of the new deadline).

14. assure/ensure: 'Assure' means to tell someone something positively to dispel their doubts (ex: The supervisor assured the transcriptionist that the workload would decrease), while 'ensure' means to make certain (ex: The transcriptionist checked the report twice to ensure accuracy).

15. awhile/a while: 'Awhile' means for a short time (ex: The transcriptionist worked awhile before taking a break), 'a while' means a period of time (ex: The transcriptionist rested for a while before resuming work).

16. bare/bear: 'Bare' means uncovered or naked (ex: In a medical report, it might be used as "The patient had a bare arm for the injection"), while 'bear' means to carry or endure (ex: The transcriptionist could hardly bear the workload).

17. bazaar/bizarre: 'Bazaar' is a market (not typically used in medical transcription), while 'bizarre' means very strange or unusual (ex: The transcriptionist came across a bizarre medical case).

18. between/among: 'Between' is used when referring to two things (ex: The transcriptionist had to choose between two templates), while 'among' is used when referring to three or more things (ex: The transcriptionist was among the best in the team).

19. borrow/lend: 'Borrow' means to take something from someone with the intention of returning it (ex: The transcriptionist had to borrow a medical dictionary from a colleague), while 'lend' means to grant to someone for temporary use (ex: The transcriptionist lent her medical dictionary to a colleague).

20. both/each: 'Both' refers to two things together (ex: Both the transcriptionist and the editor worked on the report), while 'each' refers to two or more things seen as separate individuals (ex: Each member of the transcription team was given a task).

21. brand name/generic: A 'brand name' is the trade name of a drug marketed by a specific company (ex: The report mentioned the brand name of the drug), while 'generic' refers to the common name of a drug that can be manufactured by any company (ex: The transcriptionist was familiar with both the generic and brand names of common drugs).

22. breath/breathe: 'Breath' is the air taken into or expelled from the lungs (ex: The patient's breath was labored), while 'breathe' is the action of taking in and expelling air (ex: The patient was struggling to breathe).

23. carat/carat/carrot/karat: 'Carat' is a unit of weight for precious stones and pearls (not typically used in medical transcription). A 'carrot' is a vegetable (also not typically used in medical transcription). A 'karat' is a measure of the purity of gold (again, not typically used in medical transcription).

24. cite/site/sight: 'Cite' means to mention or refer to as an example or proof (ex: The transcriptionist had to cite the correct medical term), 'site' refers to a location or place (ex: The surgical site was mentioned in the report), and 'sight' refers to the faculty or power of seeing (ex: The patient's sight was improving).

25. coarse/course: 'Coarse' means rough or loose in texture (ex: The transcriptionist noted the description of the patient's skin as coarse), while 'course' could mean a direction (ex: The course of the disease was unpredictable) or a study program (ex: The transcriptionist took a course in medical terminology).

26. collaborate/corroborate: 'Collaborate' means to work jointly on an activity or project (ex: The transcriptionist had to collaborate with the medical coder), whereas 'corroborate' means to confirm or give support to a statement, theory, or finding (ex: The lab results corroborated the initial diagnosis).

27. compliment/complement: 'Compliment' is a polite expression of praise or admiration (ex: The transcriptionist received compliments for her accuracy), while 'complement' means to complete something or bring it to perfection (ex: The doctor's notes complemented the transcription).

28. comprise/compromise: 'Comprise' means to include or contain (ex: The medical report comprised patient history, examination findings, and a treatment plan), whereas 'compromise' means to settle a dispute by mutual concession or to expose to risk (ex: Errors in medical transcription can compromise patient safety).

29. desert/dessert: 'Desert' can be a waterless, barren area, or to abandon (not typically used in medical transcription), while 'dessert' is the sweet course eaten at the end of a meal (ex: The patient was restricted from eating dessert due to diabetes).

30. differ/defer: 'Differ' means to be dissimilar or distinct in nature from another (ex: Symptoms of diseases can differ greatly), whereas 'defer' means to postpone or delay (ex: The transcriptionist had to defer her work until the audio file was clearer).

31. discreet/discrete: 'Discreet' means careful and circumspect in one's speech or actions, especially to avoid causing offense or to gain an advantage (ex: The transcriptionist was discreet about patient information), while 'discrete' means individually separate and distinct (ex: The transcriptionist broke down the dictation into discrete parts).

32. disinterested/uninterested: 'Disinterested' means not influenced by considerations of personal advantage, a neutral party (ex: A disinterested third party conducted the audit of the transcriptions), whereas 'uninterested' means not wanting to know about something (ex: The transcriptionist was uninterested in non-medical talk).

33. dominate/dominant: 'Dominate' means to have power and influence over (ex: In the transcription industry, accuracy and speed dominate), while 'dominant' means most important, powerful, or influential (ex: Accurate transcription is a dominant factor in patient care).

34. dual/duel: 'Dual' means consisting of two parts, elements, or aspects (ex: The transcriptionist was skilled in dual languages). 'Duel' is a contest with deadly weapons arranged between two people to settle a point of honor (not typically used in medical transcription).

35. e.g./i.e./etc.: 'e.g.' stands for 'exempli gratia', Latin for 'for example' (ex: The transcriptionist transcribed reports for various specialties, e.g., Cardiology, Neurology). 'i.e.' stands for 'id est', Latin for 'that is' or 'in other words' (ex: The transcriptionist worked for an MTSO, i.e., a Medical Transcription Service Organization). 'Etc.' stands for 'et cetera', Latin for 'and other things' or 'and so on' (ex: The transcriptionist needed various equipment like a computer, headphones, etc.).

36. elicit/illicit: 'Elicit' means to draw out a response or fact from someone (ex: The doctor's questions were designed to elicit specific health information). 'Illicit' means forbidden by laws, rules, or customs (ex: Sharing patient information is illicit).

37. emergent/urgent: 'Emergent' refers to conditions that are arising suddenly and need immediate attention (ex: The patient had an emergent condition that required surgery). 'Urgent' describes a situation or condition requiring immediate action or attention (ex: The patient had an urgent need for medication).

38. eminent/imminent: 'Eminent' means distinguished or outstanding in a particular field (ex: The transcription was for an eminent surgeon). 'Imminent' means likely to occur at any moment or impending (ex: Due to the patient's condition, surgery was imminent).

39. envelope/envelop: 'Envelope' is a flat paper container with a sealable flap, typically used to enclose a letter or document. 'Envelop' means to surround entirely (ex: The mist seemed to envelop the mountains, not typically used in medical transcription).

40. everyday/every day: 'Everyday' (as one word) is an adjective that means ordinary or commonplace (ex: Transcription is part of the everyday workflow in healthcare). 'Every day' (as two words) means each day individually (ex: The transcriptionist worked every day).

41. expression/impression: 'Expression' refers to the process of making one's thoughts or feelings known (ex: The doctor's expression of concern was well-noted in the report). 'Impression' typically refers to an idea, feeling, or opinion about something or someone (ex: The initial impression of the patient's condition was noted by the doctor).

42. farther/further: 'Farther' refers to a greater distance (ex: The farther progression of the disease was noted in the follow-up report). 'Further' is used to denote extension of time or degree (ex: Further examination is needed to determine the cause of the symptoms).

43. fatal/fateful: 'Fatal' means causing death (ex: The accident resulted in fatal injuries). 'Fateful' describes something that has significant consequences (ex: The fateful decision to delay treatment resulted in complications).

44. flaunt/flout: 'Flaunt' means to show off (ex: Not typically used in medical transcription). 'Flout' means to openly disregard (ex: Patients who flout medical advice may see a worsening of their symptoms).

45. foul/fowl: 'Foul' typically refers to something that is offensive to the senses, particularly smell, or an unfair play in a game. 'Fowl' is a bird, particularly a chicken or duck. Both are rarely used in medical transcription.

46. heroin/heroine: 'Heroin' is a drug that is often the subject of substance abuse (ex: The patient admitted to heroin usage). 'Heroine' is a female hero (ex: Not typically used in medical transcription).

47. idea/ideal: 'Idea' is a thought or suggestion (ex: The doctor had an idea for a new treatment plan). 'Ideal' refers to something considered perfect or the standard of perfection (ex: The ideal outcome was for the patient to fully recover).

48. lay/lie: 'Lay' is to put down, especially gently or carefully (ex: The nurse will lay the patient's arm flat to administer the injection). 'Lie' means to be in a flat position on a surface (ex: The patient was advised to lie still during the procedure).

49. lose/loose: 'Lose' is the opposite of win, and it can also mean misplacing something (ex: The patient did not want to lose any more weight). 'Loose' is the opposite of tight (ex: The bandage was too loose on the patient's wound).

50. may/might: 'May' is used to express possibility (ex: The patient may need surgery). 'Might' is also used to express possibility but often in a more speculative or uncertain sense (ex: If the medication doesn't work, the patient might require more intensive treatment).

51. moral/morale: 'Moral' relates to principles of right and wrong (ex: The doctor faced a moral dilemma about the treatment plan). 'Morale' refers to the state of spirit of a person or group (ex: The morale of the medical team was high despite the long hours).

52. palate/palette/pallet: 'Palate' is the roof of the mouth (ex: The surgeon examined the patient's palate). 'Palette' is a range of colors or elements (ex: Not typically used in medical transcription). 'Pallet' is a flat wooden structure (ex: Not typically used in medical transcription).

53. past/passed: 'Past' refers to a time gone by or beyond (ex: The patient's medical history includes past surgeries). 'Passed' is the past tense of pass (ex: The patient passed all physical examinations).

54. perspective/prospective: 'Perspective' is a point of view (ex: From a medical perspective, the patient is improving). 'Prospective' refers to something that is expected or anticipating to happen in the future (ex: Prospective studies will be required to confirm this treatment's effectiveness).

55. practice/practise: In American English, 'practice' is used as both a noun and a verb (ex: The doctor's practice is in New York / The nurse will practice the procedure). In British English, 'practice' is the noun, and 'practise' is the verb.

56. pray/prey: 'Pray' means to speak to a god either privately or in a religious ceremony (ex: Not typically used in medical transcription). 'Prey' refers to an animal that is hunted by another for food (ex: Not typically used in medical transcription).

57. precede/proceed: 'Precede' means to come before something in time, order, or position (ex: Preliminary testing will precede the surgery). 'Proceed' means to begin or continue a course of action (ex: The doctor decided to proceed with the treatment).

58. prescribe/proscribe: 'Prescribe' refers to recommend a medicine or treatment (ex: The physician prescribed antibiotics for the infection). 'Proscribe' means to condemn or forbid something (ex: Not typically used in medical transcription).

59. principal/principle: 'Principal' means first in order of importance or the person with the highest authority (ex: The principal investigator of the study is a renowned cardiologist). 'Principle' refers to a fundamental truth or proposition serving as the foundation for a system of belief or behavior (ex: The principle of first do no harm guides medical ethics).

60. prostate/prostrate: 'Prostate' is a small gland present in men, which secretes part of the semen (ex: The patient was diagnosed with prostate cancer). 'Prostrate' means to lay oneself flat on the ground face downward, especially in reverence or submission (ex: Not typically used in medical transcription).

61. quite/quiet/quit: 'Quite' is a bit or to a slight degree (ex: The patient was quite anxious about the procedure). 'Quiet' means making little or no noise (ex: The patient was asked to remain quiet before the procedure). 'Quit' means to leave a place, usually permanently (ex: Not typically used in medical transcription).

62. recent/resent: 'Recent' refers to something that happened not long ago (ex: The patient's recent tests show improvement). 'Resent' means to feel bitterness or indignation at a circumstance, action, or person (ex: Not typically used in medical transcription).

63. remuneration/renumeration: 'Remuneration' refers to money paid for work or a service (ex: The remuneration for medical transcription work varies by experience and location). 'Renumeration' is not a word in English, it is often mistakenly used instead of 'remuneration'.

64. role/roll: 'Role' refers to the function assumed or part played by a person or thing in a particular situation (ex: The role of a transcriptionist is critical in medical documentation). 'Roll' means to move in a particular direction by turning over and over (ex: Not typically used in medical transcription).

65. seam/seem: 'Seam' refers to the line where two pieces of fabric are sewn together in a garment or other article (ex: Not typically used in medical transcription). 'Seem' means to give the impression of being something or having a particular quality (ex: The patient seemed to be in a lot of pain).

66. sew/sow: 'Sew' means to join, fasten, or repair (something) by making stitches with a needle and thread or a sewing machine (ex: The surgeon will sew the incision closed). 'Sow' is to plant seed by scattering it on or in the earth (ex: Not typically used in medical transcription).

67. stationary/stationery: 'Stationary' means not moving or not intended to be moved (ex: The patient was asked to remain stationary for the scan). 'Stationery' refers to the items needed for writing, such as paper, pens, pencils, and envelopes (ex: Not typically used in medical transcription).

68. taunt/taut: 'Taunt' is a remark made in order to anger, wound, or provoke someone (ex: Not typically used in medical transcription). 'Taut' means stretched or pulled tight, not slack (ex: The bandage was pulled taut over the wound).

69. tenet/tenant: 'Tenet' is a principle or belief, especially one of the main principles of a religion or philosophy (ex: Confidentiality is a key tenet of medical ethics). 'Tenant' is a person who occupies land or property rented from a landlord (ex: Not typically used in medical transcription).

70. than/then: 'Than' is used in comparisons (ex: The patient's condition is better than it was yesterday). 'Then' is used to refer to a certain time in the past or future (ex: The patient was then referred to a specialist).

71. to/through: 'To' is used to express motion in the direction of a particular location (ex: The patient was admitted to the hospital). 'Through' means moving in one side and out of the other side (ex: The surgeon made an incision through the skin).

72. too/two: 'Too' is used to indicate that a certain degree or extent is reached or exceeded (ex: The medication dosage may be too high). 'Two' is the number following one (ex: Two nurses were present during the procedure).

73. wary/weary: 'Wary' means feeling or showing caution about possible dangers or problems (ex: The doctor was wary of possible side effects). 'Weary' means feeling or showing tiredness, especially as a result of excessive exertion or lack of sleep (ex: After a long day of work, the transcriptionist felt weary).

These are just a few examples of commonly confused words in English. By understanding the differences and correctly applying them in your transcriptions, you can greatly increase the accuracy and quality of your work. Mastering these nuances not only makes you a better transcriptionist, but also enhances your overall communication skills in the English language.

1. Association for Healthcare Documentation Integrity (AHDI): This organization offers resources for medical transcriptionists including certification programs, an annual conference, and a variety of learning resources.

Website: http://www.ahdionline.org/

2. Medical Transcription / Healthcare Documentation (MT/HDS) Forum: This forum is a great place to ask questions and learn from experienced medical transcriptionists.

Website: http://www.mtstars.com/

3. MedlinePlus: This website, run by the U.S. National Library of Medicine, offers a comprehensive database of health topics, which can be very helpful for understanding medical terminology and conditions.

Website: https://medlineplus.gov/

4. Medical Dictionaries and Reference Materials: Books such as "Stedman's Medical Dictionary" and "The AAMT Book of Style for Medical Transcription" can be extremely useful for understanding and correctly transcribing medical terms.

5. Health Information Privacy (HIPAA): The U.S. Department of Health and Human Services offers resources about the Health Insurance Portability and Accountability Act, which is crucial for all medical transcriptionists to understand.

Website: https://www.hhs.gov/hipaa/index.html

6. Merck Manuals: An invaluable resource for understanding medical topics in depth. Both professional and consumer versions are available online for free.

Website: https://www.merckmanuals.com/

Remember, the field of medical transcription requires continuous learning. Therefore, stay updated, keep expanding your knowledge base and improving your skills.